The Maltreatment of Children

TO

May, Benjamin and Michelle

The Maltreatment of Children

EDITED BY
Selwyn M. Smith

Psychiatrist-in-Chief
Royal Ottawa Hospital
and
Director, Department of Forensic Psychiatry,
Faculty of Medicine, University of Ottawa, Canada

MTPPRESS LIMITED *International Medical Publishers*

Published by
MTP Press Limited
Falcon House
Lancaster, England

ISBN 978-94-011-6164-0   ISBN 978-94-011-6162-6 (eBook)
DOI 10.1007/ 978-94-011-6162-6

Text set in 11/12 pt Photon Imprint, printed by Redwood Burn Ltd., Trowbridge
and bound in Great Britain at The Pitman Press, Bath

Contents

List of Contributors   vii

Foreword   ix
Gerald J. Sarwer-Foner

Preface   xi
Selwyn M. Smith

1. Introduction – a child speaks   1
   Myre Sim
2. Child abuse and neglect – medical aspects   9
   Christine E. Cooper
3. Radiological and pathological aspects of the battered child syndrome   69
   J. M. Cameron
4. Management of the problem   83
   A. White Franklin
5. The epidemiology of child abuse   96
   J. E. Oliver
6. The extent of child abuse   121
   J. E. Oliver, Jane Cox and Ann Buchanan
7. The psychiatrist's viewpoint   175
   P. D. Scott
8. The psychological aspects of child abuse   205
   D. R. Henry
9. The needs of children   221
   Mia Kellmer Pringle
10. Child abuse, neglect and deprivation and the family   245
    J. Jacobs
11. Medical-legal and societal problems involving children – child prostitution, child pornography and drug-related abuse; recommended legislation   317
    Judianne Densen-Gerber and S. F. Hutchinson
12. The contributions of the social agencies and the social worker   351
    Sheila M. Noble

13. The emergence of the child as a legal entity   393
    D. Ford

    Appendix   415
    J. E. Oliver

    Index   449

List of Contributors

Buchanan, Ann
        Research Social Worker
        Burderop Hospital
        Wroughton, Swindon, England

Cameron, Professor James M., M.D., Ph.D., M.R.C.Path., D.M.J.Path.
        Professor of Forensic Medicine
        The London Hospital Medical College
        London, England

Cooper, Christine, E., M.D., F.R.C.R.
        Consultant Paediatrician
        Newcastle, England

Cox, Jane, B.Sc.
        Sociologist and Teacher
        Burderop Hospital
        Wroughton, Swindon, England

Densen-Gerber, Judianne, J.D., M.D., F.L.C.M.,
        Director, The Odyssey Institute
        New York City, New York, USA

Ford, Donald, M.A., J.P.
        Chief Magistrate, Bow St. Court
        London, England

Henry, Donald R., Ph.D.
        Clinical Psychologist
        Department of Forensic Psychiatry
        Royal Ottawa Hospital
        Ottawa, Canada

Hutchinson, Stephen, F., J.D.
        The Odyssey Institute
        New York City, New York, USA

Jacobs, Joseph, M.D., F.R.C.P., F.R.C.P.(C), D.C.M.
  Professor of Paediatrics
  McMaster University
  Hamilton, Canada

Kellmer Pringle, Mia, C.B.E., B.A., Ph.D., D.Sc.
  National Children's Bureau
  London, England

Noble, Sheila, J.P., M.A.
  Department of Economics and Social Science
  City of Birmingham Polytechnic
  Birmingham, England

Oliver, Jack E., M.B., B.S., M.R.C.S., M.R.C.Psych.
  Consultant Psychiatrist in Mental Handicap and Child Psychiatry
  Burderop Hospital
  Wroughton, Swindon, England

Sarwer-Foner, Gerald J., M.D., F.R.C.P.(C), D.A.B.P.N., F.R.C.Psych.,
  F.A.P.A., F.A.C.P., F.A.C.O.N., F.A.C.Pn., F.A.A.Sc., F.I.C.P.M.
  Chairman, Department of Psychiatry
  Faculty of Medicine and Psychiatrist-in-Chief, Ottawa General
    Hospital
  University of Ottawa
  Ottawa, Canada

Scott, Peter D (Deceased), C.B.E., M.A., M.D., F.R.C.P., F.R.C.Psych.
  Formerly Consultant Psychiatrist
  The Maudsley Hospital
  London, England

Sim, Myre, M.D., F.R.C.P., F.R.C.Psych., F.R.C.P.(C), D.P.M.
  Professor of Psychiatry
  Faculty of Medicine
  University of Ottawa
  Ottawa, Canada

Smith, Selwyn M., B.S., M.D., M.R.C.Psych., D.P.M., F.R.C.P.(C)
  Associate Professor, of Psychiatry Faculty of Medicine
  University of Ottawa; Director, Department
  of Forensic Psychiatry, Royal Ottawa Hospital
  Ottawa, Canada

White-Franklin, Alfred, M.B., F.R.C.P.
  Consultant Paediatrician
  Harley St., London, England

Foreword

The maltreatment of children is an issue that has always been with us and civilized societies provide a range of services both social and medical to care for the children and families afflicted. In recent years, greater attention has been drawn to the medical aspects by competent authorities in the fields of forensic medicine, forensic psychiatry, epidemiological psychiatry, child psychiatry and family psychiatry; as well as the social aspects by those child welfare and child care agencies who have the difficult and distasteful task of removing children, with the help of the courts, from parents who can abuse them and are not able to care for them adequately. A multitude of social agencies, whose range of activities involve both the care and, where possible, the social betterment of afflicted families are now involved.

Not least in importance is an increase in our global knowledge to help in the prevention or better treatment of these problems. This means more information on familial and genetic factors in human central nervous system development in its broadest sense. This would include how the central nervous system originates, mediates and controls the build up, speed of development and impulsive release, mastery and direction of aggressive drives and impulses. Very little is so far known about these factors.

The proper application of existing psychiatric knowledge about stress imposed on mothers' passive-dependency needs by the demands of mothering a child, particularly when the mother is a single parent, or inadequately nurtured with love by a mate, or is unwilling or ambivalent about being a parent mother, whose security, in terms of a constant object relationship is being threatened, is an important area that can be improved by the application of existing psychiatric expertise. Similarly, application of existing psychiatric data and knowledge on family dynamics, the psychodynamics of aggression and rage and the eruption of uncontrolled, impulse ridden anger and aggression can be helpful in understanding and dealing with the behaviour patterns of mothers and fathers, or of men living with women who have very young children and who have very limited tolerance for children.

The importance to all who deal with children in trouble of knowing that men and women, who have themselves suffered from inadequate 'mothering' and 'fathering' have difficulties in relating to others, including violent outbursts towards their own children when they themselves mate, is obvious. The teaching of the dynamics of projective self envy, as it is felt towards their children, at having parents, etc., is another factor that is often lacking or is poorly done. The details of which psychopathology determines which type of reaction and which outcome, the problems of the build up of aggressive impulse and its expression, the problem of how to control and handle these factors, are areas that merit much-needed further study.

The virtue of this book is that it brings together recognized authorities in the field of paediatrics, law, forensic and epidemiological psychiatry, social work, social work agencies, and psychiatry in its broadest sense and collates the knowledge on these issues in well-balanced discussions. These excellent contributions by themselves would not have the general impact that has been achieved by the careful selection and editing of Dr Selwyn Smith, Director of Forensic Psychiatry, University of Ottawa, Faculty of Medicine.

Gerald J. Sarwer-Foner

Preface

'The weight of this sad time we must obey;
Speak what we feel, not what we ought to say.'
King Lear: Act V, Scene III

It is a fact that throughout recorded time, the killing, maiming, abandonment, starving, neglect, cruel punishment and sexual exploitation of children have been a feature of the life experience of every generation. Sometimes it has been given sanction by tradition and ritual usage; more often, it has been a matter of private acts committed in shameful secrecy. Only very recently, in historical terms, has any concern been voiced about the problem of maltreated children. Indeed, the child has only recently emerged in history with an identity of its own. Children have been acceded few rights and these rights have neither been properly determined nor defined. The child's dependency has always made him or her a potential victim of adults. Several committees of inquiry into fatal incidents of maltreatment have repeated the familiar charge that society as a whole must bear the ultimate blame. Unfortunately, in many instances, it has been the professionals who have failed.

The idea for this book was conceived in England in the summer of 1975. I wanted to put together a text that would review comprehensively the subject of maltreatment of children from the fields of paediatrics, pathology, psychiatry, psychology, law and social work. Journal articles, monographs and books on the subject have mushroomed throughout the last decade. I approached leading workers in the field who were willing to write original, up-to-date and comprehensive chapters which would critically review and integrate the literature that has been accumulating in diverse publications. Each contributor had the added advantage of also drawing upon a wealth of first-hand experience of the problem. Each believes passionately in the rights of children and has written and spoken extensively on some aspects of this phenomenon.

I will be eternally grateful to the authors for their hard work, perseverance, cooperation and tolerance of some of my editorial suggestions and proddings. It is with considerable sorrow that I have to report that one of the contributors, Dr P. D. Scott, died on August 6, 1977. I would also like to acknowledge the patience of MTP Press Limited for tolerating the delays that inevitably occurred when I took up residence in Canada. I am also grateful to the Editor of the *British Journal of Preventive and Social Medicine* for allowing publication of some material in Dr J. E. Oliver's chapter. Miss Pat Pottie typed and collated, with great care and diligence, the final chapters.

I sincerely hope this text will provide a useful resource for students and professionals engaged in the field. Overcoming the problem of maltreated children has become a burning issue. Governments and agencies have become engaged in a rush to try to understand the causes of child abuse and to solve the problem. The rapid increase of publications on the topic shows little sign of abatement. Hence, there will be new developments. This book cannot be the final word, but it can serve as a relatively complete reference for what has been achieved so far. I hope it will provide a guide for the future.

Selwyn M. Smith

1 Introduction – a child speaks

MYRE SIM

'Out of the mouths of very babes and sucklings hast thou ordained strength, because of thine enemies: that thou mightest still the enemy, and the avenger.' Psalm VIII, 2

Maltreatment of children exposes a sizeable section of the child community to serious physical and mental dangers and to death itself. I can do no less than offer this introduction in the words, as it were, of one of the victims—a maltreated child.

We are all very small and helpless. Many of us have not learned to walk, let alone run and most have not even learned to talk. We cannot therefore run out of harm's way, we cannot summon the help of a neighbour and we cannot 'phone for help, if only because many of our homes do not possess a telephone.

This problem of maltreated children is not new and no longer takes people by surprise, yet the number of instances keeps rising and many of us are murdered or seriously maimed. We appreciate the concern of society which has set aside funds, passed legislation, trained people and sponsored research, but it all does not seem to help. There have been public enquiries into the abuse of a particular child, usually when it results in death and almost invariably the social or welfare services that are designed to deal with the problem have been found wanting or negligent. This does not mean that these people were not well-intentioned; just incompetent.

I, therefore, welcome this opportunity to put our view forward for we are the victims who are exposed to the risks and can see the relevance or otherwise of existing and proposed measures. We may not, and probably cannot, provide all the answers but I feel that our comments may help and it is in this spirit that they are offered and I hope you will not forget that for us it is often a matter of life and death.

One aspect which troubles us is the lack of a sense of urgency, not on the

1

part of the public, but on the part of many of the agencies involved. I must be careful not to single out any special agency, for I know how touchy professionals can be, but in this instance most are to blame. If it is strongly suspected by a doctor that one of us is being abused there should be no delaying of action because of reasons of exercising discretion or waiting for stronger evidence, which means that a child has to be more severely battered. If there were reasonable grounds for suspicion that lead concentration in a factory was potentially dangerous, one would not wait for the grosser signs of lead poisoning before one took action.

Child care and other social services which employ some of the kindest and most concerned people have a peculiar way of reacting to a notification of suspected child abuse. They hold a case conference, which will rarely take place in less than a week after the notification and frequently after much longer. It would be considered ridiculous if a fire brigade adopted such an attitude even following a false alarm from a hoaxer, or if the police failed to respond immediately to a call from a concerned citizen. I wish to stress that for us these matters are desperately urgent and the machinery of child care and such services which were developed to deal with long-standing problems of minor morbidity are entirely inappropriate in our case.

Neither do we wish to be the victims, literally, of theorizing in child psychology. A slavish devotion to Bowlby's views on attachment and loss has unfortunately led to just that, attachment and then loss, and the loss has been the life of a baby. I therefore beg those agencies to be practical and see the realities of a situation and if they find that what expertise they possess does not help them to act immediately and constructively, or may even prevent them from so doing, they should admit it and not pretend to answers they do not possess. If the battered and abused baby syndrome has revealed deficiencies in professional training and competence, it calls for a reappraisal and not a retreat into perseverance with outmoded or inappropriate theory and practice. And, please, do not get involved in 'inter-union' strife as to which professional group our problem belongs. A very wise man once saw clearly that haggling over a child could only result in the death of that child and put it to the warring parties in a most dramatic way. Whoever is capable of acting quickly and decisively is most likely to save us from further harm.

In any case, if the battering does not stop and even if I am not killed, my severe injuries will result in charges being made against one or both of my parents with resulting prison sentences and a break in this sacred cow 'attachment' which so many people worship. Even though I have suffered terrible pain and injury I have a lot of love for my parents as they are not always bad and I do not wish to see them continue on a course which will lead to their severe punishment and the total break-up of our home. If prompt and effective action were taken with a temporary separation, my brothers and sisters and I could have been reunited with our parents at a later date.

It is, I hear, a hotly debated issue as to which social agency should be first involved and which should be given the responsibility to provide the necessary social manipulation to correct this problem. As there are, I understand, no clear-cut answers, this is where I can help. As a very young baby, neglect and injury can be difficult to detect when I am fully dressed. The social worker who sees my parents as her clients is disinclined to be mistrustful for she has been taught that this would destroy the relationship and so she is easily fobbed off with false information. I recall when I was burned with cigarette ends and had some bruising that nothing was suspected until my arm was broken and I had to be taken to hospital.

The district nurse is very different and my fellow victims also tell me that things are different when she gets involved. She undresses them and has a good look at them with a clinical eye and has no hesitation in calling in the doctor or taking the child herself to hospital. I have heard it said that these district nurses know nothing of family dynamics or family therapy and are therefore not suited for this problem. The former may be so but they have had a good clinical background and know when a child is not well. They weigh us regularly and know if we are not thriving, they examine us all over and can spot bruising and can make a fair guess as to what is an accident and what is a deliberate injury. Most important, in this clinical area they know their limitations and when to call the doctor. Many of my fellow victims' lives have been saved when they were promptly taken to the doctor and, unfortunately, many have died when they were not.

The nurse has authority and can exercise it on our behalf. These other ladies, I hear, are frequently anti-authority because they confuse this with their creed of anti-authoritarianism. It has been said that they regard the police as enemies of society and doctors as purveyors of a medical model which fails to appreciate that most human behaviour can be corrected by helping people to express their feelings. All my injuries were sustained when my parents were expressing their feelings and I noticed no reduction in their behaviour after their 'emotion letting' in the group or personal sessions they attended.

This may not be fashionable, but at times I have prayed for a policeman to come in and save me. To me, he would not and could not be a 'male chauvinist pig' but a knight in shining armour who would protect me from harm. I would feel safe when the nurse called for she was practical and would get me to the doctor quickly. In fact, when she became involved, my parents' behaviour improved without the benefit of 'emotion letting' sessions. They seemed relieved now that somebody was really in control and they turned to her as a good and capable person who would not be easily fooled and whose language they could understand. I must confess that I was a bit anxious when she told them she was going to take a course in family therapy. I can only hope it does not make her and them worse.

But it is not merely a matter of early detection and firm decisions to remove us from the danger area. That is still a risky game, for us. We must try and prevent the growth of this problem by tackling the root causes and then society may be able to reduce it to its absolute minimum. I would like to abolish it entirely but I realize that there are rare instances after childbirth when a mother loses her reason and destroys her baby. Even then I understand that if these unfortunate women had been treated properly by a competent psychiatrist, these causes would also disappear. It is getting more difficult for competent psychiatrists to exercise their competence for there are a lot of people, these days, who say that mentally deranged people are entitled to be free to do exactly what they want and that action can only be taken when they have broken the law. That can only mean that these civil libertarians, if that is the correct term, are quite prepared to see a number of babies murdered when treatment promptly applied could have saved these lives and saved the mother from a lifetime of anguish spent in a penal psychiatric institution or in the security ward of a mental hospital. Two to three weeks of in-patient treatment would have done the trick but the forces against this humane measure are now so strong that many doctors are showing greater reluctance to treat and governments are largely on the side of the civil libertarians. Many of these women commit suicide so that the remaining children are motherless and the husband has lost a first-class partner who could have been quickly restored to perfect health to him and his children, and the child would not have been murdered.

They tell us that law reformers are busy, with considerable success, persuading governments to make it even harder for psychiatrists and other doctors to treat people with recoverable disease and that there are lots of profound arguments in favour. Do dead babies and dead or permanently incarcerated mothers not matter? It seems to me as if reason is being stood on its head. I know that I will be told I know nothing of these matters, for I am too young. We babies and children will no longer accept this admonition and there is a good precedent as is evidenced by the quotation at the beginning of this chapter. In fact, I strongly suspect that the generous doctor who let me do this Introduction for him had this quotation in mind when he made the decision.

Historians tell us that maltreatment of children is of very long-standing. This is no doubt true, but it is equally true that many cultures had a very low incidence, but in others the incidence was high and it is certainly high in so-called Western society. While this is a deplorable state, it also offers some hope, for what is culturally determined can also be culturally erased. Some people think the world is a terrible place now with battered babies and other violent crimes, high rates of suicide, divorce, abortion, drug-addiction and alcoholism. I take some comfort in the reasonable deduction that the world must have been in an even worse state when Moses brought down the Ten Commandments from Mount Sinai. The people then had to be told that it was wrong to murder and steal and tell lies; that it was right to honour your father and your mother and that workers and beasts of burden were entitled to regular rest periods. Some cynic may say that things are not very different now, but at least these admonitions are no longer necessary even though there is a minority who would challenge them.

What has happened to a society when a baby's life is endangered, and by its own parents? We are here immediately in the realm of speculation by social scientists and others. These people are generally not at risk and are therefore regarded as more objective observers as they have no interest to declare. I am at risk and therefore declare my interest but rather than weakening my observations, I consider it strengthens them. Like the man in the condemned cell, my mind is probably more concentrated. It has just occurred to me that perhaps I should have added a footnote to the term 'condemned cell' to explain that it was the cell the convicted murderer occupied prior to his execution. While most people would not want a poor wretch to hang, it strikes me as strange that those who clamoured most vociferously against the death penalty or its reintroduction should be so cavalier about life in other respects, such as that of an unborn child who is sometimes only weeks younger than some battered babies and the elderly who may not be that much older than some pop stars. I am sure that a psychiatrist could explain it by saying that these people have identified strongly with the murderer and in their other causes, like the murderer, they show little respect for human life. Like most interpretations this is speculation, but the vehemence of the opposition to it from some quarters makes one wonder whether there may not be more than a grain of truth in it. The over reaction certainly carries some of the hallmarks of Freudian psychopathology. A psychiatrist told me that when he put this view forward to a group of Freudians, he was met with the revealing statement that 'even the Devil will quote the Bible'.

Lots of reasons have been offered and the one that is currently stressed is that battered babies are unwanted babies and that the best answer would be to abort them early in pregnancy. Obviously, this argument stems from the pro-abortion lobby. There is confusion here, probably deliberate, between the unwanted pregnancy and the unwanted baby. The former is extremely common; the latter is extremely rare. It is a plausible argument were it not for the fact that most battered babies are not unwanted; many are over-wanted. The mother, who herself may have had a deprived background, is intent that her baby be perfect, in behaviour, in appearance and in achievement. It is when the baby fails to meet these expectations that the mother becomes exasperated and loses control. This also explains why many of my fellow victims still love their mothers who have mutilated them. They know that there is a lot of love there too for they have experienced it. An even stranger argument is that a baby should be aborted in its own interests. I fail to see how destruction of an unborn child has anything to do with helping that baby. It presumes that it will otherwise certainly be destroyed in infancy by its parent or parents. If prediction had reached such a high state of certainty, which it has not, the proper course would be to have the baby delivered and use the interim to initiate these most effective social and psychological strategies of which we hear so much.

In psychiatry, it is well known that the least effective psychiatrists are those who resort too readily to the gynaecologist to treat the most minor degree of psychiatric morbidity during pregnancy. It is likely that the same criticism holds for those 'allied professionals' who clamour for abortion to prevent battered babies, and nearly every other social disability, as soon as a prospective new baby appears on the horizon. They cannot have much confidence in their professional skill. A psychiatrist who would not abort on psychiatric grounds, said: 'The day has not come when I must ask a gynaecologist to treat my psychiatric patients'. He was able with this consistent policy to see many mothers with severe psychiatric disabilities safely through their pregnancies and beyond, and with no detriment to the developing children, for he followed them all up, in some instances for as long as 20 years. He became an expert in treating the instabilities associated with pregnancies, but as he recently wistfully remarked: 'Because of the rapid growth in abortions, it is becoming a dying art'.

As we battered babies are so close to the unborn child in age we do not see it as a thing but as a younger brother or sister. In fact I had a younger brother who was closer to me in age when he was only several weeks in my mother's womb than my elder sister and I felt I knew him from the very start. It is horrible to think that just because my mother abused me he might have been destroyed completely; I would have felt that it was largely my fault. If society, in general, does not have the highest regard for human life, how can it expect its unstable, uncontrolled and socially disadvantaged to behave differently?

It is odd that those who advocate abortion on demand and euthanasia of the elderly and the unfit call themselves humanists yet subscribe to such inhuman and anti-human philosophies. George Orwell need not have worried about his predictions for 1984. Some have already been fulfilled, especially the doublethink. I think that any erosion of respect for human life dehumanizes man and reduces the other person to a thing rather than a fellow being.

I can just see my mother in one of her temper outbursts, when I had done or not done something which exasperated her. She would storm and rage at me, 'I could easily have had you aborted; in fact the clinic advised me to, but I wanted you. I wanted to have a beautiful and perfect child on whom I could lavish all my love; give you the love I didn't have when I was a baby', and she would then beat me in her frenzy. I could then sense that she saw me not as her child whom she loved but as a thing which irritated and displeased her and a thing which these days can be so easily disposed of. Her respect for human life had been eroded by dangerous cultural attitudes. It would also affect her regard for her parents should they become infirm and burdensome.

An efficient system of tax collection to support the welfare services does not compensate for the loss of human values and yet these severe wounds to the very essence of our society are self-inflicted. Respect for human life is indivisible. It cannot be left to the whims of people or governments as to which category should be kept alive and which should be destroyed. My own instance provides an example of this. Because I am of normal intelligence and passed the tests for entry into the educational system I am given less support and protection than those so-called autistic children whose middle-class parents, by skilful propaganda, were able to mobilize for them a grossly disproportionate amount of our resources. When things have been exceptionally difficult for me, I would wish that I were an autistic child.

Maltreatment is not only physical abuse. In recent years there has been a growing interest in young children of both sexes, by sexual deviants. A common initiation into these practices is through the medium of pornographic literature yet any attempt to restrict the circulation of such literature is met with the strongest opposition by civil libertarians and of course the commercial interests that thrive on the sales. Should there be a prosecution, the court is flooded with expert witnesses who testify on oath that this literature is not only harmless but beneficial to the reader. At the most, they would say, it was a 'fantasy fodder' or 'masturbatory material' which would relieve the urge to act and thus ensure that no overt behaviour would result. We children know that this is not so, for many have been assaulted sexually and otherwise and a number have lost their lives. Some are involved in performances for the distribution of blue films and even this has been said to do us good. A psychiatrist who was frequently called for the prosecution in pornographic cases would spend more time on studying the advertisements than on the text, for these gave the lie to this type of literature being for fantasy only. All sorts of contraptions were for sale for the practice of deviant, usually sadistic or masochistic behaviour, and there were also directories of those who catered for such practices. Fantasy soon gives way to the act and children who figure prominently in this type of literature are exposed to moral, physical and psychological dangers.

Even in school, on the grounds of non-discrimination, many psychiatrists urge that a practising homosexual should not be restricted in teaching appointments. The argument is that they rarely interfere with their pupils and if they do, it does no harm. But what of the vulnerable or even seductive child? We fence off large stretches of railway line to prevent children from straying on to it, yet we refuse to take similar precautions in our schools.

We are getting more and more sex education in school and this again strikes me as odd for we are the only members of the animal world who need to get this information from books and pictures. Our illiterate cousins without these educational advantages seem to do very well and animals have no sexual problems. When I see the disproportionate time older children are spending on the sex game, I wonder whether they need turning off rather than on. Curiosity in childhood is one of the greatest assets in education for it is at the root of the spirit of inquiry and provides the motive force in application. As it is a sublimation of the sex drive, is there any real point in blocking it? This emphasis on sex education has probably contributed to the lowering of educational attainment in the school years and the need for so much adult education to teach people to read and write. At one time, adult education was almost exclusively used for those who had no educational opportunities as children and wished to catch up on these lost years. Now, most students in adult education are those who failed to take advantage of their opportunities even after attending school until the age of 18 or 19 years. All school failures are not due to sex education. Many are due to ill-conceived educational experiments where the main objectives of a sound education are lost in the labyrinth of psychological and sociological theorizing and the dominance of the cult. A small pilot scheme in several selected areas with careful evaluation of the results has given way to mass experiments which even when found harmful cannot readily be dropped because of the heavy commitment. Neither ourselves nor our parents are consulted on these matters for others claim they know best. It is obvious that they do not.

There are lots of things to put right, and though the main theme of this book is on the maltreated child with the accent on physical abuse, one should not forget that there are other equally important aspects. Dr Selwyn Smith, who has devoted a lot of time to the subject, has assembled a group of experts who deal with the various aspects. Some do not express themselves as strongly as I have done but then, as I have said, I cannot be objective about this. Nevertheless they all demonstrate an intellectual honesty in their presentation and analysis and interpretation of data and for that I am truly grateful. Whatever conclusions may be drawn, I am sure that it can only benefit maltreated children and as their self-appointed representative I can only hope that this volume will have the social as well as the academic impact it deserves.

2 Child abuse and neglect – medical aspects

CHRISTINE E. COOPER

INTRODUCTION

The medical aspects of child abuse cover a wide range of disorders from inflicted injuries, through neglect, failure to thrive and severe psychological disorders. The doctor's role includes diagnosis, treatment, prediction and prevention, side by side with colleagues in other disciplines, and may involve the doctor in Court proceedings for child protection or occasionally in criminal proceedings against the parents.[1-]

In order to understand the complex, diffuse and difficult issues involved, expertise is needed in the development of normal families and children, of how certain patterns of parenting are deviant and the effects this has on the child and on the family[7,8]. Cultural practices and attitudes also have to be understood and assessed. Doctors experienced in psychological and psychiatric medicine are required as well as those with knowledge of the types of injury children normally sustain, detailed experience of minor injuries, bruises, fractures, head injuries and their causation. Knowledge of child poisoning, suffocation, cot deaths and drowning is needed and of growth problems in general and failure to thrive from neglect and deprivation in particular. Problems of slow development, speech and language disorders, learning problems at school, are among the other disorders in which doctors must be involved with other disciplines for diagnosis, management and above all for prevention.

Children may be killed or maimed by injuries from parents or guardians but these are the minority. Far more children, who may at times show moderate or minor injuries, suffer severe psychological damage causing permanent defects in development and in personality from the abusive environment in which they live, be it violent, hostile, neglectful, cruel or a mixture of these. Children are damaged by other forms of violence than by direct physical assault, and they may be brutalized by witnessing or taking part in cruelty to other people or to animals. They may be severely restricted in growth or development by under-nutrition, lack of stimulation, affection and encouragement, and by being prevented from running about, talking, playing and exploring their environment. Such parents cannot tolerate the ordinary noise and play of children.

Some forms of abuse and cruelty to children may be subtle and hard to prove but they are none the less damaging in their effects. By improved understanding of these as well as the grosser forms of abuse from parent and family malfunctioning, knowledge will increase on the optimum care and education of all children who should thereby benefit in the long run.

Those working in this field need to examine their own attitudes and the emotions aroused towards violence and cruelty, to acceptable methods for controlling children, to corporal punishment, to the ethics of child protection including the removal of children from their parents, to the rights of children for optimum growth and development, and to prediction of abnormal and dangerous parenting and ways of preventing it.

Ethology, anthropology and sociology as well as developmental biology all have a contribution to make to our understanding of family violence. We should look at the mores of child care throughout history[9], and in different cultures, and consider the place of the family in society today[10,11] and the dimensions of parenthood[12,13]. This broader view of child abuse and neglect is essential to an understanding of the complex causes and factors involved, including those of stress within the family, wife battering and the concepts of wife and children as chattels or as human beings with rights of their own[14-16].

PREVENTION – MEDICAL ASPECTS

Since child abuse has multifocal origins there is no simple method of prevention. Many different approaches are needed to improve the mother/infant and parent/child relationship. Table 2.1 sets out the main issues. Although the doctor may be involved in all of these, the second, third and fourth affect him most. All these matters are closely inter-related.

Table. 2.1   Child abuse and deprivation – prevention

1. Education of children and youth in responsible parenthood and parentcraft
2. Diagnosis antenatally, at confinement and in early weeks of troubled families
3. Early detection of child abuse
4. Development of multidisciplinary teams for prevention, diagnosis and management
5. Study and effective use of legal system for child protection
6. Increase public understanding and encouragement of families to seek help early

Education of children and youth in responsible parenthood and parentcraft

In spite of various experiments in other ways of rearing children, the family remains the most popular and most effective way of producing stable and mature adults.

The best education for parenthood takes place in the child's home in its earliest years when the child *experiences* loving care and control. As the child grows in his family and neighbourhood he *learns the model of parenting* of his own culture. Many abusing parents have never experienced consistent loving care and concern for their welfare. The model of family life for them has been distorted and abnormal, with violence, shouting, misery, disorganization, and lack of comfort, understanding and encouragement, or it may have been quiet and cold and negative with or without outbursts of violence. No wonder they have little idea how to deal even practically with their young child and still less how to cope with their own powerful emotions aroused by the whole-time care of a young baby or toddler.

The situation of such parents has been sensitively described by a forensic psychiatrist:

'Reproduction (marriage and child rearing) is the only one of our vital activities which absolutely demands sustained generosity and selflessness; it is therefore not surprising that if either or both partners are unable to give, their handicap will inevitably be revealed, and violence is one way in which the anguish of such failure may be expressed.'

Peter Scott
The Times, August 1973

Divorce,[17-21] separations, changing consorts, frequently moving house or schools are common disrupting experiences in many children's lives producing confusion, misunderstanding, unhappiness, and damaging the child's capacity to form meaningful relationships. When grown up these young people in their turn form transient unions, often producing one or two children from each, and so the vicious circle continues through the generations. Adults, whose own needs in childhood have not been met, still seek emotional satisfactions themselves regardless of their own children's needs. They often start childbearing early[22] for status or 'to have something of my own', but their immaturity leads to conflict between their own needs and that of the child.

Persuading young people to postpone pregnancy until they themselves are ready to give time and energy to rearing a family has been successfully achieved in China, and more research is needed on this matter in the West. The children of teenage mothers are at high risk for problems of behaviour and development[22-26].

Doctors and other educators have a part to play in this and the mass media could be used more effectively than at present. The vulnerable teenagers are a special group and hard to reach but a number of experimental schemes are being tried here, in the USA and in other countries[27].

Some schools in Britain and elsewhere give simple theoretical and practical experience to adolescents in parentcraft, demonstrating details of the feeding and care of a child, and in the responsibilities of parenthood, including the psychological needs of the child and the family[28]. Visits to nurseries and health clinics, and practical handling of young children is often included and seems beneficial although evaluation of these schemes is awaited. Unfortunately at present it is often only the girls who receive such teaching, the boys doing gardening or woodwork in parallel. So far it is mainly the less able pupils who receive this instruction whereas all young people need it in these days of small families. It is all too common for parents in the West in the 1970s to approach childbirth never having seen or handled a young infant, and being quite unaware of the time and patience needed in caring for babies and children.

Doctors and health visitors are often involved in these early training schemes and collaboration with others, including psychologists, social workers and ordinary parents is valuable. Suitable books with easy texts are hard to find[29].

Diagnosis antenatally, at confinement and in early weeks of trouble families

This seems by far the most effective area, and many researches in the past 10 years have produced results which show promise. Frommer and O'Shea[30,31] have shown that girls who have experienced separation from their own families have more problems in marriage and rearing children than girls who have not. More recently Wolkind[23,24] has studied a group of British born primiparous women who have experienced separation from parents in childhood. He found they had a number of social and medical factors which are known to be common in mothers with child rearing problems. Kempe and his collaborators have demonstrated that sensitive observations in the labour room and lying in ward can detect mothers who are not bonding comfortably to their infants. They have shown[32,33] that given extra services these families have fewer problems with their infants than those without extra help and that serious physical abuse can be prevented. Klaus and Kennell, in their excellent book on Maternal-Infant Bonding[34], summarised the findings of many workers revealing that premature and sick new borns are seriously at risk for severe disorders of parenting including excessive crying, feeding problems, failure to thrive and inflicted injury. Lynch[35,36] has recently shown that there are many other indicators in the maternity unit that certain families are vulnerable to stress with a particular infant, frequently have management problems and serious abuse to the child may follow.

Parenting is a delicate art with complex origins. There are three main sources of stress in parents. The first and most important is the internal stress, resulting from emotional damage or deprivation in the individual's own childhood. Secondly, stress from immediate family problems which are often multiple. These include severe marital discord, care of elderly, infirm relatives, a handicapped child, too many young children born too close together. Thirdly social problems of many different kinds add further stress so that parents are unable to provide an affectionate concerned environment, so preoccupied are they, consciously or unconsciously, with their own problems.

Parenting capacity can be considered as a continuum with at one end parents, perhaps 10% of all, who will manage to care for, encourage and control their children exceptionally well in spite of difficulties in the children or other problems in their own lives. They can be called 'super' parents. Most families have 'good enough' parents, to use Winnicott's term[37], who manage to bring up their children satisfactorily and with enjoyment. Then come the vulnerable families, maybe another 10%, where parents only just cope and where illness or difficulties in the child, or adversities in their own lives, are likely to lead to break down in relationships, abnormal parenting practices and severe disturbances in children. We have to remember the high percentage of children, especially in inner city areas, who are already seriously disturbed on entering school at five or six years of age.

At the end of the continuum are the abusing and neglectful parents, perhaps 1 to 5%, who explode into violence frequently when stressed or who use harsh and inappropriate discipline. Others are cold or hostile to their children and show little real affection or concern. These parents may be so deprived themselves that they indulge their own interests without thought or care for the needs of their children, for example going out leaving young children alone in the house for hours on end or letting a hungry new born cry itself into an exhausted sleep while they watch television or chat with a neighbour. When eventually the child is fed, fatigue and wind may complicate the feed causing vomiting, more hunger and restlessness, and the so-called feeding problem or crying baby syndrome begins. A damaging relationship between mother and baby often starts in such a way. Treated early, by exploring the mother's feelings and giving both her and her husband insight and support the problems usually resolve. Sometimes an opportunity to catch up on sleep is what the mother most needs.

Tranquillisers for the mothers of young children with symptoms of anxiety and depression must be used with great caution. The drugs are known to enhance aggressive behaviour[38,39]. When the depression is due to abnormal interpersonal feelings, common in the post-partum period, brief psychotherapy is needed if necessary supplemented with social work help, rather than drugs[40].

Research studies on newborns increasingly show the importance of a number of delicate functions and skills which are inter-related and which highlight the marvellous mechanisms which nature has developed to ensure the safety and nurture of the human infant. The first of these is the *reciprocal relationship* between mother and baby[41,42]. It begins in pregnancy and is enhanced as the baby becomes a reality at quickening, when foetal movements are first felt, and rises to a high peak after birth especially in a conscious mother, who immediately sees, hears and touches her infant, and moments later has him naked in her arms.

The normal healthy undrugged newborn opens his eyes and looks at her and this starts the important reciprocal responses between them which promote mother/infant bonding and draw from her tender protective and nurturing actions which will give her a sense of joy and fulfilment. The infant in turn responds by suckling, by watching her, by cuddling and by thriving, and soon by smiling and vocalizing his responses as well.

Secondly there seems to be a *sensitive period for maternal bonding* in the hours immediately following birth, similar to that in other mammals and possibly related to the mother's endocrine changes, when the proximity of the newborn enhances her ability to bond with her baby, to empathize and nurture her child.

The studies of Klaus and Kennell[43-47] and of de Chateau[48-51] have emphasized the importance of close proximity of mother and infant, and of the value of including the father in the bonding process from the start, in pregnancy, during labour and in the earliest hours and days.

Thirdly *the father has a similar flood of emotional responses* to his newborn, as Greenberg and Morris[52] were among the first to show and the practice is growing up in some maternity units in the USA, Britain and Sweden, of instituting 'a fourth stage of labour' with the mother and father being alone together for an hour or so with their naked infant, in a warm room and with precautions to prevent heat loss from the infant. Fondling, suckling, cuddling or sleep may occur in any or all of the three during this time. Lyn[53] has emphasized the importance of the father's contribution to child development and family life, a neglected topic in the 20th century. His deeper understanding and helpfulness to his wife from sharing the labour and early hours of the infant's life are no small contribution to the total family welfare.

Fourthly some other important matters at this time are *awareness at delivery* for the mother, and *an undrugged newborn* and so the importance of *preparation for labour* on the one hand and *natural childbirth* on the other obviously follows[54,55,56].

Planned caesarean section under epidural anaesthesia has become routine in Sweden[57] and elsewhere so that the mother as well as the father can see and touch the newborn at once and have the baby near her in the delivery room and lying-in ward. *Rooms with the infants and mothers together should be the rule* in maternity units. The development of special care baby rooms has led to a high proportion of infants with minor symptoms being admitted there, and separated from their mothers. This is detrimental to the mother/infant relationship and much of it stems from interference with natural childbirth. At most only some 7–10% of newborns need any special care, and the ordinary lying-in ward should once more learn to deal with minor infant symptoms, so that infants are not removed from their mothers[58].

When small infants have to be taken to an incubator for special care, unless they are ill or having breathing difficulty, they should spend 10–15 minutes in their mothers' arms at birth, with precautions against cooling, before going to the nursery. The mother and father should see the baby and touch him in the incubator as soon as possible after he goes to the nursery. An instamatic photograph of the incubator newborn's face for the mother to keep beside her enhances her feelings, as does the physician and nurse who emphasize the health and strength of the child and show optimism about his chances. As soon as possible parents should participate in tube feeding and other care.

Studies on *the competence of the newborn infant, and his capacity to respond*[60,61,62] at birth to visual, auditory, olfactory and kinaesthetic stimuli are complementary to the studies on parents just mentioned but doctors and nurses need to be more aware of this and the public too. A mother's responses are enhanced when her physician or nurse confirms that her newborn can see her, hear and smell her and respond to her own particular care. When mother and infant remain together she quickly becomes the expert for her own child. The importance of adequate nutrition for the early rapid brain growth, and of play and stimulation to promote the baby's development at an early stage is only now being taught and too few are fully aware of the importance of all this.

Successful breast-feeding initiated most easily by suckling immediately after birth[63-66], promotes the physical well-being and nutrition of the baby, and protects him from immediate infection by giving him his mother's bacterial flora (rather than the hospital organisms) and from later infection by enhancing gut and other cellular immunity. It also promotes his psychological well-being and bonding with his mother if it is going well and both are enjoying it. Immediate closeness between mother and baby at birth and suckling in the first hour has been shown to lead to more successful breast feeding and to mothers who suckle for longer than when the first breast feed is postponed some hours. Encouraging frequent suckling in the first week or two also promotes successful breast feeding[67].

All of these intimate relationships and functions between mother and child, and including the father, help to promote the mother/infant relationship and the father's concern and involvement with both[68,69]. Parents and infant then thrive optimally, and when the fatigue and hard times follow the parents are more able to view and handle the infant with gentleness and patience, and put the child's needs before their own as good parents do. This optimal start in life is even more important for the vulnerable family. Continuing care and help for these families in the community, as Kempe has shown, will greatly lessen parenting problems including child abuse[32].

Early detection of child abuse

Clearly, to provide help for an abused child and his family at the earliest possible time, when the harmful attitudes or first small bruise is seen, will help to reduce further damage, will safeguard the child's development, improve the parents' nurturing functions and so their enjoyment of their family. All professionals associated with young families should have this as their aim. Adequate diagnosis of the parents difficulties and their soarces is crucial in estimating the risk of further physical abuse.

Development of multidisciplinary teams for prevention, diagnosis and management

The doctor has a leading role to play with other professionals in developing society's knowledge and understanding of prevention and in predicting vulnerable families during obstetric and newborn care. In diagnosis too his role is a leading one, though the social and educational prongs of assessment will come from other disciplines. In management the doctor's role is limited, but he must play his part in monitoring the child's and siblings' growth and development in the early years, in promoting good birth control, and in assessing accidents. As a member of the original team his view may be useful in the periodic reviews of the family where continuity of care and oversight is very valuble. The child psychiatrist has much to contribute to the team's understanding as well as helping individual families.

Study and effective use of legal systems for child protection

It is the doctor's duty to assist the child protection courts or panels in providing evidence about the child's injuries, growth, development and other health matters and about the quality of the parenting. Courts are changing their attitudes in recent years towards the rights of children, but much work needs to be done on helping the parents over the court experience, and in studying and learning with the lawyers improved ways of providing clear evidence.

Increased public understanding and encouragement of families to seek help early

Doctors as well as other professionals can increase public understanding and compassion for the problems some parents have with their children, and with the multi-faceted causes of child abuse. Good neighbour schemes and other ways of assisting families in trouble can be started so that 'help not hounding' is the attitude towards such families, to encourage them to seek relief early. Evaluation is needed for all new schemes.

Political, social and educational measures

These complex issues are outside the scope of this chapter. Rutter[69,70] has examined them and many other authors[71,72].

CLINICAL FEATURES

The main groups of conditions seen in abused children are shown in Table 2.2. Manifestations of several conditions may be seen in one child, for example injuries in addition to failure to thrive, or disordered behaviour present with the other conditions.

1. PHYSICAL INJURIES – NON-ACCIDENTAL

Physical injuries were the first signs of abuse to be recognized and to begin with were considered to be the major problem. Only later was it realized that the injuries are but a signpost to a family with severe internal stress needing urgent diagnosis and treatment. Even now there is sometimes considerable

Table 2.2 Child abuse, clinical features in the child

1. Physical injuries – non-accidental
   Bruises, weals, lacerations and scars
   Burns and scalds
   Bone and joint injuries
   Brain and eye injuries
   Internal injuries
2. Other clinical disorders
   Poisoning
   Drowning
   Cot deaths
   'Funny turns'
   Repeated problems with crying and feeding
   Overactivity and demanding behaviour
   Hysterical moods (in older children)
3. Failure to thrive without organic cause
4. Disordered behaviour (observed)
5. Sexual abuse
6. Abuse while in care

reluctance to admit that injuries are probably not accidental and that the parents' story is inconsistent with the findings on the child. Other symptoms and signs of abuse or of disordered family function will usually be found to confirm the diagnosis once suspicion is aroused.

In Newcastle, studies of child abuse began in 1966 and in the first 5 years 136 children were seen with 148 episodes of injury[5,73]. These were relatively severe with over 10% dead, nearly a half with fractures and well over one quarter with subdural haematoma (SDH). When the analysis of the second 5 years is complete there will be fewer serious injuries because the children's and family's problems are more often recognized at an earlier stage. However, although there are fewer deaths and serious injuries from the battered child syndrome, more children with moderate or minor trauma are being recognized. At the same time other disorders due to abuse are beginning to be understood.

In most of the published series the sexes are evenly represented or else, as here (Table 2.3), there is a slight preponderance of boys. The highest number of cases is seen in the early months of life. Deaths are more common in the younger children

Table 2.3 NAI 136 children (Newcastle) 1965–71.
Sex incidence

Boys	80	58.8%	
Girls	56	41.2%	136 children
Boys	91	60.8%	
Girls	57	39.2%	148 episodes

who are especially vulnerable to rough handling, particularly to shaking, which causes subdural haematoma. It is obvious to most clinicians however that a number of cases are missed especially in the older age groups where ordinary accidents are more common making the differential diagnosis harder. It may not be realized that the children are too frightened to contradict the parents' false history of the accident.

Table 2.4 shows the frequency of the major injuries. As in other published series over 90% of children being physically abused have injuries on their skin, and learning to 'read' these signs is crucial to early diagnosis. Nearly all

Table 2.4   NAI 136 children (Newcastle) 1965–71.
Frequency of injuries (148 episodes)

BRUISES including lacerations, small burns etc.	127	93.4%
FRACTURES	63	46.3%
S.D.H.	39	28.7%
OTHER abdomen, eyes, synovitis, bites	21	15.6%

children who have been killed or severely injured have had former minor injuries, especially on the face, presented to a family doctor, a child health clinic or a casualty department, and not recognized as abuse, the so-called 'open warnings' of Ounsted[74]. Nearly half (46.3%) the children in Newcastle had fractures, often clinically undetectable, and the high number (28.7%) with subdural haematoma indicates the severity of the physical abuse in these early years. Severe burns are not included in this series since the burnt children were treated in another unit.

Table 2.5 shows the outcome in the first 136 children. Death resulted in 10.3%, either from the injury first recognized or from subsequent injuries. 30% of those followed were permanently brain damaged with combinations of mental retardation, cerebral palsy, blindness, deafness and epilepsy. One mother

Table 2.5 NAI 136 children (Newcastle) 1965–71.
Outcome

DEATHS	14	10.3%
Boys	8	
Girls	6	
PERMANENT BRAIN DAMAGE		c.30% of 60 followed up
DAMAGED PERSONALITIES = MANY		
TWO MOTHERS MURDERED		

was murdered 10 days after her son by a jealous consort. Another mother and her consort were murdered by her husband who immediately shot himself, several years after their children were recognized as having non-accidental injuries.

Few long term studies on the later outcome for abused children's personality characteristics have so far been carried out. The most important work is that of Martin from Denver, Colorado, who has followed up a group of children many years after the abuse[75]. These children and their families had received various treatment regimes often including psychotherapy and were probably more thoroughly treated there than anywhere else at the time.

Nine characteristics were found in these children apart from delays in development, and each child manifested several or many of them. Clinicians familiar with abusing families know that the parents of abused children show these same characteristics, this being further confirmation, if any were needed, that they too were abused in childhood.

The characteristics most commonly noted by independent observers were:

> impaired capacity for enjoyment
> psychiatric symptoms e.g. enuresis, restlessness and tantrums
> low self esteem
> school learning problems
> withdrawal
> rebelliousness
> compulsivity
> hypervigilance
> pseudo-mature behaviour or role reversal[76].

All are handicapping conditions and impair school performance further.

Baher has also shown that although the physical abuse may stop, and after help in groups the mothers may feel and function better, the abused *children* continue with a distorted perception of the world, and markedly impaired family relationships. These were children who had attended a therapeutic playgroup for several years where a high staff child ratio and a special interest in and empathy for abusing families exist. Emer found a similar gloomy picture and so did Malone[79].

Multiple injuries

The importance of recognizing as abuse multiple small injuries to the face, mouth and head cannot be over-emphasized. It is a common place for the injuries to begin and the younger the child the more significant even one bruise may be in indicating future danger. It is often largely chance that determines the severity of the injury, although not entirely so. A mother may fling her baby down in anger, and one time he bounces on the bed, while another he skids off it on to a sharp surface resulting in head injuries and bruises.

Multiple injuries, even when minor, should be suspect, especially in young children but it can sometimes be hard to know when they are outside the normal range. Any bruising in a baby not yet mobile is suspect. An important fact is that nature has endowed small children with protective reflexes so that when they tumble or fall either they tend to curl up or they fall on outstretched hands or feet (the parachute reaction) and so sustain remarkably few bumps and bruises. Bony prominences on extensor surfaces are usually the site of 'natural' bruises, the forehead, and later on, the shins, may show small bruises from ordinary play or harmless falls. Injuries involving both sides of the body said to be caused by a fall are also suspect.

It is sometimes crucial, even when individual bruising or other injuries are minor (especially in a child under 3 years), to recognize them as part of the picture of abuse and take action in order to save a life or prevent serious injury or protect a child from other forms of abuse. The injury is the signal which alerts us to the need for enquiry and help for the family, and for the child. *Every child with a non-accidental physical injury is the victim of more or less severe psychological abuse.*

Bruises, wheals, lacerations and scars

Table 2.6 shows the frequency of bruises in the Newcastle area.

Inflicted bruises may be found anywhere, but when the face and head is in-

Table 2.6   NAI 136 children (Newcastle) 1965–71.
Bruises (148 episodes)

ALONE	48	35.3%
+ FRACTURES	45	33.3%
+ FRACTURE AND S.D.H.	22	16.2%
+ S.D.H.	9	6.6%
+ RETINAL HAEMORRHAGES	3	2.2%

volved, especially in very young children, it is particularly serious since the brain is so near and so vulnerable. Normal parents do not chastise babies, and later they avoid the face and head when physical punishment is given. Bruises may be accompanied by other injuries, Table 2.6.

Variations are seen in bruises in different parts of the body. Sometimes injuries around a joint are puzzling until the joint is put through a full range of movement when it will be seen which position the joint was in when the injury occurred. Curved surfaces such as the buttocks may also distort the pattern of the weapon, and relatively avascular areas like the soles of the feet bruise less readily. It is rare for a single accident to cause bruising on both sides of the body and when this is present the doctor should be alerted to exclude abuse.

Obviously at times inflicted skin trauma may not differ in appearance from accidental trauma, but certain bruises or patterns of bruises are typical of inflicted injury in young children[80,81].

Finger-tip bruises

These are round or oval, 0.5–2.5 cm in diameter. The skin above is intact, and there is no swelling beneath the bruise which is flush with the skin. It is caused by firm pressure, usually maintained for a minute or more. The bruises are in crops of three or four together, and there is often a thumb bruise some distance away. The little finger bruise may be faint or absent. The disproportionate size of the adult hand on a small child may lead to confusion, and the physician's hand should be fitted into the bruises to test the validity of the diagnosis. Sometimes the thumb mark is on one side of the trunk and the finger marks on the other when a baby has been held and shaken. The parent's arms may tire and as they rest awhile the baby slips through their fingers a little way. If they shake again the finger or thumb marks will occur slightly higher up the trunk, and occasionally a third or fourth series of marks are present. In other cases the finger-tip bruises can be clearly seen on the baby's face, the thumb on one side and finger tips on the other, caused by forcefully holding the baby's face or pressing it on to a firm surface while shouting at the child to 'be quiet'. They may be confined to forehead, to cheeks or to the jaw, or mixed, with, for example, the finger marks on the forehead and the thumb on the opposite cheek or zygoma. It can be clearly seen whether a right or left hand has caused the bruise pattern. Occasionally the baby has been approached from sideways or above the head and the bruise pattern varies accordingly.

The bruises from finger or thumb tip pressure are most distinct on the trunk, forehead and cheek, and less so on the lower face, chin, neck and limbs. They may be of several different ages. When on the face they can be recognized from several yards away.

Subcutaneous bruising
This indicates considerable violence to the bruised area and rupture of deeper capillaries by a fall or blow, and by pinching or kicking. Swelling is produced, with shiny skin over it, and bruises may not show for some hours until the blood tracks through to the surface. Where subcutaneous tissue overlies a bony prominence such as the shin or zygoma, this type of bruising is more easily caused and may be associated with surface marks, such as abrasions or linear marks from a hand slap or stick. Subcutaneous bruising is often seen associated with petechial or other intradermal haemorrhages.

When a fall on a rough surface such as a concrete path is alleged, there will always be a graze of the skin overlying the subcutaneous contusion, though in some cases this may be very small. When a blow has caused the injury irregular or projecting objects such as a ring on a fist, the buckle of a belt or a nail on a piece of wood, may cause a graze or laceration over or near the bruising.

Petechial or intradermal haemorrhage
Rupture of the skin capillaries from high pressure of blood within them causes skin haemorrhages, which are rarely large ecchymoses, and more usually tiny pin-point haemorrhages which may coalesce. The commonest cause is a violent blow to the skin which forces blood out of the capillaries under the area of contact into the surrounding unsupported vessels which rupture under the strain. The outline of a weapon such as fingers, belt or stick, may then be clearly seen. Rough handling of a baby's skin may cause petechial haemorrhages and

sometimes these are combined with bruises on limbs or face. Traumatic asphyxia from sudden compression of the chest or neck forces blood suddenly into the face and head, and a shower of petechial haemorrhages occurs on the face, conjunctivae and retinae. Kicking children's shins while grasping their arms is a way some parents punish children. Small irregular skin and sub-cutaneous bruises result in far greater numbers than are caused by ordinary play. Grasp or finger marks on the arms or shoulder may be present when kicked shins occur.

The mouth

Injuries to the mouth are common in child abuse cases and often multiple. Small bruises of different ages may be seen on the lips sometimes with other minor injuries to the face and chin. Bruising of the lips or gums and a torn frenulum of the upper lip or tongue should be looked for carefully in every case, everting the lips in a good light. Mouth lesions heal extremely fast and in 4 or 5 days quite extensive tears or bruises may have gone. Ramming a fist or feeding bottle on to or into the mouth of a crying child is the usual cause of the mouth injuries but occasionally a boot is involved.

Ear

'The purple ear' from petechial haemorrhage is rarely seen in ordinary ac-cidents and most commonly results from repeated blows with a hand or fist. The ear lobe itself and behind it, as well as the surrounding skin, should be carefully inspected for single or multiple tiny haemorrhages, which may be of different ages. Sometimes greenish or yellowish staining indicates resolving haemorrhage of some days earlier.

Black eyes and cheek bruises

With a large bruise on the forehead blood may trickle down into the upper eyelids, or with a fracture of the frontal bone or the back of the orbit, blood may seep through into the eyelids. Rarely a black eye is part of a haemorrhagic condition such as scurvy, haemophilia or leukaemia, or of a malignancy such as neuroblastoma. Apart from these conditions a black eye must be caused by an object which fits into the bony margin of the orbit, yet not small enough to damage the eyeball. A fist or a boot are the commonest objects. A fall on a flat surface bruises the bony margins of the orbit and rarely causes a black eye.

One black eye in the absence of the conditions described above is therefore suspect, but two black eyes is almost always abuse. Injuries on both sides of the body are rare from a single accident. Similarly the soft tissue of the cheek seldom bruises naturally at any age because it is protected by a rim of bone. Falls on a flat surface or against the edge of a table usually bruise the skin over the cheek bone or chin. A cheek bruise in a baby cannot be caused 'naturally' and trivial though it seems it is a very important sign of a dangerous situation for the child. Many children dead or permanently maimed have had a cheek bruise neglected in the past.

Bites

Adult human bites must be distinguished from those of a toddler, and rarely from dog bites or those of other animal species[82]. The bite of a young child is small and limited, usually shallow and less than 2 cm in diameter. The teeth marks when visible are tiny and the whole thing disappears in 24–48 h. The adult bite is found on any part of the body as two hemispherical linear marks usually with a gap at each end, but sometimes as a full circular bruise. There may be abrasions in the skin caused by individual teeth which later scab over, but usually petechial haemorrhages are produced at the time and in a few hours marked bruising is evident. Variation is due to the amount of tissue included in the bite, the degree of pressure, the amount of suction or tongue thrust and the individual dentition. Overlapping bites, especially those of different ages, may cause confusion.

Saliva test

In fresh cases a saliva test may be carried out for the presence of antibodies. Using forceps a square inch of cigarette paper is cut from a piece freshly removed from the packet. It should be moistened in tap water and rubbed on the unwashed skin over the bite mark. This should be done thoroughly, moving the forceps and turning the paper over so that the whole paper is covered. It should then be put into a dry container. A control area of the child's unwashed skin, some distance from the bite, should be similarly rubbed with a diamond shaped piece of fresh moistened cigarette paper held only in forceps, and put into a second dry container. Another control, this time using a circular piece of cigarette paper held in forceps, is moistened in tap water and put directly into a third dry container. *The specimens must never be touched by the fingers.* Each specimen is carefully labelled with the child's name, date, time and contents and sent to the laboratory. The service of a forensic dental surgeon is of great value in some of these cases and with photographs of the lesions and casts of the mouths of possible assailants he can often indicate who was responsible.

Grasp marks

Usually on a limb, these are irregular linear bruises caused by firm pressure and sometimes associated with one or more finger-tip bruises on the opposite side of the limb.

Bizarre skin marks

These can occur from firm pressure through coarse weave clothing or other material, where the pattern is outlined on the skin. Sometimes an unusual shaped or textured weapon causes strange marks, such as the bristles of a brush.

Ligature marks

These may be seen on arms or legs, on the neck or penis, and rarely on the trunk. String, thong and other materials are used, and a shawl may be pulled tightly round the neck to stop a baby crying. A search should be made for signs of tying up or strangulation. Chafing and bruising from string around wrists and ankles tying a child to his cot or to furniture usually leaves an area of pigmentation on the skin which takes a few weeks to fade. Strangulation marks on the neck are often quite faint, even when the baby is killed, but a careful search should be made. At autopsy inspection of the front of the larynx or trachea may reveal a tell-tale line of small petechial haemorrhages. The penis is sometimes tied up with string to prevent a child wetting his bed and bruises and abrasions may be seen or a swollen shaft and glands beyond the ligature which must not be confused with a paraphimosis.

Mongolian blue spot

These irregular patches of pigmentation in the skin are seen in babies of African or Asian extraction even when only a distant relative is coloured. They appear soon after birth and resolve by the early school years. They are slaty-grey in colour, flush with the skin, have a smooth or occasionally irregular edge and are commonest on the buttocks or lumbar region but may occur anywhere on the trunk or limbs. *They are not bruises.*

A disproportionate amount of soft tissue injury

In severe cases of battering a child's limbs, body and head may be severely bruised on both sides, and other signs such as bites, burns and neglect may be present. In all such cases the amount of injury can have only one explanation. The parents sometimes say the child fell downstairs. Even in seriously injured children with road traffic accidents such extensive bruising is never seen.

Weals

When the skin is struck by a hard object such as a stick there is considerable swelling for some hours at the site of impact, and when this goes down the outline of the weapon in petechial haemorrhages will be seen. In fresh injuries this must be borne in mind as they may look quite different a few hours later.

Lacerations, scars and scratches

Lacerations, often needing sutures, are one of the commonest accidental injuries which children sustain, and usual sites are the forehead, chin, hands and knees. Parents and the older child usually know the cause of each scar from ordinary injuries and there are not many on any one child.

Abused children's lacerations often occur with multiple bruises, and are less easily explained. A fist with a ring on it beating a child, or the buckle of a belt, may cause abrasions and violent blows from any firm weapon may lacerate the skin. Multiple scars of different ages may be seen on the face, head or elsewhere, and scars of burns or scalds may be associated with them.

Clean linear cuts with a razor blade are used as a punishment by some sadistic parents and occasionally scars several inches long are seen. Scratches may be caused by all manner of things and people, including a jealous child. When caused by finger-nails there may be two or three parallel marks sometimes repeated in a criss-cross fashion. Nail scratches may vary in width being broadest at the start and typically they have heaped up cuticle at the end. Crescentic nail marks may also be seen.

Burns and scalds

Accidental burns from open fires are greatly reduced in societies where central heating is common. Similarly scalds from falling into a bowl of hot water prepared for a child's bath are also rare when most families have a bathroom. Inflicted burns and scalds can be very difficult to diagnose but as accidental burns and scalds become rarer, each burnt child should be critically examined to see that the history really does match the clinical findings. The age and ability of the child should be remembered. The direction of splash marks should be noted in scalds. Undoubtedly some plausible stories are given about inflicted burns and scalds, which would be hard to refute, but other factors about the child or parents or a previous suspicious injury to the child or siblings may alert the doctor to make further enquiries.

Scalds

Inflicted scalds may occur around a child's mouth when hot fluid has been forced into the child. Accidental or inflicted corrosive poisoning gives rather a similar appearance. Scalds from pouring boiling water on a child may be seen, and, if his legs and feet are the target, the absence of scalds on the soles, or the great toes, and the mildness or absence of scalding on the backs of the legs should be noted. In accidental scalds the arm, hand and front of the child is predominantly the area involved, whereas it may not be so in inflicted injuries. 'Dunking' scalds of a limb or the flexed buttocks, with the glove or stocking distribution, or the 'high-water-mark' on back and thighs needs mention.

Burns

Deliberate burning of children's hands or feet by a lighter or in the fire to pre-vent them playing with matches is sometimes used as a punishment, and they may be sat on a hot plate or fire as a punishment for wetting or soiling.

Cigarette burns ('Tab' marks)

These are found to be common in abused children and the author has heard a group of delinquent 15 year olds in a special school boast how they had often seen their brothers, uncles or boyfriends deliberately burn a baby or toddler with their cigarette. They described it as commonplace and so it seems to be. A cigarette burn may be single, and anywhere on the child, but they often occur in crops. The severity depends on the depth and whether the end is moved across the skin, and the amount of secondary infection which ensues. Sometimes coalescing burns are seen, but the area will then have a scalloped edge and may have discrete cigarette burns nearby. The discrete burns heal as small circular scars about 0.5–1 cm across, and varying in depth. When full thickness skin is involved the scar has an irregular puckered appearance.

Linear burns from pokers or the bars of a fire clearly show the shape of the weapon imprinted on the skin (cf. the outline of the weapon after a violent blow). Sometimes there are bizarre shapes of hot objects which have been held on the skin. Toddlers or young children may be held near the fire by their parents to watch a loved teddy or other toys burning as a punishment. If the skin is bare, burning may occur, possibly unintentionally, although the torture involved and the totally inappropriate punishments show highly pathological parenting.

Acute staphylococcal septicaemia with bullous skin lesions in an infant or toddler may be mistaken for a burn and so too may epidermolysis bullosa. Fric-tion burns can be accidental or inflicted and are sometimes due to carelessness in play.

Bone and joint injuries

These are a very important part of the battered child syndrome and indeed it was a radiologist, Caffey[83], who in 1946 first drew attention to the occurrence of multiple long bone fractures being associated with chronic subdural haematomata in babies and young children, and postulated violence which few really believed at the time. Babies' fractures have been missed because they do not produce any clinical signs.

Because radiological lesions are common in ill-treated infants and toddlers it is mandatory to do a full skeletal X-ray survey when abuse is suspected, and to repeat it in two weeks in most cases. The skull, the ribs and the ends of the long bones need very careful examination. The pelvis may be omitted from the survey unless clinically indicated to limit exposure of the gonads to X-rays because pelvic fractures are rarely seen.

Table 2.7 shows the typical radiological features in inflicted injury in babies and young children. The injuries are often multiple, of different ages, and are unexpected and unexplained clinically.

Table 2.7   Child abuse – radiological features

Multiple injuries
In various stages of healing
Clinically unexpected and unexplained
Metaphyseal injuries
Epiphyseal displacement
Periosteal new bone formation
Thickening of the shaft
Spiral fractures

X-rays should be repeated in 2 weeks

Metaphyseal and epiphyseal injuries and displacements are seen in infants whose limbs have been pulled or twisted or shaken. They do not show up until some two weeks after the injury when healing by periosteal new bone formation takes place. Tiny metaphyseal chip fractures may be seen when careful views in different projections are made, and with macro-films of the ends of the long bones.

Periosteal new bone formation, sometimes in successive layers, produces the onion skin effect. The actively growing and loosely attached periosteum of the young child is easily bruised and stripped up by pulling and twisting forces on the limb when the child is yanked up, swung or shaken by the limbs.

Temporary thickening of the shaft of the bone occurs from repeated periosteal stripping and healing. When the trauma ceases, the bones remould to their normal shape in 6–12 months.

Spiral fractures need special mention because, although sometimes accidental, in the young child they are often inflicted and the result of a torsion injury.

A single long bone shaft fracture in a baby under walking age is highly suspect.

Rib fractures in a baby or toddler are rarely accidental as the ribs are springy to all but violent compression injuries. With lateral compression of the chest the ribs usually fracture posteriorly. Anterior posterior compression or blows may cause fractures in the axillary line.

If the above types of lesion are present inflicted injury is very likely although the radiologist alone can seldom make a conclusive diagnosis. His comments alert the physician to further enquiry clinically and socially. Silverman has stated that he feels some 25% of all fractures under 3 years are probably due to non-accidental injuries.

Joint swellings

When children are roughly pulled or yanked up by an adult producing the injuries to the ends of bones just described there is sometimes subcutaneous swelling and tenderness around the joint and there may be a small effusion into it, both of which increase the discomfort. However the child may soon use the limb in play and in a few days normal movement is resumed.

Immediate X-ray may be normal except for the increased joint space but in two weeks the damage to the epiphysis, metaphysis or periosteum will be apparent, and this is almost diagnostic of abuse. An exception is when an adult suddenly catches a limb and jerks it to prevent a child from falling, but this is a rare situation.

Brain and eye injuries

The brain

The brain may be injured by direct blows to the stationary head, as, for example, when a child is struck while lying in his cot. It may also suffer as a result of whiplash injuries, i.e. acceleration–deceleration injuries, which are caused in two ways. By far the most important is shaking the baby or young child in anger, and this probably accounts for most of the brain damage in the battered child syndrome. Secondly, the child may be flung against an object. If it is hard like a wall the skull may fracture and there may be an overlying skin bruise. If the head hits a soft surface like a bed or upholstered chair there may not be a fracture or any sign of external bruising to the head. Signs of grasping and metaphyseal injuries should be sought.

In sudden deceleration injuries the tiny veins crossing the subdural space from brain to dura are ruptured and slow oozing of blood gradually produces a subdural haematoma, usually bilaterally. There may also be small intracerebral haemorrhages, not giving rise to particular signs at the time but which may be a cause of learning problems, clumsiness or epilepsy later on. At surgery or at autopsy considerable bruising of the reflected scalp, the galea and the pericranium may be seen even though no visible bruising is present externally.

Fractured skull

If a baby or toddler falls several feet on to its head there may be a linear fracture of the parietal bone, or occasionally of the frontal or occipital bones. A subperiosteal haematoma may form causing a soft swelling under the scalp, usually with little or no bruising on the surface, depending on the nature of the site of contact (carpet, earth, concrete, etc.). There may be brief loss of consciousness from concussion.

Multiple or stellate fractures are caused by falls from a considerable height or severe blows and never from 'just rolling off the sofa'. Contusion of the brain with coma and sometimes intracranial bleeding is usually present.

Subdural haematoma

Caffey[84,85] and Guthkelch[86] have described the whiplash injuries from shaking infants. Guthkelch pointed out that subdural haematoma is a rare condition in adults although it may occur following relatively minor trauma which can often be shown to be of the acceleration–deceleration type, e.g. a bob-sled or motor car accident. In the infant and young child, especially under 2 years, however, subdural haematoma is a common condition following head injury when it is usually bilateral, associated with eye haemorrhages and is often seen without any signs of trauma to the head. There may be evidence of grasping limbs or trunk and small fractures at the ends of long bones. Some cases are unsuspected until autopsy. Confessions of shaking the infant are usually obtained and such lesions are inflicted in almost 100% of cases.

Caffey states that 'habitual manual whiplash shaking of infants is a substantial primary, frequent cause of later mental retardation and permanent brain damage'. He emphasizes the importance of vision and hearing defects following these injuries. This is therefore a major public health problem for education of parents in the newborn period and early months of life.

The baby with subdural haematoma may be unconscious and severely ill with a full fontanelle. There is little problem with diagnosis in such a case. When the damage is less and the bleeding occurs more slowly it may take several days of slow oozing of blood to form the subdural clot. The baby then presents with a feeding problem, vomiting, irritability, lethargy and sometimes unexplained fever and an enlarging head. Once subdural haematoma has been thought of and the limbs and fundi carefully examined, followed by diagnostic needling of the subdural space, there is little diagnostic difficulty. With a very slow onset the diagnosis may be missed, and then a large clot expanding from osmotic attraction of surrounding fluid may eventually be found with damage to the cortex from pressure.

Table 2.8 shows the combination of SDH with other injuries in the Newcastle series.

Table 2.8   NAI 136 children (Newcastle) 1965–71. Subdural haematoma (148 episodes)

ALONE	4	2.9%
+ BRUISING and FRACTURES	22	16.2%
+ BRUISING	9	6.6%
+ FRACTURE(S)	4	2.9%

Usually bilateral
All but one had retinal haemorrhages

Damage to the eyes and vision

Table 2.9 shows the lesions which may occur[87,88].

Table 2.9   Child abuse – damage to the eyes and vision

Peri-orbital bruising
Conjunctival and sub-conjunctival haemorrhages
Anterior segment injuries: hyphaema
                                    traumatic mydriasis
                                    sub-luxation of the lens
Intra-ocular haemorrhage: retinal
                                    pre-retinal
                                    vitreous
Retinal detachment
Optic atrophy
Cortical blindness
Squint
'Conjunctivitis'

Peri-orbital bruising causing black eyes has already been dealt with in the section on bruising, p. 22.

Conjunctival and sub-conjunctival haemorrhages are uncommon and heal quickly. They may be caused by direct trauma, or following fractures of the anterior cranial fossa, or from chest compression. Violent coughing, especially with pertussis in young children, may be a cause.

Anterior segment injuries. This is rare in battered children but hyphaema, traumatic mydriasis and sub-luxation of the lens have been described.

Intra-ocular haemorrhage. Retinal, pre-retinal and vitreous haemorrhages are by far the most important eye lesions in cases of abuse. They are usually caused by shaking but sometimes arise from chest compression, and then some sign of traumatic asphyxia on the face and head will probably be present. Retinal and pre-retinal haemorrhages alone are the commonest finding, and may be multiple, few or single, and large or small. They commonly absorb completely in 1–6 months leaving no visual impairment. If macular scarring has occurred from fibrosis in the retina a central field defect will be present.

When the haemorrhage is large it may break through into the vitreous and then visual impairment is likely, either from retinal fibrosis or from a traction detachment of the retina. In severe cases complete detachment may occur. Patches of choroido-retinal scarring may also be seen, especially in the lower temporal quadrant of the fundus following child abuse.

Retinal detachment. This is rare in infancy and childhood and may be caused by a tumour or by other hereditary retinal disease. However, trauma should always be considered and other injuries sought, because organization and fibrosis of large intra-ocular haemorrhages can lead to detachment.

Optic atrophy. This is a late sequel either due to intra-cerebral damage, to haemorrhage into the optic nerve itself or to severe intra-ocular injury. Macular damage and scarring may also occur.

Cortical blindness. The commonest cause of permanent visual defects is damage to the visual cortex or the visual pathways in the brain, but it may also follow the retinal or vitreous damage already described.

Squint. This may be seen as a transient paralytic squint in the presence of the subdural haematoma. Later on with visual defects from severe retinal damage, optic atrophy or macular scarring, a squint usually develops. It is important to establish the cause since orthoptic treatment would be useless in the presence of a damaged eye.

'Conjunctivitis'. Sometimes parents instil an irritant substance into the child's eyes and then complain of the redness and lacrymation. This can be seen as another cry for help or 'open warning'[89].

Internal injuries

Abdominal injuries

The second most common cause of death, after brain injury, is abdominal injury which may result in rupture of intestines or liver, or more rarely spleen, kidneys or bladder. An acute abdominal emergency is presented. Less severe injuries may result in haematomata in or around these organs with varying degrees of shock, pain and dysfunction. Intestinal obstruction, partial or complete, from a haematoma may lead to severe dehydration and vomiting, and is sometimes misdiagnosed as a 'tummy upset' until the child is very ill[90,91].

It is important to remember that there may be *no abdominal bruising from a blow to the relaxed abdomen.*

Thoracic injuries

Blows or compression injuries to the thorax may fracture the ribs, and in a few cases damage the lungs, or more rarely the heart or great vessels. Haemothorax, pneumohaemothorax, haemopericardium and intra-pulmonary haemorrhage may be seen although they are rare in abused children, and their immediate diagnosis and treatment is the same as for those conditions following severe accidental injury. Proper attention to the history and to the family situation should help to avoid missing cases of child abuse.

Spine and spinal cord injuries

These are rare but serious, and possibly under diagnosed. Swischuk[92] described 7 cases all under 3 years old.

2. OTHER CLINICAL DISORDERS

Poisoning

Since accidental ingestion of drugs and of domestic substances is a common reason for a child attending Casualty or being admitted to a paediatric ward, it is surprising that so few studies have been done on the characteristics of the child and of his home. The hazard from large quantities of dangerous drugs now prescribed for families, and their careless storage was highlighted by Jackson[93]. Craft and Sibert[94] have summarized the present position with accidental poisoning indicating that stress factors in the family and the personality of the children are more important than availability of drugs. Sibert showed the importance of children taking poisons in homes other than their own.

Margolis[95] in a follow-up study showed that children with poisoning of the so-called accidental type could be differentiated from control subjects some years later. They were seen as more defiant by their mothers and teachers. Significant problems included destructiveness, hyperactivity, uncooperative behaviour and fighting. They did not continue to poison themselves, to have other accidents or problems with academic performance. It is against this complex situation that deliberate poisoning must be assessed. In these children self-poisoning was the result of purposeful behaviour by the child in response to a frustrating parent/child relationship. It seemed to result from misdirected anger due to the child's conflicts about aggression and was a developmental phenomenon of the pre-school child emphasizing the importance of the toddler's oral exploratory behaviour, negativism and mimicry.

Sometimes deliberate poisoning presents as any other case of ingestion and only odd behaviour or comments by parents or child may arouse suspicion. Another alerting sign may be that severe *symptoms* of poisoning lend more weight to the likelihood of abuse, since toddlers rarely swallow enough accidentally to cause severe poisoning.

Paediatricians increasingly realize that bizarre complaints about young children not confirmed in hospital or recurrent 'attacks' of various kinds may be due to certain forms of abuse, including poisoning. Salt, hypnotics and tranquillizers are commonly incriminated. Rogers *et al.*[96] have recently reported seven cases of mothers repeatedly poisoning their children, highlighting the need to be more aware of this syndrome, and to deal with it radically or death may ensue from further episodes. A high index of suspicion is the first essential and then biochemical and toxicological studies of blood, urine and gastric washings on admission. It may be necessary after initial biochemical studies to do special tests for particular drugs suggested by the chemical findings. Phenformin, for example, or diuretics may be administered, and more than one substance may be used.

The authors stress the need to examine the parental and marital situation carefully since severe disorders in family relationships are present, and legal protection for the child side by side with treatment for the family is mandatory.

More use should be made of toxicological studies of blood, urine and stomach contents.

Drowning

Three situations need thought in making the diagnosis of deliberate drowning or threatened drowning. The first is that 'fell into the water' should really be 'dropped (or pushed) into the water'[97]. Secondly, the mother may present with a desperately ill or moribund baby saying 'I only left him in the bath a few minutes while I went downstairs to let my friend in'. She seems genuinely surprised on her return upstairs to find her baby, 6 weeks old, under the bathwater! After a number of discussions the mother of such a baby said 'I couldn't even answer the door to my friend without that bloody baby needing me!' indicating her unrealistic expectations and her incapacity to cope with the feeling, common to many young mothers, especially of a first child, that the infant engulfs the mother leaving her no time to pursue her own life or interests, or even, at times, to catch up on much needed sleep. Here is an example of the need for careful preparation of parents pre- and post-delivery for the immediate powerful emotions which caring for a baby arouses. It also illustrates the need for all parents to plan for physical help to be available through a relative, friend or neighbour should it be necessary in the weeks after delivery. When this is not available the public health nurse should be aware of it and remain extra sensitive to the possible consequences for the mother.

The third situation where 'drowning' is involved is less often recognized. Parents may punish a child by pushing his face in a bowl of water or under the bath water or even down the lavatory. The terror of suffocation may only be revealed later when the child is in a safe place. Some mothers do eventually talk about such problems and ask for help.

Cot deaths

It is surprising how often the abused child's history reveals a previous cot death in the family or in close relations. As Emery[98] has shown the family factors tend to be similar in a high proportion, but by no means in all families. Smothering with a pillow or a plastic bag leaves little evidence, and at autopsy can be difficult to differentiate from the sudden infant death syndrome. Families are on record where more than one child has been dealt with in this way. Poisoning which kills the child may be unsuspected and passed off as a cot death. A very careful immediate history and inspection of the home is needed as well as a careful assessment of all past events to the child and siblings. The nature of the parent/child relationship also needs careful study[99]. When in doubt a skeletal survey should be done post-mortem and samples of blood, stomach contents and urine should be saved for toxicological study.

Certain children may be more vulnerable, and in this connection when 'too many girls' arrive in an Asian family, they may have to be considered to be 'at risk'.

The enquiries made must be extremely delicate because the sudden death of an infant, regardless of cause, is an exceedingly traumatic event. It is helpful for all parents after a sudden infant death to talk at length about their feelings and the family social and medical factors which need study. Such a discussion should be part of the treatment of the shocked family and not an intrusive enquiry. Most parents readily discuss every detail and reassurance is some comfort. There may be subtle indications that the account is not straightforward.

'Funny turns'

Complaints by a mother that her child has changed colour, stopped breathing, choked or is having attacks of various vague symptoms should alert the doctor to episodes of abuse by shaking, smothering, poisoning or other means.

Repeated problems with crying and feeding

Much more notice should be taken of the severe problems with crying and feeding in the baby about which a number of mothers complain. For some it is merely that mother and child have not quite settled down together, the baby being easily roused and perhaps the mother, fatigued by having to face other family problems, finds insufficient time to tend to the infant. In such cases simple help and advice will soon solve the problems.

Abused children have a much higher incidence of crying and feeding problems in the early weeks and months, and when the infant does not respond to ordinary measures and the mother remains stressed urgent help should be forthcoming especially when risk factors are present in the mother's or infant's history. This will often call for a few days observation in hospital for the baby, to be quite sure there is no underlying painful lesion and to lessen his tension. The mother will enjoy some rest and refreshment at home in this period. Sometimes such babies are found to have already suffered injury with healing fracture of ribs or metaphyses. In others a medical condition such as hiatal hernia, anal fissure or too concentrated feeds may be the problem. A further spell of observation of mother and child together either by a paediatric nurse at home or by admitting the mother with the child should usually follow. Opportunities to observe and discuss the mother/child relationship will often reveal underlying problems between mother and baby or in the marital relationship. A child psychiatrist is a helpful colleague in this situation in which abuse can be prevented by suitable help at this stage. Involvement of the father or cohabitee is important. Very close follow-up is needed and help to the parents at home. Occasionally the mother clearly shows at this stage that her relationship with the child is not likely to improve and she may consent, with relief, to permanent placement away from home. Many risk factors which have prevented bonding are usually clearly demonstrable. In a few other cases, as time goes on, the symptoms continue and the mother's attitudes and behaviour with the baby indicates considerable rejection which is not responding to psychiatric help, yet she will not consent to relinquishment. It may be necessary to protect such a child from serious maldevelopment by Care Proceedings after a suitable trial of support and treatment has been unsuccessful. Repeated periods in voluntary care are often used in this situation, but represent further abuse of the child and should be avoided. The mother's capacity to mother and care for her young baby is damaged by separating her from the infant, except for a short time (2 or 3 days) for her to catch up on her sleep, or for tension in the infant to be lessened. The infant and toddler removed into care 'to give the mother a break' is very much damaged by repeated disruptions in relationships. He may also be upset with grief and missing his warmer foster-mother when he returns home and be even more difficult for his own mother. If a single such placement has been deemed necessary it is crucial for the mother to take over the child's care again gradually by visiting him and restoring some degree of mutual relationship before removing the child from his present security.

Over-activity and demanding behaviour

When the parents have been unable to satisfy the emotional needs of the infant or toddler he may increase his attachment behaviour with clinging and demanding behaviour and, once mobile, over-activity is often characteristic. The lack of organization of the family's day, and unpredictable response to the child's cries to have his needs met, result in a chaotic state for the child where over-activity signals a state of persistent tension. If anger, hostility and unreasonable demands for obedience are the parents' reponse a vicious circle results, with more and more restlessness and demands from the child, and increasing frustration and lack of warmth from the parents. Such behaviour may persist throughout the school years and greatly impedes learning and general development.

Hysterical moods (in older children)

In some abused school children it will be apparent that mood swings are excessive, and that on some days the child is exceedingly edgy and easily moved to tears or anger. In between his mind may be far away. Such a child is unlikely to be making good academic progress and may often be at odds with his teacher or peer groups. In other cases the child is lonely and isolated, and passive in the classroom. Outbursts of hysterical crying or negativism may also occur after family rows or violence.

It is important for teachers to realize that all is not well with such a child and between teachers and parents it should be agreed that help is needed for him. Parents in the throes of severe family problems often deny that there is any secondary effect on the child or children but they are wrong. The child is caught up in an anguish of divided loyalties and muddled understanding. If actual abuse of the child, whether physical or mental, is involved this too may present in the same way, and hysterical outbursts follow on an attack. These should be investigated by a full psycho-social study of the family. Many more school children need our help and protection.

3. FAILURE TO THRIVE WITHOUT ORGANIC CAUSE. DEPRIVATION DWARFISM OR THE MATERNAL REJECTION SYNDROME

The excellent review on this topic by MacCarthy[100] highlights its importance, and it is clear that it is under-diagnosed at present because growth charts are not regularly used on children. The growth retardation is more easily demonstrated during the rapid growth period in the first 3 years. It should be remembered that while physical growth is most easily measured and demonstrated, growth and development of the other systems is equally damaged so that the intellectual, emotional, social and moral aspects of growth are all affected (Table 2.10). Speech and language are markedly delayed and on recovery seems to remain immature as it does in cases of physical abuse[101].

Table 2.10   The five aspects of growth and development

PHYSICAL:	increase in size and function
INTELLECTUAL:	capacity to learn and to adapt behaviour
EMOTIONAL:	capacity to form relationships and empathize
SOCIAL:	capacity for:
	self care
	useful work – or play for children
	appropriate social behaviour (with family, friends, society)
MORAL:	knowledge of right and wrong through the child's developing conscience

Remember considerable interdependence between all 5 aspects

Lacey and Parkin[102] drew attention to the need to look at the psycho-social environment of children who are not growing properly. That the parents are small too is often given as a reason for not investigating the child but it is often the case that the parents are small for the same psycho-social reasons. During a period of hospital investigation or while on a convalescent holiday it can be shown that these children have a marked growth spurt which usually relapses when they return home. The important features of the condition are shown in Tables 2.11 to 2.14.

The appearance of the child is very characteristic when the fully developed picture is present, dejection and apathy being striking. His height is below the 3rd centile for his age and birth-weight, and he is usually thin and sometimes even emaciated. His proportions are infantile for his age, with the shorter legs of the much younger child. He has a pot belly and some hypotonia shown in his

posture. There may be episodes of diarrhoea and occasionally typical malabsorption stools. Tension and misery seem to be the cause of these loose motions
which are similar to those seen in normal people before examinations or interviews. The skin is dull, pale and cold with mottling of the extremities and

Table 2.11   Deprivation dwarfism   1. Child's appearance

Short stature
Usually thin
Infantile proportions
Pot belly (with episodes of diarrhoea)
Skin dull, pale and cold
Extremities pink or purple, cold and mottled
Oedema feet and legs, sometimes hands and forearms
Poor skin care, excoriations, abrasions and tiny ulcers
Sparse dry hair
Patches of alopecia
Dejection and apathy
May have bruises, small cuts, burns or scars

sometimes little sores and abrasions. Hypothyroidism may be suggested from
the skin and sparse dry hair. Sometimes there are patches of alopecia.

Vascular skin changes may be present in advanced cases and then the hands
and feet, and sometimes the legs and forearms, are reddish or purplish, cold and

Table 2.12   Deprivation dwarfism   2. Child's behaviour

passive ± catatonia
Rocking or head-banging
Retarded speech and language
Delayed development
Solitary and unable to play
Easily bullied
No separation anxiety
Gorging food and scavenging from dustbins or gutters

swollen. Since blushing is a vascular skin change entirely caused by emotional
stimuli, it is possible to believe in the emotional origin of these vascular
changes even when they are severe. These signs clear up rapidly in hospital and
recur when the child is returned to the mother. The neural and vascular pathway is
probably via the thalamus, hypothalamus and posterior pituitary where the release

Table 2.13   Deprivation dwarfism   3. Child's progress in hospital

Rapid recovery of growth and liveliness
Slower progress with speech and language
Affection seeking but   { shallow
                         { promiscuous
Attention seeking
Severe tantrums at slightest frustration
Rocking and head banging when upset
Remains greedy and scavenges food

of vaso-pressin takes place. There is usually evidence of deficient hygiene and care with inadequate clothing, although siblings may look normal. There may be bruising, lacerations, small scars or burns to suggest some degree of physical abuse as well in some cases.

Table 2.14   Deprivation dwarfism   4. Child's later behaviour

Speech and language immaturity
Gorging food may last 6 months +
Restless with short attention span
Rocking and head banging if stressed
Difficulties with ⎰ peer group
⎱ learning at school
Soiling and wetting
Stealing and lying
Tantrums and aggression

Such a clinical picture is quite a clear entity and even when only five or six of these twelve signs are present the child should be admitted at once for study.

In the ward the child's behaviour (Table 2.12) will be seen to be disordered, and passivity is the striking feature, sometimes progressing to catatonia. The mother has usually complained bitterly of how the child sits or stands for hours on end, perhaps rocking himself, and refusing to play. She refers to him as dull and stupid, words which a normal loving mother never uses about her child even when she knows he is mentally retarded. Speech and general development are much retarded from under-nutrition, lack of stimulation, and by a pervading atmosphere of rejection and hostility present in most mothers with such children. The child shows no separation anxiety and remains indifferent to his mother's presence or absence. He tends to gorge food or scavenge from dustbins or gutters even when plenty of food is provided, and this is another symptom which angers and frustrates his mother. Whitten et al.[103] have shown that deprivation of adequate food has been a long standing problem whatever the mother may say. The interia and depression in the fully established picture further interferes with appetite and reduces food intake.

Once admitted to a paediatric ward where a stimulating and affectionate regime is provided with plenty of attention, carrying about and frequent feeding, the child improves rapidly. The growth spurt, sometimes after a few days initial delay, is marked, liveliness returns, and development advances rapidly, but demanding behaviour follows with shallow and promiscuous affectionate responses from the child[104]. Speech and language develop more slowly. The child remains greedy for some months and usually develops severe tantrums with minimal frustration. Later on, either in a children's home or foster home there may be problems with wetting and soiling and with stealing and lying in the school years. Difficulties in peer relationships and in learning at school are common. With help in a good foster-home these troublesome symptoms[105] do resolve.

Attention must be given to the mother and her relationship with the child and also the father's attitudes and the condition of the siblings. Usually only one or two children are rejected, while others seem to do better in the family. Rejection may have begun at conception or in the early hours of life, or more subtly when the infant reminds the mother of the 'bad' parts of herself, the child's father or some other close relative. The mother has often been rejected herself. Careful psychiatric study of the parents is essential for a complete diagnosis.

In the newborn period or the early weeks of life, puerperal depression may lead the mother to reject her child and treatment will reverse this process in many. A profound rejection by the mother over many weeks or months usually lies behind the clinical picture. Investigation, treatment and support may improve the relationship in milder cases, but when the full-blown picture is present these children do not do well at home and fostering is needed for them[105]. The foster mother may also need help in coping with the behaviour disorders in the ensuing months.

4. DISORDERED BEHAVIOUR (OBSERVED)

This refers to behaviour of the child which is repeatedly seen to be abnormal by professionals trained and experienced with children, such as a health visitor, teacher or children's ward nurse. Passivity is the main feature causing alarm, and indifference to separation or to painful stimuli are others. A negative relationship with the mother may be noted, where neither child nor mother enjoy each other, and where affectionate, playful exchanges do not occur. Fear of one or other parent and refusal to be cared for by them is unusual in hospital and when shown by a young patient it needs assessment. Open hostility, physical or verbal between child and parents sometimes highlights the issues. Hysterical attacks or severe mood changes are other behavioural signs requiring careful investigation.

5. SEXUAL ABUSE

The frequency of sexual encounters between adults and children is not known but is probably much more common than has been realized. Incest may be the pattern or sexual activity outside the home. Boys and girls are involved as active or passive partners, in various combinations although mother–son incest is probably rare.

Apart from violent sexual assaults on children, the upset which follows the investigations may sometimes be more damaging to the child than the experiences themselves and this should always be borne in mind. Reviews of sexual exploitation of children by Burton[106], Farm[107], Schecter and Roberge[108] have emphasized the need for more research. Burton's own study revealed a greater need for affection and fear of rejection in the affected children, but no significant degree of emotional trauma seemed to result. This is also the view put forward by Schecter and Roberge concerning non-violent sexual activities with children. Giarretto[109] describes the humanistic treatment of father-daughter incest.

The law in England did not protect children from sexual assault until 1869 and various laws have been made since. The Sexual Offences Act 1956 consolidated the previous legislation and set out five offences:

1. Unlawful sexual intercourse with a girl between 13 and 16 years.
2. Sexual intercourse with a girl under 13 years.
3. Incestuous sexual intercourse.
4. Buggery.
5. Indecent assault on females.

These categories are self-explanatory and will not be further discussed. The last category covers all sexual advances or practices with children not included in the other four.

Most of these sexual encounters remain hidden for years. The vast majority come to light after pregnancy is discovered or following a family row when a parent, who has known about and condoned the sexual acts before, reports them, usually to gain an end of their own unrelated to the child. In other cases incest or other sexual activities during childhood are revealed during psychotherapy with adults. History taking in such cases has already been referred to, and only research and careful follow-up will give understanding of the effects on the child and the best forms of management.

6. ABUSE WHILE IN CARE

Rarely the child may provoke abuse from his foster-parents or house-parents and this has to be monitored carefully in some of the very disturbed abused children. The commonest form of 'abuse' in care, however, is the failure to make permanent long term plans for a child for continuity of care, either in a foster home or by rapidly getting him back to his family. As a result the child is often moved about from one home to another and his capacity to form meaningful relationships is thereby damaged, often irreparably. He remains in limbo[110–112].

When a baby or young child is placed in foster care with a view to returning home, it is crucial that his mother visits him at least weekly and that she takes part in his care by feeding and bathing him, as well as playing with him, as the physical caring is a vital part of a mother/child relationship at this stage. Work towards getting him home should be begun with the parents at once, and they must understand that if they are not capable of having him home within a few months he will have formed strong attachments to his foster-parents and that disruption of this relationship will be damaging to the child.

The Courts are beginning to recognize this and to make judgements in favour of a child remaining with foster-parents under these circumstances.

> My mother does not love me,
> I feel bad,
> I feel bad because she does not love me,
> I am bad because I feel bad,
> I feel bad because I am bad,
> I am bad because she does not love me,
> She does not love me because I am bad.
>
> *R. D. Laing*

THE HISTORY FROM THE PARENTS IN CHILD ABUSE CASES

In cases of injury or accident

Features in the history of the 'accident', of the child and of his family, as detailed below, should be obtained in a concerned and sensitive way by the doctor who should be very alert to the parents' feelings and to what they do *not* say, as well as to what they tell. Preferably the doctor should be senior and experienced in talking to parents and children. Once a thorough history has been taken and then the parents' and child's personal biographies have been obtained, *a critical path* can be constructed for the family. It may be necessary to consult with the family doctor, public health nurse, paediatrician or others to gain leads in understanding family stresses which may have led to abuse.

To keep on asking questions about an injury is non-productive, as most parents will repeat the story they have given, whether true or false, and the more often they do so, the more anxious and annoyed they will become at having to repeat it again. In no other situation in medicine is the physician's skill, enhanced by experience in the psychological and psychiatric fields, more necessary than in showing empathy with these troubled parents and helping them to reveal, to a sympathetic ear, their own personal and marital problems which have led up to abuse of their child. Needless to say a non-accusatory and non-condemning approach is essential.

It is important to remember that not all abusing parents have obvious personal, family or social stresses such as low income, disordered family care, criminality, etc. Some are apparently warm and loving parents, perhaps very adequate in home care and in their jobs. The baby may have immaculate care physically. Nevertheless abusing parents carry over from their own upbringing and life experience, problems in parenting. They also have difficulty in impulse control with the aggravations normal to all parents in caring for babies and young children. Their attitudes to controlling and punishing infants and toddlers may be unrealistic too.

Because it takes time to go into details, to assess the 'accident' and injuries, to ponder on the family psychodynamics, to empathize with parents, many paediatricians are content to turn a blind eye to a probable case of inflicted injury once a negative history has been obtained. The same paediatrician may think nothing of spending many hours during the night or over several days investigating, with colleagues, a newborn baby with, for example, congenital heart disease, when there is only a 5 or 10% chance of a live, healthy child at the end of it. Yet the abused child is potentially normal and healthy. Establishing the diagnosis should lead to the promotion of adequate nurturing care for him in the future. Untreated, the abusing environment will continue, in most cases, to damage the child psychologically if not physically and permanently retard his full development. The parents too need help.

A brief account of some of the particular features of the history is needed because, with experience, doctors and others can become more sensitive to factors which ought to alert the physician to the risk, if not the fact, of abuse.

In injured children
Parental reactions

Two opposite extremes may be seen in the parents' attitudes while giving the history, although some abusing parents show more or less normal attitudes and responses at this time. The doctor can be alerted when the parent is excessively tearful and distressed, overconcerned or agitated about trivial injury in a child who appears more or less comfortable and contented. In spite of this anxiety in the parent there may also be some vagueness over the actual cause of the injuries.

Other abusing parents, whose child may be mildly or seriously injured, are extremely vague and elusive about how the injury occurred or in describing the child's usual state of health. At hospital they may disappear, leaving the child in the ward, before the doctor arrives to make the clinical notes. Sometimes they send a neighbour or an 11 or 12 year old sibling up with the child, and when asked to come themselves leave it several days before they appear on the ward. Abusing parents telephone enquiries to the ward are usually much more concerned with the expected date of the child's discharge (and so their feeling of being safe from further enquiries) than with their child's condition or happiness. This is all in striking contrast with normal parents who show much anxiety and concern for the child who is injured, asking many questions about the treatment and prognosis, staying with the child, telephoning frequently, giving much detail about how the injury occurred and blaming themselves for letting it happen.

Detailed questioning

When being questioned in detail about the circumstances of their child's injuries and the accident which caused them, most parents these days are aware of greater care being taken by medical staff and others not to miss cases of inflicted injury. They are less aware of the paediatrician's great concern to understand the causes of all accidents in order to teach prevention, first in this family in the future, and secondly for all children. To this end detailed enquiries *should* be made in all cases of accidents. Parents can see more relevance in these enquiries in the case of an ill child or a head injury than in the presence of more minor injury but it is nevertheless important.

The doctor should ask in whose care the child was at the time, who else was about, what was going on immediately before the episode, how the child was injured and what the various people present did after that.

Accidents don't just happen

Even accidental injuries seldom happen by chance. They are related to personal, family or environmental stress in the majority of cases. It is therefore important for doctors to help the parents understand how and why the accident *was caused* rather than 'happened' and therefore be more aware of how to prevent future accidents. Example: A sensible mother was icing her 6 year old's birthday cake with her 3 year old fussing around the kitchen. There was a sense of urgency to get finished to collect the elder child from school on time. Rather exasperated the mother firmly told the 3 year old to go and ride his tricycle in the back yard until she had finished and then he would have the dish to lick. He began to cry but went down the step and onto his tricycle, pedalling it vigorously amid his tears. He rode straight into the clothes prop holding up the washing on the line. The prop fell onto him, causing a minor skull fracture and brief concussion. The mother, quite rightly, blamed herself for her impatience which led, unintentionally of course, to the 'accident'.

The discrepant or unrealistic history

Failure to realize that the parents' history is false is the chief reason why the whole subject of battered children was unrecognized for so long. Doctors, especially in busy surgeries or casualty departments, were more concerned with emergency care and treatment or with reassurance about minor injuries than with matching up the injury with the history of how it happened. Knowledge of physical child abuse has thrown a great burden on all doctors who see children, and alerted them to the need to be aware of this diagnosis. It is a doctor's usual custom to listen and take careful note of what parents tell him about their child, and it is distasteful to be distrustful, but this is necessary on occasions.

Great care should always be taken to match the injury with the history, and this is particularly important in the younger children first because the risk of serious injury or death is much greater if the doctor makes a mistake; secondly because such injury is the signal of a child and maybe his siblings in danger of poor development, and of family stress, often intolerable, which urgently needs investigation and treatment.

A boy of 17 months was admitted with facial and thigh bruising after being some hours alone with the mother's consort. She explained the extensive scarring on his back was due to a severe scald 4 months earlier when he pulled a kettle over himself. He had just been home two weeks after treatment in a burns unit in another hospital. Both parents were 17 years old.

It was noted that the scalded area was confined to his back, and examination of the burns unit notes confirmed this, so the history seemed discrepant, as it was unlikely a 13 month old boy would pull a kettle over and only scald his back. Next day the mother admitted that she knew her consort had scalded the child deliberately when the baby was crying and toddling around him when he was getting ready to go out for the evening.

In another case a first degree scald on the chest of a 13 month old girl had faint splash marks *above* it which seemed wrong for the history that the child had reached up and pulled the cup over. Next day a 5 year old sibling confirmed the doctor's suspicion by telling her teacher 'Our baby's gone to hospital because Mum threw a cup of tea at her'. This trivial injury, noted by the social worker at a routine visit, was important in enabling legal action to be taken on all the children in a very disturbed and violent family where adequate evidence for a Court had been hard to establish before. The family doctor, health visitor, social worker and paediatrician had known for some time that abuse was occurring. Normally the family did not answer the door to officials, but on this occasion one of the children let the social worker in!

The changing history

Sometimes the parents have told one story at home and another when they reach the hospital, or they may produce several different stories in as many days. Allowance must be made for inarticulate people expressing things differently at different times. Parents usually collude, and the glances, nudges or knee pressure they exchange when jointly describing the events can be very telling. Writing down the account at once is of crucial importance, particularly if it is to be used in Court and the parents own words should be quoted.

The truth but not the whole truth

With inflicted injuries, when parents or others falsify the history, they often tell the truth, but not the whole truth, and this may seem confusing. There are often witnesses to prove the part of the story they tell. For example, an 11 month old boy came in with obvious linear finger marks on his cheek and forehead and deep bruising over the zygoma. The step-father, alone with him at the time, insisted the injury was caused when he crawled to a small coffee table and upset it and himself down the steps between the sitting room and kitchen. The overturned table was there when the mother came in a few minutes later, and they both insisted that bumping his face on the carpeted steps had caused the linear marks. Eventually the step-father admitted to hitting the child for crying after the table episode. In another case a child of 4 years had a badly bruised face and sundry other limb and trunk bruises especially on the top of his arm, alleged to be caused by falling downstairs. Various relatives and neighbours confirmed the fall. They omitted to reveal the severe family row which preceded the child's fall, and that on the top landing the child had been severely chastized and was more or less pushed downstairs. It is important to remember that ordinary childhood falls in the house do not result in much bruising as a rule, and falling downstairs, an excuse often given by battering parents, seldom causes more than an odd bruise next day over a bony prominence, as most parents know from experience. Falls from the bed or from tipping over the pram are other explanations which are quite inconsistent with severe bruises, fractures or head injury.

'No there has been no injury' or 'He must have done it himself'

Not infrequently even intelligent parents whose young infant has a few bruises, one or more fractures or even a head injury will insist that 'nothing has happened', that there has been no injury or accident, and that furthermore the child has not been out of their care at all. They may insist the infant 'banged his face with his hands' or fractured his arm 'turning himself over' when they are quite well aware that the baby is much too young to turn over. There seems to be a dissociation in their minds, perhaps a defence mechanism after a sudden impulsive act which they now strive to deny. It seems to be more subtle than simply telling a lie, and the best ways of breaking down these defences need sensitive consideration.

Delay in reporting the injury

Another problem in the history is parents who bring a child saying they 'just noticed the bruise (or swelling or pain) today' when examination and/or radiology reveals the injuries have been there some time. Often multiple small fractures of several different ages are seen when a baby with a minor bruise or two is X-rayed. It seems that many parents really do not experience the usual very protective attitudes normally shown in handling a young baby, and when rough or casual with their infant they do not know their own strength. Others, of course, are deliberately lying.

'He bruises very easily'

More research is needed on the easy bruising of young children in the absence of a coagulation defect. This is frequently what abusing parents report, and yet when the same child is in hospital or a nursery no such ease of bruising is noted. Normal parents rarely mention easy bruising in their children in routine visits to health clinics. Doctors and nurses who examine many hundreds of babies and young children seldom see significant bruising on them, and when they do normal parents readily explain it.

Restless, overactive children, usually from unsettled homes, may show slightly more bruising than the average, even in a nursery, but the bruises are usually on the forehead and lower legs. These children are more prone to minor bumps and falls due to lack of early care and gentleness producing poor co-ordination.

What the child will tell

It is often asked 'Why doesn't the child who can talk tell how he got his injuries?' There seem to be many reasons. Fear of further abuse; loyalty to the family; feeling he deserved it; being overwhelmed by the assault and then by the medical attention; or not having an adequate vocabulary. He may have no experience whatever of tender care or being able to trust an adult. He may feel that assaults from adult to child are part of existence, as indeed they are in some families.

Some weeks after the child is moved from the family, and when he can feel himself in a caring and safe environment, then he may begin to talk to a trusted adult about what happened. Sometimes the episodes of assault come out in nightmares long after the child is in a loving environment. When an older child *is* able to talk about it, and accuses someone of causing the injuries it is important to pay special attention to all the details, since a child could fantasize about what happened, although the author has not yet had experience of this.

Injury from siblings

Undoubtedly siblings do sometimes injure the baby but watchful parents in a normal family usually prevent all but an occasional scratch or bite. The toddler is the usual offender since older children have learnt to control their aggressive impulses towards the baby. The power of a toddler to harm an infant is limited. He has little weight in his arm, belying the history, sometimes given, that a toddler has bruised the baby by hitting it. It is important therefore to examine the history in detail when a young child is said to have caused the injury.

Injuries caused by older siblings are more often accidental than deliberate, and it is important to question the child about the details if he is alleged to have assaulted a younger sibling. Prompting by the parents must be watched for and as little time as possible should elapse before the child is seen. Sometimes it is more appropriate for the police to be involved in this type of enquiry if serious injury has been caused.

Collusion between parents

Collusion is usual between the parents who are caught up in a knot of family stress and do not know how to seek help. Often both parents are injuring the children, but where it is only one, the other covers it up, denies it or actively promotes it as punishment for imagined misdeeds. Wife battering is common in these families too, and condoned or subtly encouraged in many cases by the wife. When her tolerance snaps or after a particularly severe beating of herself or the child she may present one or other for medical care, and her story then is often exaggerated.

Previous injuries or admission to hospital of child or siblings

The parents often conceal the fact of previous injuries and should be asked about them and about former hospital admissions of this child or others in the family. In suspicious families the answers should be cross-checked with the family doctor, health visitor, and if necessary with inpatient or casualty records at other hospitals. Variations or changes in the child's surname, frequent changes of address, lack of a family doctor or failure of medical records to catch up with them are problems which make tracing these families very difficult. They may even be deliberately evasive and elusive.

Previous admissions for other conditions may be more readily revealed and failure to thrive, crying or feeding problems are common in the child or his siblings.

Enquiries about injuries, deaths and other health problems or hospitalizations in the siblings should also be made as it is well known that they are also at risk for abuse, and it is the family as a whole which needs diagnosis and treatment.

In cases of failure to thrive

In cases of poor growth and development due to lack of loving care and concern, the parents usually show little interest and may actively resist any investigations. This is in striking contrast with normal parents who unconsciously monitor their child's size at different ages, and when the child is noted to be much below average for his age they tend to seek help or reassurance early.

Children who are small and thin from neglect and lack of affection usually have other symptoms. In severe cases the child is withdrawn and passive and unable to play, may seem to over-eat and may have bouts of diarrhoea. Earlier he may have had sleeping or feeding problems or restless demanding or clinging behaviour. Although the mother may report the child as greedy and always hungry, research into the feeding habits in such families reveals striking underfeeding much of the time. One child in a family may be the subject of such neglect and want of concern, whereas others thrive well, the so-called scapegoated child. The disturbances in mother–child relationship in such cases are sometimes florid and easy to diagnose. In other cases it may be very subtle, and while talking to the mother or parents careful observation should be made of the way the mother describes the child, the words she uses, and how she nurses or responds to him as he sits on her lap or plays beside her. Normal parents avoid such words as 'stupid' or 'ugly' even if they think their child is retarded, whereas abusing parents often use derogatory expressions about their child. While history taking the doctor may observe a lack of tender glances and physical contacts and instead cold or hostile attitudes from mother to child. Unrealistic demands for good behaviour and obedience are often striking too. Experience with mothers and young children is essential in noting these subtle differences from the normal, and sometimes this begins in the labour ward or lying-in department. Improved awareness of the mother's problems at this stage by sensitive observation and then treatment can do much to prevent the later problems of abuse and poor care[32].

Psychological problems

When children are being abused by cold and hostile attitudes and unrealistic expectations, a variety of behaviour disorders, speech and learning problems result. In taking the history such disorders will be noted. Often they are the presenting feature, with the mother or father or both seeking help for a child's annoying behaviour. Their attitudes to and expectations of the child need careful assessment. They are often glaringly abnormal but subtle, although no less damaging attitudes to the child are harder to define.

The parents' background

The history is not complete without an account of the parents' own childhood experiences, although it may not be appropriate to discuss these matters at the first consultation. This personal biography should include the number of children in the family and the individual's place in the sibship, their own parents' marriage, their attitudes to the children, their discipline, schooling, holidays and treats. The work record since leaving school should be noted. Any health or behaviour problems, school difficulties or court appearances should be noted, and whether any separation of the parent from his family occurred. A parent should be asked about his own views on his family and his upbringing and how much contact he has now with members of the family. When early life has been difficult a parent may feel unable to reveal this at first until a more trusting relationship has grown up with the interviewer. In other cases a parent may say they come from a home which is 'all right' or where they had good care. Later it may be revealed that violence, instability and criminal behaviour was the common pattern in the childhood home. 'You get used to it' one mother said, and knowing no other type of family behaviour, such individuals model their own on similar lines and so the cycle of deprivation and disadvantage continues.

The history in sexual abuse

Occasionally the mother will describe sexual activity in the family, usually between father and daughter but it may be father and son, brother and sister or between other relatives or a lodger and a child. The revelation often follows a family 'row', the mother having condoned the behaviour until then. Sometimes a child himself or herself will reveal unwanted sexual advances, and occasionally a toddler or pre-school child reveals it in his play or behaviour. The parents often try to deny such activity or cover it up. Sometimes quite young children are involved in group sexual activities with adults or in pornographic exercises. Although such facts are hard to uncover they may be revealed in play or during psycho-therapy.

Bizarre attacks or apnoeic attacks

When a parent or caregiver presents a child with a confused or extraordinary story, such as choking, peculiar 'turns', changing colour, stopping breathing, becoming unrouseable, it may be due to equally bizarre happenings such as shaking the child, attempts to smother, drown or poison him, and in one case to ramming a pacifier down the child's throat.

EXAMINATION OF THE CHILD

This will be done by a doctor, preferably one experienced with children and with the kind of minor injuries normally seen in children of different ages. Sometimes a nurse at a nursery, a school or a clinic may make the preliminary examination. In hospitals, the casualty officer may be the first person to see the child, but if he has strong suspicions of child abuse, either because of injuries, stunted growth, slow development, neglect, or for other reasons, he should immediately contact the consultant paediatrician or his deputy to examine the child with him, and if the suspicions continue, to arrange for the child to be admitted to the paediatric department. Here the multi-disciplinary team of paediatrician, family doctor, health visitor and social worker, perhaps with the teacher, psychologist or child psychiatrist as well, will at once be involved, and steps to confirm or refute the diagnosis of abuse will be taken immediately. When serious injury is present, care of the child's medical or surgical problem obviously takes precedence over all else.

The child should generally be examined in the presence of one or both parents, except in an emergency. Where strong suspicion of abuse exists and the parents are known to be very difficult it is sometimes appropriate to make a preliminary examination, for example in a school or nursery, before sending for the parents to assist in completing the consultation. Their account of how the injuries or other signs have been caused should be very carefully noted in writing. A young child should generally be examined on the mother's lap if he seems comfortable there, and this will give the doctor an increased opportunity to observe the mother–child relationship. A warm room is essential.

It should go without saying that a gentle approach to the child and the parents is essential, and every effort should be made to produce a relaxed atmosphere and to diminish fear and anxiety of parents and child using, where appropriate, smiling, playing, toys, sweets or soft drinks for the child, tea or coffee for the adults, for example. The doctor and the parents, as well as anyone accompanying them, should be seated, and an unhurried approach used. This is even more important if the parents *have* injured the child, as they will usually be even more anxious and afraid than the parents of a child accidentally injured. Treatment of the sick family of the abused child begins with the first contacts made with them. If these are hostile or unfeeling even more damage will occur to the family and to the child.

The child should be completely undressed and examined in a good light. The adequacy of the clothing and hygiene should be noted. Obvious bruising or other signs should be looked at first, and discussed with the child, if old enough, and with his parents. It is important to observe how the child answers, and with what degree of hesitation, fear or communication with the parent. Careful note should also be made of the way in which the parent or parents describe the accident or other matters in the history, whether they are vague and confused, or clear and detailed and obviously accurate. The amount of anxiety for the child's state and concern for his comfort should also be noted.

In examining the child steps must be taken to exclude medical and surgical disorders, especially neurological abnormalities. After looking at the obvious signs for which the child is referred (injury, poor growth, etc.) a careful search of the whole body for some of the minor but classical signs of non-accidental injury should be sought, including petechial haemorrhage or bruising around, inside or behind the ear, bruising of the lips or gums, a torn frenulum of the upper lip or tongue, conjunctival or fundal haemorrhages, marks around the back or front of the neck, bite marks, cigarette burns fresh or scarred, anal or vulval bruising, napkin rash, faint ligature marks on neck or limbs, curved nail imprints, scratches. A list of every positive sign should be made at the time, with the size, shape and colour noted. An outline diagram should also be used to indicate the site of all the signs. At this point an overall assessment of injuries should be made, their extent, their distribution and their probable age, and this compared with the history given.

Next the child should be weighed, and then measured for length or height and skull circumference. The percentiles of growth in these three parameters should be noted. The child's birth weight and the parents' height and weight should also be noted, especially if the child is at all undersized. Infantile proportions, vascular skin change, pot belly and hypotonia should be looked for and the quality of skin and hair. A rough assessment of the child's development in locomotion, manipulation and in speech should be made and recorded, mainly on observation but partly on discussion with the parents if the child is young or badly hurt. A more detailed developmental assessment will be completed later.

The child's mood and behaviour and his attitude to parents and other adults should be carefully noted. The passive withdrawn child or the over-friendly promiscuous one, or the child afraid of, or indifferent to, a parent should be looked for. Failure to thrive, other signs of neglect or severe emotional disturbance, if present with inadequately explained injuries, further strengthen the doctor's suspicion of abuse.

Admission to hospital

At the end of the examination the doctor may want to talk to other professionals who have accompanied the child or who are involved with the family. He may also want to telephone the paediatrician to discuss the case at this stage or for advice on procedure. He will then formulate his views on the likelihood of child abuse and if this seems probable will arrange for further investigation in the paediatric department of the hospital. With a young child the mother should be admitted too whenever possible.

When obvious signs of inflicted injury are present it may be necessary to mention this to the parents there and then before admission. It is important not to suggest *who* may have 'been rough with the child', but simply to state that the injuries appear to be inflicted and further tests are needed. In other cases, where the diagnosis of abuse can only be made after further investigation and assessment in hospital, it should not, of course, be mentioned to the parents at this stage. (Similarly, if a doctor in family practice or in casualty is concerned that a child might have, say, leukaemia he does not mention this to the parent then but waits for the diagnosis to be confirmed after further investigation in hospital.)

Where a parent is reluctant for a child to be admitted, the doctor can explain that the signs are puzzling to him, he is not sure of the diagnosis or appropriate treatment, and he needs his specialist colleague to perform further tests and to give his opinion before the diagnosis can be made. When bruising is part of the symptomatology, the need to exclude haemophilia or leukaemia, among other things, may need to be mentioned to a reluctant parent. If fractures are suspected the possibility of brittle bones or other pathology can be mentioned. Few parents refuse admission at this stage if sympathetically handled, and if the doctor is obviously concerned to help them and their child. Sometimes the parents themselves may mention 'battered children' at this point, very difficult and aggressive parents may do so in a threatening way to the doctor. It is important to remain quiet and calm and to attempt further discussion, asking the parents why they have raised it. If pressed the doctor can say that in all injuries to children, inflicted injury is a possibility that must go through the doctor's mind, just as underlying pathology is considered as well. He should reaffirm that he is puzzled by the signs and feels certain the child should be admitted. He should further reassure the parent that all paediatric departments (at least in Britain and the USA) have free visiting and the parents will be able to stay all day with the child if they wish or be admitted with him if he is young. They will be able to discuss all the details with the paediatrician and other specialists concerned, day by day.

If the parents still resist admission the family doctor may consider inviting the paediatrician to join him on a domiciliary visit to assist in diagnosis and handling the parents. The other alternative is to discuss with a senior case worker from the department of social services, the NSPCC or with the police, the need for a 'Place of Safety Order' being obtained from a magistrate, or, outside Britain, for some sort of formal Child Protection Order to be made. This ensures that the child shall be properly investigated in hospital with blood tests, X-rays or studies on poor growth, slow development, emotional or other problems as the case may be. The psycho-social study of the family by the multidisciplinary team will be initiated after admission if abuse still seems likely. The very fact of refusing admission at once highlights parents as unusual and probably 'scared', since normal parents, although naturally reluctant, do not refuse admission for their child when a doctor has carefully explained the need for it. With patience, perseverance, skill and experience, doctors find a decreasing need to invoke the law in order to have the child admitted.

After admission a similar examination will be made by the hospital staff, together with a list of the injuries and an outline chart, which should be signed and dated. Further investigations are dealt with in the next section.

IN THE PAEDIATRIC UNIT

Ten or fifteen years ago the staff of paediatric units found it hard not to show anger and disgust when a child was admitted with inflicted injury, neglect or other forms of abuse. Experience teaches that the parents are but victims of similar experiences in their own childhood, that they do love their children in most cases and want to care for them well. Their own intolerable internal stresses, often combined with ignorance and severe social and marital problems, have led up to the child's plight. With this knowledge and experience, all the ward staff, from the senior to the junior, including the auxiliaries and domestics, can be brought to understand that abundant concern and compassion for the parents is needed as well as for the child. Regular staff discussions are needed to emphasize these points.

Abusing parents may be frightened and difficult and patience can be tried to extremes by aggressive, complaining, demanding, dirty or drunken parents. Staff should learn to call assistance when their own reserves are exhausted. It has to be remembered that parents who abuse or neglect their children have exceptionally low self esteem and poor self confidence however much they may try to dominate in the ward. Their capacity to trust anyone has been damaged severely and often irreparably in their own childhood, and staff need to learn not to lose their equanimity with such parents when they are exhibiting trying behaviour. The parents are extremely sensitive to criticism and often imagine it where none exists. A sense of humour, together with a motherly caring attitude and some firmness, usually succeeds in restoring peace and order when such parents make a scene. If parents threaten to remove the child before the investigations and plan of management are complete, persuasion by senior and experienced members of staff is usually effective. If not, a Place of Safety Order (or other legal measure outside Britain) will be considered at any time of the day or night by calling the senior case worker on duty, or the NSPCC.

Having the parents of abused children seen by an experienced and sympathetic social worker as a member of the team as soon after admission as possible helps the parents to find someone with whom they can share some of their anxieties in an on-going therapeutic relationship. Having this worker for themselves will help them to face the reality of their situation, while the child's investigations and the family study is being made.

The objects of the hospital admission are:

1. To treat the injuries or other conditions present.
2. To make a complete assessment and diagnosis of the child's state of health, of growth and development, of injury, disease, mental or emotional problems.
3. To formulate a prognosis for the child and outline his treatment needs.
4. To assess the parental and family capacity, and their problems in health, social, marital and personal spheres.
5. To decide whether the parents and family at home can meet the child's needs, with or without help from outside agencies. The needs of the siblings will be considered too.
6. To plan help for the parents and child or children at home, including any special medical, educational, psychological or psychiatric treatment for any family member or for the family as a unit.
7. To consider the need for Court Proceedings.
8. To consider short or long term placement of the child away from the family.

A multidisciplinary team, always including doctors and social workers, will be needed to make the psycho-social study of the family. The paediatrician usually welcomes the help of a child psychiatrist as well as the family doctor and health visitor. The head of the child's nursery or school and perhaps a probation officer or worker from a voluntary agency already involved with the family should also be asked to collaborate where relevant. The paediatrician will be responsible for seeing that the parents are kept fully informed about the child's condition from day to day, and for discussing abuse or rough handling with them once that diagnosis has been confirmed. The social worker and child psychiatrist will usually be much involved at this stage as well.

In some cases after tests have been made and the family assessed, abuse will seem unlikely although social and emotional problems in child or family may need treatment in order to promote the child's and sibling's better health and development. The child should not be sent home until the family doctor, health visitor, social worker and where relevant school doctor all agree and understand the plan of management. Case conferences are normally the way in which the various workers meet to discuss and make the major plan and decisions.

In case of injury

The full examination of the child has already been described, and the importance of making a list of the injuries and an outline chart. Photographs of the child and his injuries should now be made, in colour and in black and white, and full skeletal X-rays in all babies and young children where abuse is being considered and in most cases the films are repeated in two weeks. When school age children are concerned, selective X-rays, where clinically indicated, will be adequate except in exceptionally severe cases of cruelty.

Studies of blood coagulation must be done in all cases where bruising or bleeding is present, including a blood film, platelet count, bleeding time, prothrombin time, partial thromboplastin time and thrombin time. In selected cases a Factor VIII assay will be needed. It is important not to miss rare cases of, for example, von Willebrand's Disease, or other similar disorder (Table 2.15).

Table 2.15   Clinical diagnosis of child abuse

COAGULATION STUDIES

Blood film	Prothrombin time
Platelet count	Partial thromboplastin time
Bleeding time	Thrombin time
(Factor VIII assay)	

When the child is able to run about and play or with the normal handling of a baby, the frequency of falls and small bruises should be noted. Abusing parents often say the child bruises easily, although this is usually not confirmed in the ward.

Failure to thrive

After a full history and examination of the child with careful charting of his growth and development some basic investigations such as a haemoglobin, blood count and film, urinalysis and culture, urine chromatogram, sweat test, chest X-ray, skull X-ray and bone age estimation should be carried out. If these are negative further investigations should be delayed for observation of the child's appetite, behaviour, growth and development on the ward. Changes in infant formula should not be made but the infant or toddler should be encouraged to feed *ad lib* on a normal diet suitable for his age. In cases of neglect and rejection growth is usually quickly resumed in the ward, where the loving care of the nurses, even in the institutional setting, promotes the child's capacity to thrive. Rapid catch-up growth is seen on the chart and even the head circumference increases fast. These children often have a head circumference at or below the 3rd centile and on recovery from marked dwarfism in the first two years or so, before the skull bones are fully united, a rapid increase in skull circumference may be seen to the 50th centile or more, sometimes associated with temporary widening of the cranial sutures[113–116]. No further biochemical or other investigations, tiresome for the child, are needed, but the psycho-social study of the child and family must be thorough and detailed.

Meanwhile the parents are encouraged to visit and care for the child, emphasis on nutrition, play and physical contact being stressed. Careful observation of parental capacity to love and care for the child is essential with praise and encouragement of unskilful parents by the ward staff. The relationship of the child with his parents must be closely observed. The multidisciplinary team may need to meet two or three times to plan continuing care after discharge and to decide whether the parents should continue to look after the child. Where the parents insist on taking the child home before a planned discharge programme is arranged, and it is felt that an immediate order for child protection is scarcely indicated, the child's growth and development should be carefully monitored at home with a weekly assessment of weight and monthly of height or length. Some children die of starvation, cruelty and neglect unless urgent measures to monitor the child's progress after leaving hospital have been taken[117]. It is crucial to *see* the child, not only his face, which is the last to waste, but his limbs and body too. When a visiting nurse or social worker calls and is told the child has 'gone away' it is important to follow this up and arrange for a visit in the child's new locality. Refusal by parents to have the child seen or to take him for further medical assessment should not be passed by and if necessary a Court Order should be obtained.

If the catch-up growth, begun in hospital, is not maintained at home, readmission is usually indicated after a few weeks and after two or three weeks only in a baby. When further catch-up growth occurs in the ward, which is an institution where well cared for children do not thrive better than at home, placement of the child in a foster home will usually be needed. The profound disturbance in mother–child relationship which leads to severe failure to thrive, is rarely fully curable, even with prolonged psychotherapy[100–105]. An exception may be found in the early weeks of life in a mother with puerperal depression, when adequate treatment may quickly resolve the problem. In other cases it is better to 'divorce' the mother and child at an early stage than allow the baby or toddler prolonged undernutrition and poor development, which have permanent long term effects on ultimate physical growth, intelligence, emotional and social development.

If the child is placed in a foster home, decisions will need to be made about visiting by the parents. Unless a temporary fostering for a few weeks is part of planned rehabilitation, it may be better not to press the mother or parents of a failure-to-thrive baby to visit but to leave it to her own inclination, facilitating transport if she wishes. Many mothers are content to fall out of the picture, and they need much support to do this, and encouragement and help to resume their own lives in a more effective and meaningful way. Adoption for the child will then be possible, and is desirable to promote his security in the future[110,118,119].

The choice of foster or adoptive homes for failure-to-thrive children must be very carefully made, because disturbances in behaviour on recovery are usual, and for weeks or months can be quite severe, as has been described earlier. The foster parents will need to understand this and be prepared to deal gently with tantrums, overactivity, gorging food and rather promiscuous friendliness in the child. Periods of stealing and lying in the school years may also be a feature of the earlier disturbance, and sometimes a stormy adolescence will occur. As long as the new parents can accept realistically the possible need for psychiatric help for their child from time to time, and the child and new family accept each other well in the early weeks after placement, there should be no anxiety for the child's future well-being.

for weeks or months can be quite severe, as has been described earlier. The foster parents will need to understand this and be prepared to deal gently with tantrums, overactivity, gorging food and rather promiscuous friendliness in the child. Periods of stealing and lying in the school years may also be a feature of the earlier disturbance, and sometimes a stormy adolescence will occur. As long as the new parents can accept realistically the possible need for psychiatric help for their child from time to time, and the child and new family accept each other well in the early weeks after placement, there should be no anxiety for the child's future well-being.

Long-term management – medical aspects

Whether the child returns to his family, or goes to a nursery, children's home or foster home, regular assessment of growth and development, and of school progress will be needed, and this should be reviewed three monthly at first and later six monthly or annually. The team involved with the original study may continue to monitor progress, and should meet at intervals to discuss further treatment needs. It is often necessary for the paediatrician and social worker to help the foster parents through a phase of difficult behaviour after placement to prevent the fostering breaking down, especially in the case of very young children. The social worker, paediatrician, and in some cases child psychiatrist, should plan the programme of follow-up care so that their work and visits are co-ordinated.

In some children the injuries will need regular review and where head injuries have occurred, clumsiness, epilepsy and learning problems may ensue and need appropriate management. These assessments could be done in a Child Health Clinic, a Child Development Unit or even by the family doctor if he is trained and interested in developmental and psycho-social assessment. Close liaison with the social worker is essential, and in many cases family therapy in a child psychiatric unit will be extremely valuable, complementing the work of the paediatrician and social worker.

The importance of making long term plans for the child cannot be over-emphasised. The young abused child should either be returned home or placed in a long term foster home within 6 months. Little children cannot wait a number of years for parents to mature. Their need for warm parental care is immediate and their time sense is based on the urgency of the instinctual and emotional needs.

Delaying, or moving a child from one placement to another, thus repeatedly breaking affectional bonds is disastrous for the child's mental health.

When rehabilation is the plan parents have to understand the urgent need for them to work hard with the therapeutic team to resolve their problems so that the child can return to them in 3 to 6 months. During this period they should have frequent contact with their child.

Much research is needed on the sometimes conflicting needs for contact between parents and child in a long stay home. With very young children parental 'visiting rights' should not over-ride the child's need for stability. Young children should not be expected to go off alone for hours with relative strangers. Too many young foster children, already vulnerable to stress, are torn, crying, from their foster mother to see their family. They return several hours later. The visit being followed by several days of moody, difficult behaviour, wet beds, nightmares and other difficulties. What does this do to the child's sense of trust, to his self confidence to his faith in the future without which a child's development is at risk?

The child psychiatrist

It is always valuable for the paediatrician and child psychiatrist to share the burden of helping and understanding these difficult and sometimes puzzling families. With very disturbed, deprived and psychopathic or subnormal parents response to psychiatric skills may be minimal, and then a plan for maximum help from community services may be the best policy. It may be necessary for the child or children of such families to be removed after Court Proceedings. Nevertheless the parents and family will still require continued support.

In families who seem, on the surface, to be functioning reasonably well, and yet a child has undoubtedly suffered inflicted injuries which the parents continue to deny, it should be mandatory for the child psychiatry team to be involved in the family assessment. Few paediatricians or social workers have the time or skills necessary to uncover the parents' deepest anxieties and conflicts which lie at the root of the family problems, and which may be largely unconscious. It may be dangerous to return a child to such a family until the conflicts have been brought out into the open and to a great extent resolved.

The police

The role of the police is still a matter for debate in all countries concerned with services for abusing families. Many areas in, for example, the USA, Britain, Holland and Scandinavia have included senior police officers in the team for assessment and planning management in confirmed cases of child abuse, especially when a non-accidental injury to a child has occurred. In cases of mild injury in reasonably functioning families the police are content to keep a watching brief. Where serious injuries or neglect have occurred the police will naturally interview the family, and may prosecute one or both parents. The Courts are more inclined to impose probation orders on offenders so that they can continue with the treatment programme unless they are known violent or criminal types.

DIFFERENTIAL DIAGNOSIS OF CHILD ABUSE

Injuries

When confronted with an injured child the physician has to differentiate four situations:

'accidental' injury
carelessness
neglect
inflicted injury

Since 'accidental' injury usually has a cause in preceding stress of some kind, and since a good many of the frequent minor accidents to children are due to carelessness or neglect, whether momentary or long-standing, it can be a little difficult to determine which of the first three situations a particular child is in. The younger the child the more it is the parents' responsibility to protect him from harm.

It is not always easy to be sure about inflicted injury either, especially when the injuries themselves are slight.

Six studies are needed to help the physician (or nurse or other professional) clarify the issues involved (Table 2.16):

Table 2.16   Six studies for differential diagnosis of child abuse

---

1. Assess injuries, growth, development and general health of child, including X-rays, blood studies and photographs.
2. Obtain full history of injuries, how and why they occurred, and subsequent action and attention given.
3. Enquire about child's personal history from conception and histories of siblings.
4. Observe personality, attitudes and behaviour of parents.
5. Formulate a personal biography of each parent, and note details of marriage relationships.
6. Note social circumstances of the family.
↓
THE CRITICAL PATH CAN THUS BE DEMONSTRATED

---

(1) *Assess injuries, growth, development and general health of child, including X-rays and blood studies.* After a full examination, skeletal X-rays and blood tests are done as already described. If bites, cigarette burns, fingertip bruises, eye haemorrhage, metaphyseal or epiphyseal lesions are found abuse is almost certain. Any bruising on a baby and any fracture under 2 years is very suspicious. Black eyes, facial bruising, ear and mouth injuries and bruising on

both sides of the body from ordinary falls are also very suspicious. Poor hygiene, small stature and unattended health problems are common on some abused children.

(2) *Obtain full history of injuries, how and why they occurred, and subsequent action and attention given.* This history must be carefully matched with the injuries and the doctor should not be gullible about fabricated stories when he sees an obviously abused child.

(3) *Enquire about child's personal history from conception and histories of siblings.* This may reveal relevant factors commonly associated with abuse such as unwanted pregnancy, requests for abortion or adoption, a premature, small or sick newborn, feeding, crying and sleeping problems, repeated accidents to this child or to siblings, death of a sibling from an accident.

(4) *Observe personality, attitudes and behaviour of parents.* Very often the appearance of the child and the behaviour of the parents are the two clues to diagnosis, and this has already been discussed. Vagueness and evasiveness about the history, coldness, indifference or anger with the child, aggressive and argumentative behaviour, or disappearing and sending a young sibling along with the child all arouse suspicion.

(5) *Formulate a personal biography of each parent, and note details of marriage relationships.* This includes their care in childhood, their health, education, family attitudes when small, discipline and punishment, separations, divorce of parents, family violence, difficult behaviour, Court appearances, jobs held, the stresses and strains in their lives, and whether they now have helpful contact and support from family members. The nature of the marriage relationship, how it has developed, which are the stressful areas, needs exploring. The parents' feelings for the children from conception onwards should be noted. Loneliness, anxiety, fatigue and ill-health in the mother are potent factors which may bring her to breaking-point leading to the injuries, or one or other parent may see the child as abnormal or bad or be acting out painful unresolved family conflicts. It is feelings rather than facts which are being studied here.

(6) *Note social circumstances of the family.* This will include problems over poor housing, over-crowding, money, unemployment, divorce, changing consorts, illegitimacy, violence, criminality, dull intellect, too many children too soon, etc.

With these six studies the doctor should know how the parents see the child, whether they expect too much of his performance, whether they had depriving or violent experiences growing up, whether they have helpful support from family or friends to act as a life-line. Usually there is a crisis with the child, such as continual crying, messing or difficult behaviour, before the assault, and when this follows a domestic crisis control may snap.

As Lynch and Ounsted[23] have emphasized the build-up of stresses from the parents' own background together with marital problems, subsequent medical and social pressures and then a child's behaviour which they see as difficult or unrewarding leads down the critical path to abuse[120]. There have usually been several warnings when one or other parent has unsuccessfully sought help before the child is assaulted.

An evaluation of this kind can be done superficially in a few minutes by an experienced doctor in many cases of abuse. In others a few days are needed to look into the various factors in detail. The grey area of 'I don't know' should be very small when such a thorough assessment is made, using the multi-disciplinary team.

Failure to thrive

The study proceeds as for injury, but dwelling also on the history of the child's feeding and care and on symptoms of ill-health or difficult behaviour. The child's, the siblings' and the parents' biographies and social factors are assessed as before, and a clear picture of the critical path of the multiple stresses can usually be built up. Intrauterine growth retardation may need to be excluded and, very rarely, progeria. It is the associated parental attitudes and the recovery in hospital which distinguish abuse.

Psychological abuse

Here detailed attention is needed to the parents' biographies and their feelings about the child from conception onwards. Empathy and gentleness with parents which will allow them to reveal problems and show their hurt and unhappy feelings is essential in making these studies to reveal the extent of the abusive environment.

Medical conditions to be excluded

With bruising

When bruises or bleeding are present the coagulation studies will exclude various forms of purpura, haemophilia, von Willebrand's disease and other conditions which interfere with blood coagulation. In difficult cases a paediatric haematologist will be helpful and a full consultation should take place.

With skeletal lesions

With regard to the bones, birth fracture is sometimes difficult to exclude in a young infant, and the obstetrician, midwife, radiologist and paediatrician need to discuss this together. In birth fracture a traumatic delivery and signs of fracture with swelling and disuse are usually obvious in the first week of life.

Syphilitic osteitis is usually easy to exclude but pyogenic osteitis is not. Redness, swelling, heat and pain may be present over a large sub-periosteal haematoma in an infant, and there may also be a mild fever and a moderately elevated ESR. If chip fractures are seen trauma alone is likely although rarely the haematoma can act as a nidus for the staphylococcus. Unless the infant is ill with probable septicaemia it is wise to withhold antibiotics for 12–24 hours for a more thorough assessment. Once used it will probably be impossible to be sure that the periosteal reaction is due to trauma when treated osteitis remains a possibility.

Traumatic haemarthrosis may simulate pyogenic arthritis, and coagulation studies will be needed to exclude haemophilia. Scurvy is a rare possibility. Rickets from nutritional neglect may co-exist with physical abuse and this can be confusing. Hypervitaminosis A can cause tenderness and swelling of the tibiae with secondary periosteal reaction. Secondary deposits, usually from neuroblastoma, are rare and usually multiple. Osteopetrosis and histiocytosis X may cause fractures. Fragilitas ossium (osteogenesis imperfecta) in its milder form is often impossible to exclude on the X-rays alone, although metaphyseal injuries by themselves would be rather against it. Diligent history-taking and assessment is needed to exclude other signs, including mild deafness in the child or family. The finding of obvious parental factors associated with abuse usually helps to settle the matter. Infantile cortical hyperostosis (Caffey's disease) is another condition of infancy which can cause difficulty, but the jaw swelling, rare in abused babies, is helpful.

With skin disorders

Eczema and thrush skin lesions should not be confused with neglect. Epidermolysis bullosa is rare but important to exclude, and toxic epidermal necrolysis and impetigo may simulate burns. The Ehlers Danlos syndrome with scarring and bruising is rarely a real problem, as the associated factors in abuse cases usually confirm that problem. Mongolian blue spots in babies of African or Asian descent may be confused with bruises. Loose threads in mittens or socks sometimes cause constriction on a digit.

THE DOCTOR AND THE JUVENILE COURT

When Court Orders for child protection are being sought the paediatrician and social worker between them usually have the task of presenting the main evidence[121]. Five points of importance are:

1. It is extremely helpful if the paediatrician writes a full medical report on the child's injuries (if present), his opinion as to their cause, the child's general health, growth and development, and the parents' attitudes and capacity to care for him. Much time is needed to ascertain facts and feelings and to formulate these views in the multidisciplinary team before the medical report is composed. At times the paediatric ward sister and child psychiatrist will also need

to be witnesses and should then present reports as well, so that the lawyers and social work team can study them when formulating policy in the Court and afterwards. Charts to show deviations in growth curves are valuable evidence to the Court and so are photographs of injuries or of the child's growth and proportions.

2. Time should be spent with the lawyer beforehand to make sure he understands the implications of the paediatric evidence, particularly with regard to growth, developmental and behavioural signs in the young child, and to the facets of parenting capacity.

3. It is particularly helpful if the paediatrician discusses his evidence with the parents on several occasions before the court hearing. Most of the facts will have been talked about already in the day to day discussions in hospital. The parents should realize that no-one is on trial, that the Court is concerned with the child's care, and that they have had problems with this about which they will now be receiving help. In some 20% or so of cases, where rehabilitation of the child into the family is considered unwise, the social worker and doctor will be working towards helping parents relinquish the child.

4. In giving evidence the doctor should be firm in his opinions, which should be given slowly and clearly in lay terms. He should avoid being led away from the particular case by vigorous cross examination! To questions such as 'But surely, doctor, a baby of this age could fall off a chair and sustain these injuries?', the answer should not be 'Well, perhaps' but 'In my opinion *this* baby did not sustain his injuries falling off a chair', making it quite plain to the Court.

5. Observations on the parents' behaviour and their attitudes and feelings towards the child are important evidence too, based on seeing and talking to them and watching them with their children. Insight into their situation can also come from understanding their individual biographies and studying reports about them from family physicians, public health nurses, schools and other professional services where relevant. Some prediction about their future capacity based on their abilities and functions to date is justified from an experienced and concerned paediatrician or child psychiatrist.

Perhaps paediatricians need to consider more often whether the rights of the child patient should be protected by law when the parents are unable or unwilling to meet his needs for affection, security, new experiences, encouragement, control and independence. Doctors tend to identify with the adults, and a voice for the child is not raised often enough. The legal processes are complicated to learn, consume time and energy and are usually emotionally unrewarding to the doctor. Nevertheless they should be studied in order to help children[122,123,124].

Paediatricians tend to turn a blind eye to a great deal of childhood suffering which it is in their power to alleviate through the Courts, in co-operation with child protection agencies. The first essential is to recognize the problem, and the second to consult with the relevant agencies.

Kempe's dictum on child abuse can be stated again here:

> 'The definition of child abuse and neglect is not
> what the doctor thinks it should be, or what the
> social worker thinks it is, but is actually what
> the Court says it is. The Court is of course
> influenced by the public and its definition will
> change from time to time and may be different
> in different localities, based on the emotional
> climate of the cities in that area.'
>
> *C. Henry Kempe, 1973*

Looking at the results of long term studies on abused children should alert us to the wisdom of protecting their interests—their need to grow and develop in an affectionate and encouraging home in order to break the vicious spiral of transmitted deprivation and abuse in the next generations.

The end of a poem by a member of Parents Anonymous in the USA poses the question:

> Why couldn't others understand
> What I suffered at my parents' hands
> Until finally I became
> The things they called me
> Every name.
>
> In a life devoid of love
> I became what I was told I was
> I am what I was taught to be
> Why couldn't others help and see
> Instead of simply hating me?

REFERENCES

1. Renvoize, J. (1978). *Web of Violence.* (London: Routledge & Kegan Paul)
2. Oliver, J. E. and Taylor, A. (1971). Five generations of ill-treated in one family pedigree. *Br. J. Psychiat.,* **119,** 473
3. Oliver, J. E. and Cox, J. (1973). A family kindred with ill-used children: The 'burden on the community'. *Br. J. Psychiat.,* **123,** 81
4. Smith, S. M. (1975). *The Battered Child Syndrome.* (London: Butterworth)
5. Cooper, C. E. (1970). Battered babies. *J. Med. Wom. Fed.,* **52,** 93
6. Ackley, D. E. (1977). A brief overview of child abuse. *Social Casework,* **58**
7. Anthony, E. J. and Benedek, T. (1970). *Parenthood—Its Psychology and Psychopathology.* (Boston: Little, Brown and Co.)
8. Mahler, M. S., Pine, F. and Bergman, A. (1975). *The Psychological Birth of the Human Infant.* (London: Hutchinson)
9. Rapoport, R., Rapoport, R. N. and Strelitz, Z. (1977). *Fathers, Mothers and Others.* (London: Routledge & Kegan Paul)
10. Elliot, K. (1970). *The Family and its Future.* (London: J. & A. Churchill)

11. Vaughan, V. C. and Brazelton, T. B. (1976). *The Family—Can It Be Saved?*. (Chicago: Year Book Medical Publishers, Inc.)

12. Department of Health and Social Security (1974). *The Family in Society. Dimensions of Parenthood*. (London: HMSO)

13. Pringle, M. Kellmer (1975). *The Needs of Children*. (London: Hutchinson)

14. Steinmetz, S. K. and Straus, M. A. (1974). *Violence in the Family*. (New York: Dodd, Mead & Co.)

15. Flynn, J. P. (1977). Recent findings related to wife abuse. *Social Casework*, **58**, 13

16. Elbow, M. (1977). Theoretical considerations of violent marriages. *Social Casework*, **58**, 515

17. Anthony, E. J. (1974). Children at risk from Divorce: a review. In: *The Child in His Family*. Vol. 3: *Children at Psychiatric Risk*. (E. J. Anthony and C. Koupernik; eds.), p. 461. (London and New York: John Wiley & Sons)

18. Wallerstein, J. and Kelly, J. (1974). The effects of parental divorce: the adolescent experience. In: *The Child in His Family*. Vol. 3: *Children at Psychiatric Risk*. (E. J. Anthony and C. Koupernik; eds.). (London and New York: John Wiley & Sons)

19. Wallerstein, J. and Kelly, J. (1975). The effects of parental divorce: experiences of the preschool child. *J. Am. Acad. Child. Psychiat.*, **14**, 4

20. Kelly, J. and Wallenstein, J. (1976). The effects of parental divorce: experiences of the child in early latency. *Am. J. Orthopsychiatry*, **46**, (1), 20

21. Wallenstein, J. and Kelly, J. (1976). The effects of parental divorce: experiences of the child in later latency. *Am. J. Orthopsychiatry*, **46**, (2), 256

22. Lynch, M. A. and Roberts, J. (1977). Predicting child abuse: signs of bonding failure in the maternity hospital. *Br. Med. J.*, **1**, 624

23. Wolkind, S. N., Kruk, S. and Chaves, L. P. (1976). Childhood separation experiences and psycho-social states in primiparous women: preliminary findings. *Br. J. Psychiat.*, **128**, 391

24. Wolkind, S. N. (1977). Women who have been in care – psychological and social status during pregnancy. *J. Child Psychol. Psychiatry*, **18**, 179

25. Oppell, W. C. and Royston, A. B. (1971). Teenage births: some social, psychological and physical sequelae. *Am. J. Public Health*, **61**, 751

26. Osofsky, H. J. and Osofsky, J. D. (1972). The low income adolescent factors related to overall prognosis and infant development. In: *Psychosomatic Medicine of Obstetrics and Gynaecology*. Proceedings of the 3rd International Congress, London (1971). (Basel: S. Karger)

27. Ayond, C. C. and Pfeifer, D. R. (1977). An approach to the prophylaxis of child abuse and neglect. *Child Abuse and Neglect*, **1**, 71

28. Reynolds, C. (1978). Can good parenting be taught? In: *Child Abuse: Prediction, Prevention and Follow-up*. (A. White Franklin; ed.), p. 80. (London: Churchill-Livingstone)

29. Baldwin, D. (1975). *Understanding Your Baby: A Course in Child Development 0–3 Years*. (London: Ebury Press)

30. Frommer, E. A. and O'Shea, G. (1973). Antenatal identification of women liable to have problems in managing their infants. *Br. J. Psychiat.*, **123**, 149

31. Frommer, E. A. and O'Shea, G. (1973). The importance of childhood experience in relation to problems of marriage and family building. *Br. J. Psychiat.*, **123**, 157

32. Gray, J. D., Cutler, C. A., Dean, J. G. and Kempe, C. H. (1977). Prediction and prevention of child abuse and neglect. *Child Abuse and Neglect*, **1**, 45

33. Kempe, C. H. (1976). Approaches to preventing child abuse. *Am. J. Dis. Child.*, **130**, 941

34. Klaus, M. H. and Kennell, J. H. (1976). *Maternal Infant Bonding*. p. 3. (St Louis: C. V. Mosby & Co.)

35. Lynch, M. A. (1975). Ill health and child abuse. *Lancet*, **ii**, 317

36. Lynch, M. A. and Roberts, J. (1977). Predicting child abuse: signs of bonding failure in the maternity hospital. *Br. Med. J.*, **1**, 624

37. Winnicott, D. W. (1965). *The Maturational Processes and the Facilitating Environment*. p. 145. (New York: International Universities Press)

38. L. A. (1975). Tranquillisers causing aggression. *Br. Med. J.*, **1**, 113

39. Lynch, M. A., Lindsay, J. and Ounsted, C. (1975). Tranquillisers causing aggression. *Br. Med. J.*, **1**, 166

40. Cookson, I. B. (1975). Tranquillisers causing aggression. *Br. Med. J.*, **1**, 266

41. Brazelton, T. B., Koslowski, B. and Main, M. (1974). The origins of reciprocity in mother–infant interaction. In: *The Effect of the Infant on its Caregiver*. (M. Lewis and L. A. Rosenblum; eds.). (London and New York: John Wiley & Sons)

42. Ainsworth, M. D. S., Bell, S. M. and Stayton, D. J. (1974). Infant–mother attachment and social development: socialisation as a product of reciprocal responsiveness to signals. In: *The Integration of a Child into a Social World*. (M. P. M. Richards; ed.). (Cambridge: Cambridge University Press)

43. Klaus, M. H., Kennell, J. H., Plumb, N. and Zuehike, S. (1970). Human maternal behaviour at the first contact with her young. *Paediatrics*, **46**, 187

44. Klaus, M. H., Jerauld, R., Kreger, N. C., McAlpine, W., Steffa, M. and Kennell, J. H. (1972). Maternal attachment: importance of the first post-partum days. *N. Engl. J. Med.*, **286**, 460

45. Kennell, J. H., Jerauld, R., Wolfe, H., Chesler, D., Kreger, N. C., McAlpine, W., Steffa, M. and Klaus M. H. (1974). Maternal behaviour one year after early and extended post-partum contact. *Dev. Med. Child Neurol.*, **16**, 172

46. Ringler, N. M., Kennel, J. H., Jarvella, R., Navojosky, B. J. and Klaus, M. H. (1975). Mother to child speech at 2 years: effects of early post-natal contact. *J. Pediatr.*, **86**, 141

47. Hales, D. J., Lazoff, B., Sosa, R. and Kennel, J. H. (1977). Defining the limits of the maternal sensitive period. *Dev. Med. Child Neurol.*, **19**, 454

48. de Chateau, P. and Wiberg, B. (1977). Long-term effects on mother–infant behaviour of extra contact during the first hour post-partum. 1. First observations at 36 hours. *Acta Paediatr. Scand.*, **66**, 137

49. de Chateau, P. and Wiberg, B. (1977). Long-term effects on mother–infant behaviour of extra contact during the first hour post-partum. 2. A follow-up at three months. *Acta Paediatr. Scand.*, **66**, 145

50. de Chateau, P. and Wiberg, B. (1978). Long-term effects on mother–infant behaviour of extra contact during the first hour post-partum. 3. A follow-up one year later. In: *Psychosomatic Medicine of Obstetrics and Gynaecology*. Proceedings of the 5th International Congress, Rome (1977). (Basel: S. Karger)

51. de Chateau, P. (1977). The importance of the neonatal period for the development of synchrony in the mother-infant dyad – a review. *Birth and Family J.*, **4**, 1, 10

52. Greenberg, M. and Morris, N. (1974). Engrossment: the newborn's impact upon the father. *Am. J. Orthopsychiatry*, **44**, 520

53. Lynn, D. B. (1974). *The Father: His Role in Child Development*. (Monterey, California: Brooks/Cole Publishing Co.)

54. Doering, S. G. and Entwistle, D. R. (1975). Preparation during pregnancy and ability to cope with labor and delivery. *Am. J. Orthopsychiatry*, **45**, 825

55. Kitzinger, S. (1971). *Giving Birth: The Parents' Emotions in Childbirth*. (London: Gollancz)

56. Chard, T. and Richards, M. P. M. (1978). *The Benefits and Hazards of the New Obstetrics*. Clinics in Developmental Medicine. (London: William Heinemann Medical Books, Ltd.)

57. Winberg, J. (1977). Personal communication

58. Richards, M. P. M. and Roberton, N. R. C. (1978). Admission policies for special care nurseries. In: *Early Separation and the Special Care Nursery*. (F. S. W. Brimblecombe, M. P. M. Richards and N. R. C. Roberton; eds.). Clinics in Developmental Medicine. (London: William Heinemann Medical Books, Ltd.)

59. Klaus, M. H. and Kennel, J. H. (1976). *Maternal–Infant Bonding*. Chapter 4. (St Louis: C. V. Mosby & Co.)

60. Stone, L. J., Smith, M. T. and Murphy, L. B. (1974). *The Competent Infant*. (London: Tavistock Publications)

61. Bower, T. (1977). *The Perceptual World of the Child*. (London: Fontana Open Books

Publishing Co. Ltd.)

62. MacFarlane, A. (1977). *The Psychology of Childbirth*. (London: Fontana Open Books Publishing Co. Ltd.)

63. Kennel, J. H., Fiauze, M. A. and Klaus, M. H. (1975). Evidencefor a Sensitive Period in the Human Mother. In: *Parent–Infant Interaction*. (R. Porter and M. O'Connor; eds.), p. 59. (Amsterdam: Excerpta Medicine)

64. Gunther, M. (1973). *Infant Feeding*, p. 59. (Harmondsworth, Middlesex; Penguin Books Ltd.)

65. Gunther, M. (1976). The new mother's view of herself. In: *Breast Feeding and the Mother*. CIBA Symposium 45. (K. Elliott and D. W. Fitzsimmons; eds.), p. 150. (Amsterdam: Elsevier-Excerpta Medica)

66. de Chateau, P., Holmberg, H, Jakobsson, K. and Winberg, J. (1977). A study of the factors promoting and inhibiting lactation. *Dev. Med. Child Neurol.*, **19**, 575

67. Stanway, P. and Stanway, A. (1978). *Breast is Best*. Chapter 7. (London: Pan Books Ltd.)

68. Stern, D. (1977). *The First Relationship: Infant and Mother*. (London: Fontana Open Books Publishing Co. Ltd.)

69. Rutter, M. (1975). *Helping Troubled Children*. (Harmondsworth, Middlesex: Penguin Books Ltd.)

70. Rutter, M. and Madge, N. (1976). *Cycles of Disadvantage: A Review of Research*. (London: Heinemann)

71. Birch, H. G. and Gussow, J. D. (1970). *Disadvantaged Children: Health, Nutrition and Social Failure*. (New York: Grune & Stratton, Inc.)

72. Wedge, P. and Prosser, H. (1973). *Born to Fail*. (London: Arrow Books)

73. Cooper, C. E. (1975). The doctor's dilemma – a paediatrician's view. In: *Concerning Child Abuse*. (A. White Franklin; ed.). (London: Churchill Livingstone)

74. Ounsted, C. and Lynch, M. A. (1976). Family pathology seen in England. In: *Child Abuse and Neglect: The Family and the Community*. (R. E. Helfer and C. H. Kempe; eds.). (Cambridge, Mass.: Ballinger Publishing Co.)

75. Martin, H. P. and Kempe, C. H. (1976). *The Abused Child*. (Cambridge, Mass.: Ballinger Publishing Co.)

76. Morris, M. G. and Gould, R. W. (1963). Role reversal: a necessary concept in dealing with the battered child syndrome. *Am. J. Orthopsychiatry*, **33**, 298

77. Baher, E., Hyman, C., Jones, C., Jones, R., Kerr, A. and Mitchell, R. (1976). *At Risk: An Account of the Work of the Battered Child Research Department*. (London: NSPCC-Routledge & Kegan Paul)

78. Elmer, E. (1977). A follow-up study of traumatized children. *Pediatrics*, **59**, 273

79. Malone, C. A. (1966). Safety first: comments on the influence of external danger in the lives of children of disorganised families. *Am. J. Orthopsychiatry*, **36**, 6

80. Hall, M. H. (1974). The diagnosis and early management of non-accidental injuries in children. *The Police Surgeon*, No. 6 (October 1974)

81. Hull, D. (1974). Medical diagnosis. In: *The Maltreated Child*. (J. Carter; ed.). (London: The Priory Press)

82. Furness, J. (1974). Bite-marks in non-accidental injuries of children. *The Police Surgeon*, No. 6 (October 1974).

83. Caffey, J. (1946). Multiple fractures in the long bones of infants suffering from sub-dural hematoma. *Am. J. Roentgenol.*, **56**, 163

84. Caffey, J. (1972). On the theory and practice of shaking infants. *Am. J. Dis. Child.*, **124**, 161

85. Caffey, J. (1974). The whiplash shaken infant syndrome. *Paediatrics*, **54**, 396

86. Guthkelch, A. N. (1971). Infantile subdural haematoma and its relationship to whiplash injuries. *Br. Med. J.*, **2**, 430

87. Mushin, A. S. (1975). The ego of the battered child. In: *Atlas of the Battered Child Syndrome*. (J. M. Cameron and L. J. Rae; eds.). (London: Churchill Livingstone)

88. Harcourt, R. B. and Hopkins, D. (1973). Ophthalmic aspects of the battered child syndrome. In: *Neuro-ophthalmology*, No. 7. (J. L. Smith; ed.). (St Louis: C. V. Mosby & Co.)

89. Taylor, D. and Bentovim, A. (1974). Recurrent non-accidentally inflicted chemical eye injuries to siblings. *J. Pediatr. Ophthalmol.*, **13,** 238

90. Touloukian, R. J. (1968). Abdominal visceral injuries in battered children. *Paediatrics*, **42,** 642

91. Gornall, P., Ahmed, A., Jolleys, A. and Cohen, S. J. (1972). Intra-abdominal injuries in the battered baby syndrome. *Arch. Dis. Child.*, **47,** 211

92. Swischuk, L. E. (1969). Spine and spinal cord trauma in the battered child syndrome. *Radiology*, **92,** 733

93. Jackson, R. H., Walker, J. H. and Wynne, N. A. (1968). Circumstances of accidental poisoning in childhood. *Br. Med. J.*, **4,** 245

94. Craft, A. W. and Sibert, J. R. (1977). Accidental poisoning in children. *Br. J. Hosp. Med.*, 696

95. Margolis, J. A. (1971). Psychosocial study of childhood poisoning: a 5-year follow-up. *Paediatrics*, **74,** 439

96. Rogers, D., Fupp, T., Bentovim, A., Robinson, A., Berry, D. and Goulding, R. (1976). Non-accidental poisoning: an extended syndrome of child abuse. *Br. Med. J.*, **1,** 793

97. Pearn, J. and Nixon, J. (1977). Attempted drowning as a form of non-accidental injury. *Aust. Paediatr. J.*, **13,** 110

98. Emery, J. L. (1976). Unexpected death in infancy: early recognition of the 'at risk' situation. In: *Recent Advances in Paediatrics*. (D. Hull; ed.). London: Churchill Livingstone)

99. Hick, J. F. (1973). Sudden infant death syndrome and child abuse. *Paediatrics*, **52,** 147

100. MacCarthy, D. (1974). Effects of emotional disturbance and deprivation (maternal rejection) on somatic growth. In: *Scientific Foundations of Paediatrics*. (J. A. Davis and J. Dobbing; eds.). (London: Heinemann)

101. Blager, F. and Martin, H. P. (1976). Speech and language of abused children. In: *The Abused Child*. (H. P. Martin and C. H. Kempe; eds.), p. 83. (Cambridge, Mass.: Ballinger Publishing Co.)

102. Lacey, K. A. and Parkin, J. M. (1974). The normal short child. *Arch. Dis. Child.*, **49,** 417

103. Whitten, C. F., Pettit, M. G. and Fischoff, J. (1969). Evidence that growth failure from maternal deprivation is secondary to undereating. *J. Am. Med. Assoc.*, **209,** 1675

104. Silver, H. K. and Finkelstein, M. (1967). Deprivation dwarfism. *J. Pediatr.*, **70,** 317

105. Fischoff, J., Whitten, C. F. and Pettit, M. G. (1971). A psychiatric study of mothers and infants with growth failure secondary to maternal deprivation. *J. Pediatr.*, **79,** 209

106. Burton, L. (1968). Sexual assault in childhood. In: *Vulnerable Children*. (L. Burton; ed.). (London: Routledge & Kegan Paul)

107. Farn, K. T. (1975). Sexual and other assaults on children. *The Police Surgeon*, No. 8, 37. (October 1975).

108. Schechter, M. D. and Roberge, L. (1976). Sexual exploitation. In: *Child Abuse and Neglect: The Family and the Community*. (R. E. Helfer and C. H. Kempe; eds.), p. 127. (Cambridge, Mass.: Ballinger Publishing Co.)

109. Giarretto, H. (1976). Humanistic treatment of father-daughter incest. In: *Child Abuse and Neglect: The Family and the Community*. (R. E. Helfer and C. H. Kempe; eds.), p. 143. (Cambridge, Mass.: Ballinger Publishing Co.)

110. Rowe, J. and Lambert, L. (1973). *Children Who Wait*. (London: The Association of British Adoption and Fostering Agencies)

111. Page, R. and Clark, G. A. (1977). *Who Cares? Young People in Care Speak Out*. (London: The National Children's Bureau)

112. Andreu, N. (1977). *Child of a System*. (London: Quartet Books)

113. Winick, M. and Rosso, P. (1969). Head circumference and cellular growth of the brain in normal and marasmic children. *J. Pediatr.*, **74,** 667

114. De Levie, M. and Nogrady, M. B. (1970). Rapid brain growth upon restoration of adequate nutrition causing false radiologic evidence of increased intracranial pressure. *J. Pediatr.*, **76,** 523

115. Winick, M. (1969). Malnutrition and brain development. *J. Pediatr.*, **74,** 667

116. Pearl, M., Finkelstein, J. and Berman, M. R. (1972). Temporary widening of cranial sutures

during recovery from failure to thrive. *Clin. Pediatr.*, **11,** 427

117. Godber, G. (1975). Report of the Review Body appointed to enquire into the case of Steven Meurs. (Norwich: Norfolk County Council)

118. Kadushin, A. (1970). *Adopting Older Children*. (New York: Columbia University Press)

119. Tizard, B. (1977). *Adoption: A Second Chance*. (London: Fontana Open Books Publishing Co. Ltd.)

120. Lynch, M. (1976). Child abuse: the critical path. *J. Maternal Child Health*. p. 25. (July 1976)

121. Cooper, C. E. (1978). Preparing the paediatrician's evidence in care proceedings. In: *Child Abuse: Prediction, Prevention and Follow-up*. (A. White Franklin; ed.). (London: Churchill Livingstone)

122. Godfrey, G. (1975). *A Report by Justice: Parental Rights and Duties and Custody Suits*. (London: Stevens & Sons)

123. Hoggett, B. (1977). *Parents and Children*. (London: Sweet & Maxwell)

124. Goldstein, J., Freud, A. and Solnit, A. J. (1973) *Beyond the Best Interests of the Child*. (London: Collier Macmillan)

3 Radiological and pathological aspects of the battered child syndrome

J. M. CAMERON

Part I – RADIOLOGICAL ASPECTS

Radiology plays an essential part in the investigation and diagnosis of non-accidental injury in children (battered children). By such an examination a radiologist should be able to state that not only are certain skeletal injuries caused by non-accidental injury, but that such injuries had been caused in a certain way and are of a certain age.

There is no standard appearance of the progress and consolidation of new bone so that one can only give a rough estimate as to the age of the injuries according to one's experience[1].

It is the custom nowadays to radiograph the whole body prior to autopsy and then to dissect out and re-radiograph any bone that appears to be damaged. This makes it possible for the smallest of injuries to be detected in detail and even take macro-radiographs. The radiographic study of the 'dead battered child' has helped to piece together a comprehensive picture of the type of skeletal injuries that one should look for in the live suspect battered child where the small injuries may not be so clearly demonstrated radiographically. There are two principal reasons why one wishes to understand the mechanism by which these injuries were caused: firstly to establish where possible and confirm the diagnosis in cases in which there is a discrepancy between the history as given and the radiographic findings; secondly, one should in most cases be able to give an opinion as to how such injuries were caused. Any unusual skeletal injury or an injury, the severity of which is not consistent with the history given, *demands* a complete radiographic skeletal survey. This establishes the full extent of the injuries with special reference to the metaphyses and ribs; and ascertains whether there are any old injuries, indicative of previous trauma.

The presence of multiple fractures of the long bones in various stages of healing, implying more than one traumatic incident, may suggest to the experienced eye a case of child abuse but this need not necessarily be definite proof alone of non-accidental injury. One must exclude natural bone disease which can resemble non-accidental injury.

When the periosteum has been lifted from the underlying bone by a haematoma, periosteal new bone formation occurs normally and can be seen in over 40% of such cases within 7 days. In a case of injury, a distinction must be made between the normal bone layer and the pathological new bone resulting from the trauma. In the case of trauma, the normal layer may be interrupted by a fracture or by haemorrhage. When the pathological new bone forms later it will be as a continuous, unbroken layer superimposed upon the normal one. This distinction is of importance when estimating the age of the injury. Deformities resulting from metaphyseal injuries may persist for some time and it is important that they should be recognized. In a case of non-accidental injury to children any deformity, however slight, should not be disregarded. The older the injury the less noticeable will the deformity become. Any metaphyseal injury may be so small as to be considered of no importance, but it cannot be emphasized too strongly that any injury in the region of the metaphysis – be it a crack or a small piece of detached bone in a suspected case of child abuse – should in the first instance be regarded as a result of non-accidental injury.

It is unusual for a baby to sustain multiple fractures of the ribs merely by falling from a cot or a pram or by being dropped and it is very rare to sustain multiple fractures. Multiple fractures can occur in automobile accidents and in cases where there is a pathological lesion, such as osteogenesis imperfecta ('brittle bone disease'). In cases of child abuse, a common site of these fractures is in the posterior aspect of the rib often close to the spine and frequently bilateral which are caused by direct violence against the ribs. Fractures of the costochondral junctions may be associated, though less commonly, and are caused frequently by violent squeezing of the chest from side to side. The reason for this action is that it tends to make the ribs spring and fracture at their fixed points. Antero-posterior compression is more likely to cause fractures underneath the armpits (i.e. in the mid-axillary line) but one must remember that fractures can also occur as a result of cardiac resuscitation. Direct violence, as distinct from compression, can also cause fractures of the ribs, such as striking the chest with the fists, with a boot or by swinging the child by the foot and causing the chest to come into contact against some hard object. The site of a fracture caused in this way will usually be at the point where the violence is applied and is usually associated externally by a bruise. Many cases when first radiographed show multiple fractures of the ribs in varying stages of healing, indicative of more than one traumatic incident[1].

As further healing takes place, the nodules (callus formation) become contracted and less dense. They may even become almost indistinguishable from normal. It is well known that cases return to normal some six months after an injury, although in some cases they may well retain the fracture deformities. In some cases it must be noted that recent fractures are not demonstrated unless a number of views are taken from varying angles, hence the reason for removing the rib cage on death following alleged non-accidental injury and violence so that the rib cage itself can be radiographed in three dimensions. In every case of suspected Battered Child Syndrome where there are no obvious fractured ribs, the whole length of the rib should be carefully examined for evidence of old fractures. The presence of multiple rib fractures must be considered as having resulted from non-accidental trauma after the exclusion of such causes as a vehicular accident or manual compression in an attempt to revive the child either by a doctor or by a parent. *Proven bone disease must also be excluded, but it should be remembered that even a baby with a bone disease can be battered or subjected to non-accidental violence.*

A fracture of a long bone occurring as the only skeletal injury in suspected battering usually cannot be distinguished from one resulting from an accident, such as falling from a cot, but when it occurs in conjunction with a metaphyseal injury or with multiple rib fractures, it should be considered as non-accidental injury, unless there is definite proof to the contrary. The age of the injury and the mechanism by which it was caused are important in establishing the diagnosis, particularly in cases where legal proceedings have been instituted. The type of fracture of a long bone sustained as a result of falling from a cot or by being dropped can be spiral or transverse. The spiral fracture or oblique fracture occurs when the baby falls with the limb under the body and then rolls over so that a torsion force is applied. This fracture may be transverse if the limb strikes a hard, projecting object during the fall. The spiral fracture is more common than the transverse in cases of accidental trauma. It is the view of the writer that any fracture occurring in a child under eighteen months that is of the spiral variety in the long bone should be regarded as being suspicious until proven otherwise, for such a fracture can be caused by a torsion force applied to a limb as when a baby is forcibly jerked upwards and rotated whilst held by the wrist or ankle. Similarly, when a spiral fracture of the humerus occurs, this may result when the wrist is held or a fracture of the femur when the child is held by the ankle. In the absence of any corroborative evidence, one cannot, however, say how this type of fracture was caused but the presence of an associated metaphyseal avulsion injury, as in the wrist, is conclusive evidence of non-accidental trauma. A transverse fracture usually is the result of a direct blow. Avulsion of a muscle from its attachment to a long bone can result in the so-called traumatic myositis ossificans, which is ossification of a periosteal haematoma.

As regards the estimation of age of the fracture of a long bone, the same criteria apply as in the case of a metaphyseal injury and in multiple rib fractures; that is callus is not visible on the radiograph for seven to ten days following the injury and the subsequent estimation of age becomes a matter of natural experience. In a case of a fracture of the skull, it is unusual for any notable healing change to take place for four to six weeks following the injury. The fracture may become more definite in the days following the injury, especially if increased intracranial pressure in the form of a subdural haematoma develops. A fracture of the spine may also occur more often than one would give it credit for and, if it is an isolated injury, it may not be diagnostic, as it will not differ from that sustained by accidental injury. If, however, it is associated with other skeletal injuries, the diagnosis of abuse will probably be made in the presence of these injuries and particularly if associated with a heel mark in the back of the child.

DIFFERENTIAL DIAGNOSIS

There are several diseases where bone injuries can simulate those seen in non-accidental cases in children but, in most of these, the clinical examination should establish the diagnosis. It is important, however, that the medical practitioner should be conversant with these radiological appearances when examining a suspected case of non-accidental injury and when giving evidence in a court of law on such a case.

Osteogenesis imperfecta

In the majority of the cases, the diagnosis is not in doubt and in the neonatal type there are multiple fractures of the tubular-shaped long bones or multiple fractures where the bones are thin and bowed. In the severe cases the bones may be thin and not fractured. Cases which simulate the Battered Child Syndrome are those when the bones appear normal and fractures occur several months later and, although a special test has been described in which the collagenous tissue of the body is examined, this is of negative value because it provides only negative proof. It is, however, frequently found where a suggestion is made to the court that the case could be one of 'brittle bone disease' in spite of the fact that the children concerned improve on hospital therapy, and sustain fractures only when at home. It should be noted, however, that the fractures of the long bones involve the diaphyses and not the metaphyses, as occurs in the avulsion-type injury. These are not avulsion fractures, but fractures occurring in porotic bones, either spontaneously or as a result of slight trauma. A similar type of fracture is seen in the porotic bones of a case of spina bifida, although exuberant callus is seen to be a feature of 'brittle bone disease' (osteogenesis imperfecta). Nevertheless, one must state categorically that excessive new bone formation is not an uncommon feature following injury to the distal end of the femur in a case of spina bifida. It can occur in cases of osteomyelitis involving the metaphysis and also in cases of non-accidental injury to children in which there has been no immobilization. There are, however, other features which are diagnostic of osteogenesis imperfecta such as blue sclerotics and a mosaic pattern in the posterior aspect of the skull. The possibility that skeletal injuries in the case of osteogenesis imperfecta may have resulted from non-accidental trauma should, however, not be overlooked because even children suffering from abnormal bone disease can be battered.

Scurvy

The changes occurring in scurvy with the fractured metaphysis and calcification in the subperiosteal haematoma closely resemble the appearances of metaphyseal injuries in non-accidental injury. In theory, however, there is a generalized osteoporosis and the metaphyses of most of the long bones will be involved.

Congenital syphilis

In congenital syphilis there may be a fractured and separated metaphysis of a long bone with periosteal new bone along the shaft. Extensive periosteal new bone is a common feature of the shafts of the limb bones and this tends to be symmetrical. It tends to extend the metaphysis, though the bone adjacent to the metaphysis is often porotic. There are no changes in the metaphysis as would be seen in cases of an avulsion injury. Occasionally, however, the metaphyseal border may be eroded by the syphilitic inflammation and in such a case it may be difficult to exclude superimposed trauma.

Infantile cortical hyperostosis of Caffey

In this condition periosteal new bone forms along the shafts of several long bones. Where this new bone extends to the metaphyses, it may occasionally resemble the periosteal new bone resulting from an avulsion injury, especially when the injury involves the proximal and distal metaphyses of the long bone. In Caffey's disease, the metaphyses will show no evidence of injury. One will see, however, a fracture of either a short oblique or transverse type and the callus is more localized. In a large proportion of Caffey's disease the mandible will show cortical thickening.

Osteomyelitis

When the metaphysis of a long bone is affected by osteomyelitis, the appearances resemble those of metaphyseal avulsion injury. The metaphysis may become irregular and periosteal new bone may form along the shaft. In some cases there may be excessive calcification of the surrounding soft tissues resembling a severe avulsion injury. Such deformity resulting from the osteomyelitis in the region of the metaphysis, with thickening of the cortex, could in some cases simulate the thickened cortex of an old subperiosteal haematoma.

There is, however, no metaphyseal damage and the soft tissue swelling would probably be more extensive than that resulting from a haematoma.

Spina bifida

In cases of spina bifida where the legs are paralysed and the bones are porotic, very slight trauma can cause a fracture, but it is usually transverse at the distal end of the shaft of the femur or causes a dislocation of the epiphysis with associated damage to the metaphysis. These injuries are frequently accompanied by excessive haemorrhage and subsequent new bone formation in the adjacent soft tissues. This creates an appearance not unlike that seen in a case of child abuse, except that this degree of dislocation of the epiphysis is uncommon as a result of non-accidental injury. As in 'brittle bone disease' (osteogenesis imperfecta), the fact that the slight trauma can be non-accidental should not be overlooked. It should also be remembered that fractures in both these diseases can occur spontaneously.

Part II – PATHOLOGICAL ASPECTS

If anyone has a right to be loved, a baby does. We all know how vital it is for a human being to have a good start in life and for this it is essential that one should be wanted and loved when one first enters the world, frail and helpless. People sometimes think that they have a right to be loved and that it is the duty of their husbands, wives, children, parents and friends to love them. Frequently they expect this to happen without any effort on their part to make themselves loveable. Asked about this, many of those who complain of being unloved would be horrified and even resentful.

Sadly, we are all somewhat afraid of one another and of being criticized and this is what sometimes makes us behave in a disagreeable or aggressive manner. On the other hand, it has some advantages because it makes us more willing to compromise in order to be accepted and wanted. As far as a child is concerned, the mother is the baby's life-line, both from the physical and psychological point of view. A baby or a small child cannot realize the effect it is having on others and it has very little control over its behaviour or emotions.

It sometimes happens that children with the most loveable natures do not get their due, whilst those less deserving receive far more than enough love, and this is by no means always fair. No-one can love to order, simply because someone deserves love or needs it. On the whole, we have to work hard to make ourselves loveable if we want to be loved! Over the age of seven this is relatively easy, but under that age a child, or baby, has no control. In a family there are, of course, natural bonds of affection between husband and wife, parents and children, and between the children themselves. At the same time one is apt to show one's worst side to one's families, e.g. children usually behave worse at home than outside; the husband and wife may exhibit less charm and grace in their home lives, particularly to their children, than they show to outsiders, for frequently those who are the life and soul of the party may be irritable and morose in the family circle. The love parents feel for their baby may not be less, but it is certainly different from the love they feel towards an adolescent or married son or daughter. In the same way children's love for the parents undergoes many changes as they develop from complete acceptance of them to the critical and independent attitude of youth.

It is in this climate that children are battered. There are still many people – doctors, lawyers and social workers among them – who even today deny that battering exists at all. (It has been estimated that 15% of children that are battered die.) They cannot bring themselves to accept that 'ordinary' people could ever attack their own children. At the start of the 1950s the American medical profession recognized that many children had definitely been attacked but not until 1962, when Professor Kempe[2] used the phrase 'Battered Child Syndrome', did the subject really become widely discussed. The safety of the child must be the primary consideration, for one must remember that 'battering parents' may and usually need help and above all a good relationship with the helping person. Priority in many cases for re-housing, a nursery placement or even temporary reception of the children in care during periods of stress and crisis can be of extreme importance. Co-operation between doctors and social agencies is essential at all stages. If a greater understanding of the cause of child abuse can be achieved there may be less need for the legislation, which many demand for the obligatory reporting of cases when a child is found to be injured – for accidents can happen.

It is well recognized that child abuse is a major problem for accident and emergency departments of children's hospitals, general practitioners, social workers, the police and many others concerned with the welfare of children. The injuries include fractures, bruises, lacerations, soft tissue swellings and burns. Ophthalmic damage can occur as a result of direct injury to the skull or by vigorous shaking, whilst laceration of the liver or perforation to the stomach or intestines, emotional deprivation, starvation, dehydration, anaemia, gross retardation of growth and development or poisoning are also recorded. A child may be poisoned by deliberate administration of a drug, or by being given an overdose, or by the deliberate act of leaving poisonous material conveniently near the child. The victims of child abuse are usually under four years of age and many are under two years of age.

The overall exact aetiology or causation factors are generally unknown. The majority of 'battering parents' are more or less normal parents who are worn out with their small children; parents who are lonely, poor, immature or under emotional or financial stress, with no-one to turn to for help. Actually it is usually the mother or father, but sometimes it can be the grandparent or other children, or even foster parents, who do the battering. If one parent batters a child the other will almost certainly know about it and aids and abets the battering[1]. The diagnosis can be difficult to reach and often impossible to prove. There may be a suspicious delay between an injury and the visit to the doctor or hospital. The story given may not agree with the physical findings and the explanation of the injuries may be vague. Suspicious indicative features can be injuries at different stages of resolution: bruises for which there is no good explanation, especially on the face; bite-marks, laceration of frenulum linguae; or a child may be distinctly apathetic. If subdural effusion is present, there are almost always retinal haemorrhages. The pathologist has to be knowledgeable to all other causes of disease, such as coagulation defects in cases of bruising, and a wide variety of conditions, particularly those relating to the bone or collagenous tissues, if the child appears merely to be failing to thrive.

In dealing with living patients the problems of teamwork between hospitals and doctors, social workers and police and of the medico-legist is essential, and precipitate unilateral action is to be condemned. Aetiology plays an essential part in the investigation and diagnosis of the Battered Child Syndrome, as it does in fact in all cases of sudden infant death. In radiological examination the radiologist should be able to state that not only are certain skeletal injuries caused by child abuse, but that these injuries are caused in a certain way and are of a certain age. One's thought that an adult in a position of trust could be directly responsible for maltreating a child is so repugnant to natural feeling, that it does not come readily to mind. Despite published reports in the lay and medical press to clarify and to define the legal and medical social-issues associated with the Syndrome, some doctors, and police officers as well, still find it hard to accept the reality of wilful abuse of children. Possibly the hardest person to persuade is the social worker[3]. Cases that come to light are merely 'the tip of the iceberg'[4].

No-one wants to believe or even think that the ordinary young man or woman one passes in the street, or sits next to in the underground or bus, could, driven by some terrible impulse, swing their infant by the ankles and dash its head against the wall or furniture; shake or jump on his or her chest until the ribs are crushed, the diaphragm torn, or the liver and intestines ruptured; or burn or knock the infant into a state of unconsciousness, and death. According to Kempe[5] every parent is a potential 'baby basher'. There can be few who at one time or another have not been exasperated beyond endurance by the behaviour of their children[6]. A pathologist who is called to see a child who has died as a result of an injury, particularly under the age of four, must always consider the diagnosis of the 'battered child', until the case is proved otherwise. Nevertheless, he should not on the slightest provocation start 'a witch hunt', for accidents do happen.

No other entity better illustrates the need for a comprehensive approach to the investigation of unnatural death than that of child maltreatment and no other calls for better 'teamwork'. No matter how straightforward the findings may appear initially, or how elaborate and complete the confession, during the gathering of all the documentary evidence at the time of the preliminary investigation, one should proceed according to an orderly pattern. An initial confession to 'baby battering' may well be thrown out or some subsequent findings in the investigation may well reverse the hypothesis which had been evolved at the initial investigation.

The absence of overt trauma on the exterior of the body should in no instance be considered a contra-indication for a full autopsy in a dead child, since it often bears no relationship to the trauma on the interior of the body. One should initially inspect the body carefully to note the nature of the clothing, the degree of its cleanliness and its state of repair or disrepair. This should be noted, together with the general external characteristics, including height, weight, state of nutrition (including any suggestion of apparent selective nutritional deficiency). Any discrepancy no matter how subtle – such as disparity between the distribution of the hypostasis and the alleged terminal position of the body; taking the body temperature and the alleged final care by the parents; or between the obvious state of nutrition and/or the well-being of the infant or child; and the alleged concern of the parents – should be carefully followed up. Photographs, with careful drawings or sketches and, in some cases, even tracing (such as in teeth marks) may afford an opportunity to reach a conclusion concerning the nature of the weapon used to inflict the wounds that are found. These may be of considerable help in the subsequent investigation. Each wound should be specifically topographically located on the body with reference to known anatomical landmarks. One must remember, however, that the umbilicus and the nipples vary regarding the position of the body. Measurements should be taken from a fixed point, namely from the heel and from the mid-line of the body in cases of autopsy, routine histological examination should be carried out on every organ in all cases and, particularly, the eyes.

Recent contributions to the literature point out the importance, in addition, of a general toxicological examination to rule out the introduction of noxious poisons or overdosage of therapeutic agents. The toxicological assay should be qualitative as well as quantitative and should be as comprehensive as the scope of the toxicological laboratory will allow. Naturally, this in part will depend on a degree or level of suspicion of the pathologist.

ASSAY OF INJURIES

In cases of subdural haemorrhage, with or without fractured skull, and injuries within the abdomen, such as rupture of the liver, or bruising of the intestines or mesentery, the diagnosis cannot be confused. However denial of any accident or explanations by the parents, such as (1) he bumped his head against the cot, (2) he bruises easily, (3) he fell down stairs, (4) he fell off the bed, (5) the swing hit him in the tummy, are frequently made. On many occasions the injuries all speak for themselves, either by their nature or pattern. In other words, the mechanism of a fracture may be capable of interpretation. Injury of the mucosa of the upper lip, seen in numerous cases, is almost diagnostic or pathognomonic of the condition. Care must always be taken in interpreting the presence of bruising, but finger-tip type bruises are always highly suggestive and one cannot take too many photographs during an autopsy because frequently one cannot go back and re-photograph.

Following an autopsy on an alleged 'battered child' one must remember, on completion of the examination, particularly after a period of, say, some twelve to twenty-four hours refrigeration, it is of value to re-examine the exterior of the child's body for, frequently, with progressing blanching of the skin, clearer demarcation of surface bruises of the skin surface can be revealed and even patterned injuries not noted on earlier examination may have become more apparent. One may fail to see bruising externally on the scalp, yet at autopsy, on reflection of the scalp, deep bruising is often detected. The limbs frequently show 'finger-tip' type bruising; commonly grouped around the elbows and knees, due to gripping of the child in order to shake or pull him or her, or to hurl him or her into his or her cot or against furniture, while more diffuse bruising may be due to blows or impacts by or against a flat surface. Bruising of the chest and trunk may be due to blows, whilst severe bruising of the abdomen is often minimal, in spite of a severe intra-abdominal injury, due to the laxity of the abdominal muscles. It is often difficult, due to shock and peripheral vascular failure, to age bruises with accuracy, and this is one advantage of using colour photography, where one can leave it for the court to decide the age of the bruising. Recently it has been shown that there has been an increasing incidence of bite-marks[7]. Radiological examination should exclude conditions in a differential diagnosis, including rickets, congenital syphilis, osteogenesis imperfecta and various other bony abnormalities which have been described elsewhere.

Analysis of the fatal injuries show predominantly that they are associated with the head or, as an alternative, with a ruptured liver. If proper objective consideration is given to this pattern, the terminal injuries are nearly always seen to be a subdural haemorrhage, with or without a fractured skull and, at the same time in many cases, compression of the chest with fractured ribs and ruptured viscera. The commonest cause of infantile subdural haemorrhage[8] is rupture of one or more of the delicate bridging veins which run from the cerebral cortex to the venous sinuses, the mode of injury being either a single acceleration or deceleration due to a heavy moving object striking the head, or the rapidly moving head being brought up against a stationary mass; multiple applications of force would increase the total strain on the bridging veins and might result in an increase in the incidence of rupture. Subdural haematoma is one of the commonest features of the 'Battered Child Syndrome' – seen in approximately 40% of cases – yet by no means all the patients so affected have external marks of injury to the head, suggesting that the child might well have been shaken, rather than struck. In such cases ophthalmic damage is far more common. Rupture of the liver and abdominal viscera with tearing of the mesentery is seen, but external bruising of the abdominal wall is not necessarily present – a reminder that a diffuse blow to the relaxed abdomen may cause severe internal injury and yet leave no mark. Explanation for the high incidence of visceral injury near a relatively fixed point in the abdomen has been offered by Haller[9] who distinguished the cause of blunt abdominal injury by the mechanism of the injury. He noted that crushing or compressing forces produced bursting injuries of the liver or spleen or they may cause perforation of distended hollow viscus, such as the stomach, intestine or bladder. Intestinal injuries are usually on the antemesenteric surface[1]. A deceleration force, such as a punch or blow, tears the mesentery and may rupture the small intestine at sites of the ligamental support. The galaxy of visceral injuries in fatally battered children fits the latter category[10]. The possibility of visceral injuries from apparent blunt trauma should be eliminated in any child with abdominal complaints who has characteristic bruising, whether or not skeletal fractures or head injury are present. Increasing observation of permanent impairment of vision affecting one or both eyes in cases of subsequently proven battered children reminds one that at autopsy one should remove the eyes for ophthalmic pathological opinion.

THE AUTOPSY

As in all medico-legal cases, photography is essential and photographs should be taken at all stages in the investigation of a suspected battered child, at the request of and under the direction of, the pathologist. Obviously, the first object is to have a photograph of both the front and the back of the child and of the facial views in case one has to damage any of the facial features subsequently. The body, having been identified by the relatives, can then be subjected to the necessary examinations as are required in all child deaths. A full antero–posterior skeletal radiological survey and a lateral view of the skull must be taken, realizing the fact that a negative radiograph of the chest need not necessarily mean that there are no fractures, either old or recent, of the rib cage. Using a diagram to assist as an *aide memoire*, the bruises and injuries, as seen externally, are noted and recorded, taking the heel and the mid-line as the fixed points of the body. Marks that resemble bite-marks should be treated as an actual bite-mark, namely a swab should be taken to test for secretor status in case the assailant is not related to the deceased[11]. Petechial haemorrhages must be looked for in the conjunctivae and externally on the face, in case there has been a constrictive element in the cause of death. After all the injuries and bruises have been noted externally and the body has been skeletally surveyed radiologically, the internal examination can commence, provided that any marks resembling those caused by human dentition have been examined by a forensic odontologist before dissection. It is of minimal value for a forensic odontologist to examine any mark resembling human dentition after any incision has been made, because such an incision might reduce the elasticity of the skin and alter the shape of the 'bite-mark'. Any unusual mark should be photographed with a scale, particularly those resembling bite-marks, which can be blown up to a 1 to 1 scale, in order that a forensic odontologist might compare it with casts of the teeth of the potential assailants.

Swabs should be taken of every orifice, as if it were a case of a sexual assault, to exclude the possibility of necrophilia or a sexual element in the cause of death. In the United Kingdom the usual Y-shaped incision from both ears to the top of the sternum should be used, extending down the mid-line to the pubis. Next, the ear to ear incision must be used for the removal of the vault of the cranium. When one reflects the skin of the scalp one can note whether there are any subaponeurotic haemorrhages, to exclude the element of asphyxia or deep bruises. Thereafter, even though the child might be under three months a saw-cut should be made around the head to remove the vault of the skull, contrary to the usual practice of incising down the suture lines. This excludes the possibility of any fractures that might have extended into the suture lines. On removal of the skull vault, if necessity arises, namely by the presence of a subdural haemorrhage or subarachnoid haemorrhage, further photographs should be taken. The brain should be removed and retained for fixation and subsequent examination. It is the writer's belief that it is far wiser to examine a 'dry' brain than a 'wet' brain.

The incisions, i.e. head and body post-mortem incisions, having met, it is relatively easy to reflect the skin of the face over to the point of the nose, thus exposing not only the angle of the jaw, the upper and lower jaw, the sublingual region, the supraclavicular region, but also around the orbit and the bridge of the nose. This makes it considerably easier to enucleate the eyes. The eyes should then be sent, after fixation, for ophthalmological pathological opinion. Such a manoeuvre can be done without defacing the face because most mortuary superintendents can correct such defects by their training and technique. The rib cage is opened by using a scalpel and by dissecting through the sterno-clavicular joint, where it can be disarticulated, thus freeing the clavicles from the rib cage, and retaining them within the skeleton.

Using the classical Rockitansky post-mortem techniques, the organs are removed *in toto* and observation can be made as to whether there is free blood or fluid, pus, or stomach contents present in the thoracic cavities or in the abdominal cavity and as to whether the diaphragm is ruptured or not. Should there be any fractures of the ribs, this should be noted. After total evisceration of the body, if any evidence of fractures of the ribs is detected macroscopically although not radiologically, the rib cage should be dissected by cutting through the intravertebral disc between the twelfth thoracic and first lumbar vertebra and between the sixth and seventh cervical vertebra and, by cutting round the body next to the skin, one can remove the rib cage intact, leaving the skin whole. The rib cage can then be X-rayed in at least three dimensions in order to visualize and confirm any fractures[1]. Such fractures should be subjected to histological examination as well as to this radiological examination, in order to age them. Histological sections must naturally be taken of all the thoracic organs. By this manoeuvre of the reflection of the skin of the face, one incorporates reflection of the 'V' of the neck, over the chin cutting through the mucosal membranes of the lips at the edges and thus exposing the inner aspect of the lips, to see whether there is any bruising of the lips following a blow or blows to the face impinging the gums against the teeth and also to see whether there are underlying bruises of the chin. It also makes removal of the tongue more easy and exposure of the neck more readily available and, in addition, samples of blood can be taken from the vessels in the neck. It is the writer's preference to take all his samples from the right side of the body, working from that side. Samples of blood should be taken as they might later prove to be of value in cases of alleged disputed paternity. Disputed paternity might well prove the exclusion of an individual from being a potential assailant.

As far as the abdominal cavity is concerned, it is very difficult to offer advice as to what should be done when there is a ruptured mesentery or ruptured intra-abdominal viscera. It is the writer's experience that it is wiser to fix the abdominal cavities *in toto* for subsequent examination should there be any possibility or question as to any ruptured viscera or mesentery. Otherwise, the organs are dissected in a normal manner, as described in any normal pathology textbook. Naturally, samples of liver blood, bile and stomach contents and the usual samples for any medico-legal autopsy are taken at the appropriate time. Should, however, there be a fracture of a limb, of which one feels, as a result of one's examination, it would be advantageous to know its age, one should remove that limb, i.e. the skeletal and muscular attachments thereof, leaving the skin to be reconstructed by the mortuary superintendent/technician, for radiological and histological examination. Whilst one realizes that such a technique is radical, one can never be challenged with being negligent in one's approach nor can the fairness of one's report and the availability of specimens (as retained in England and Wales under the Coroners' Rules 1963) be questioned. Naturally, this technique must be modified for every country in which autopsies are requested by law to be carried out in cases of alleged child abuse. By and large the technique which one does carry out in such cases can prove a guilty case. If there is any doubt, it is the duty of the forensic pathologist, or medico-legist, to give the benefit of the doubt to the accused, remembering that the autopsy room is the Temple of Truth.

References

1. Cameron, J. M. and Rae, L. J. (1975). *Atlas of the Battered Child Syndrome*. (Edinburgh and London: Churchill Livingstone)
2. Kempe, C. H., Silverman, F. N., Steele, B. F., Droegenuelleur, W. M. and Silver, H. K. (1962). *J. Am. Med. Assoc.*, **181**, 17
3. Cameron, J. M. (1977). Unpublished data.
4. Simpson, C. K. (1965). *The Battered Child Syndrome*. (London: NSPCC)
5. Kempe, C. H. (1970). Unpublished data
6. Fleming, G. M. (1967). *Br. Med. J.*, **2**, 421
7. Sims, B. G., Grant, J. H. and Cameron, J. M. (1973). *Medicine, Science and the Law*, **13**, 207
8. Guthkelch, A. N. (1971). *Br. Med. J.*, **1**, 430
9. Haller, J. A., Jr. (1966). *Clin. Pediat. (Phila.)*, **5**, 476
10. Touloukian, R. J. (1968). *Pediatrics*, **42**, 642
11. Cameron, J. M. and Sims, B. G. (1976). *Forensic Dentistry* (Edinburgh and London: Churchill Livingstone)

4 Management of the problem

A. WHITE FRANKLIN

The contents of this book demonstrate clearly the complexities of the problems presented by child abuse even to the reader who lacks practical experience. If consideration be limited to the action required when babies and children are physically battered, what remains involves a wide range of human activities. The attempt even to outline plans for general management of battered children demands of the planner not only vaulting ambition, but also unreal optimism. The injuries represent a final common path for so many and such different circumstances. Yet action is required, even urgent action and in the light of experience already gained, theoretical objectives can be described and possible methods for attaining these objectives. How far the practical application of these methods is likely to attain objectives in real life can then be discussed.

The broad objectives of management are two-fold. First, babies and children must be protected from physical injury. Secondly, the family must be rehabilitated whenever this is a practical possibility. No-one should dispute these general propositions but it must be confessed that as they stand, they are open to considerable misunderstanding and their influence over the conduct of professional workers is not and has not been uniformly good. Once non-accidental injury is known to have occurred, the protection of the child from further injury is an absolute priority. The repeated injuries produced in small babies may rapidly increase in severity and early in life a sub-dural bleed or the shaking injury to the eyes may leave the baby brain-damaged, blind, mentally handicapped and paralysed. Therefore, to await non-accidental injury is not enough. Management of the battering situation which begins after the diagnostic injury has been inflicted is not a sufficient protection so that one attaches prime importance to prediction of vulnerable families and preventive support. The special methods of prediction and prevention are not included in this discussion of general management as interpreted in this chapter, which limits itself chiefly to the management of the diagnosed rather than of the vulnerable family.

As to family rehabilitation, serious criticisms exist. Firstly, all workers agree that for a small proportion of families with profound psychiatric disturbances, no form of treatment yet practised can make these adults safe to take responsibility for the care of children. Once recognized they need to be divorced immediately from their children and ideally prevented from producing any more. There is further criticism. The crises of injury may come to an end but leave behind relationships so poor or so damaged that the baby who was physically injured lives through his early years emotionally deprived. This means that the prevention of further physical injury, a priority important though it is, is not enough. The argument cannot be allowed to rest even there, because the next question that must be answered is, would the child have suffered less if removed from the care of his biological parents? What is in issue is not the old and (hopefully) discarded concept of the blood tie, but the certainty that the care and love in the alternative environment will be good enough and acceptable enough by him to provide the growing and developing child with the caring relationship that he needs but which, in the opinion of some person or persons, he cannot be given by his own parents. Experience shows that the possibilities of rehabilitation of parents are not always correctly measured. Underestimates as well as the overestimates which attract public notice can be equally tragic.

A third general objective is to encourage all the professional workers to cooperate. The professions likely to be involved are many and various. The basic work usually falls to the lot of the social worker employed by the local health authority with responsibilities that include preparing reports at the stage of diagnosis, playing an important part in the conference that plans management and having the responsibility for surveillance and for giving practical advice and help. To these may be added preparing reports for the courts, appearing in court, making assessments of progress and deciding on the success or failure of the plans. This is indeed a formidable assignment. The probation officer sometimes is entrusted with much of this work, especially when the family or one of its members is or has recently been, on probation. The National Society for the Protection of Children and the Children's Aid Society have also an important part to play, acting in much the same way as the social worker.

Six other professions are frequently involved.

The first in time may be the *health visitor* who should in theory be a welcomed friend to all the families in her area with the routine duty of visiting the home after the arrival of the new baby and having the opportunity of regular supervision in the Child Health Clinic or at the office of the general practitioner to whose practice she may be attached. For a shorter period the *midwife* has care of the mother with opportunities to observe, especially the earlier interactions between mother and baby. She has also a profound influence on the mother's perinatal welfare, welfare both of mind and body.

The *medical profession* has taken a leading part in the elucidation of these problems and it has been only by following a medical model that the information has been collected that has made generally acceptable the present idea that non-accidental injury is caused by an adult responsible for the care of the child. For this reason the doctor is not yet able to see his duty as only repairing the damage and assisting in the making of the diagnosis. His sense of responsibility for his patient carries him on into management and surveillance. The family practitioner may become suspicious or, with physical injury occurring in an urban population, it is more likely to be the doctor in the accident and emergency department of the hospital. He may be an 'accident' surgeon or physician, or a paediatrician. Sometimes an orthopaedic surgeon is in charge of the department or is invited to supervise the fractures. In other cases, the child with a head injury is brought to a neurosurgeon or with an eye injury to an ophthalmologist. All of these doctors must be sensitized to the possibility of non-accidental injury and abuse.

Besides doctors and those who work alongside doctors – and mention should be made of hospital nurses – three professions with no direct involvement in medical matters are also concerned. The first in time may be the *police*. The family may have become known to the police through anti-social behaviour, including being drunk and disorderly, causing grievous bodily harm or causing an affray. The reason for this is the connection between aggressive behaviour and non-accidental injury. Or it could be that the police are called to a dead child. As will be seen, the question of police involvement in general management does not follow a universally accepted pattern in the United Kingdom or in North America.

The *legal profession* and the law are concerned with child neglect as well as with criminal assault. This brings in the magistrate and the clerk to the magistrates court, who is sometimes a key figure, together with solicitors, barristers, and even Judges when crown court or the Ward of Court procedures become involved.

Finally in the *educational service* the school teacher assisted by the education welfare officer and the school doctor has the opportunity to observe the child and to note injuries, general hygiene, educational progress, school absence and, when necessary, growth and general health.

This long list has been detailed because when the plea is made for co-operation, coupled usually with advice about mutual trust and the sharing of information, the plea is being made to a large number of individuals. When the scene is thus surveyed, the tendency towards difficulties in communication can be more readily understood.

In considering general management, some attention must also be paid to the influence of the public as exercised both in an individual capacity and also collectively through the media. This influence reaches its peak during enquiries into the tragic histories of children who have died. Nothing can more effectively destroy confidence, weaken resolve and warp judgement than the worker's realization that fixed upon him is the public eye with its compulsion for and delight in identifying a scapegoat. The revelation that certain members of the public have made their own diagnosis and often informed against the abusing families, seemingly without effect, illustrates the need for improvements in relationships between the social workers, who usually become the scapegoats because they have a statutory duty of protection, and the public on whose behalf they seek to discharge these obligations. It can be reasonably claimed that while in the final analysis the fault lies with the parents, responsibility for failure to prevent the tragedies must be shared between a number of people in more than one profession, most of whom did at one time or another miss the opportunity to help the family to avoid the catastrophe. This assumes that prevention is always a practical possibility. Those most closely concerned with these families realize that this is not so. While every effort must be made to prevent child abuse, the public would be wrong to expect total success and to insist that when tragedies do occur blame can be affixed to some one person.

The broad strategy outlined above has led to many tactical recommendations. In the United Kingdom the Department of Health and Social Security has accepted the responsibility for laying down plans in considerable detail for the commanders in the field although, with the usual expected modest courtesy, recognizing the rights of the troops in the field to make their own modifications. These plans may be found in many publications by the Department itself[1], by the Tunbridge Wells Study Group[2], by the British Paediatric Association with the British Association of Paediatric Surgeons incorporating the Newcastle recommendations on management[3] and in many documents issued by Health Areas. It is not proposed here to repeat these recommendations but simply to make some general comments about their virtues and their faults as revealed by time and experience. Planning is one thing, practice another.

As a principle, everyone accepts the wisdom of the admission to hospital of any child about whom the suspicion of battering arises. The obvious advantage for the child is to remove it from a potentially dangerous environment. At the same time the necessary thorough investigation of the child becomes easy, not only for the exclusion of bone disease by radiological study or of some coagulation defect or of any defect of growth (height and weight), but also for the recognition of previous injuries and for an assessment of mental development and of emotional reactions. The value of a psychiatric assessment of the parents, mentioned in other chapters, is clear. There is time also for the hospital social worker to gather information about the family and the home. At this point an exchange of information should take place between all those with direct knowledge of the family including its past history and the way in which it has been developing. This preliminary case conference should be exploratory but because the child's admission is frequently part of a family crisis, contingency plans should be agreed and one person should be given authority to take any necessary action.

The index of suspicion has become very high. This inevitably causes loving parents to be somewhat apprehensive about reporting accidents to their young children and it also will probably produce a backlash so that social workers as well as doctors will find increasing difficulty in translating suspicion into action. As regards the knowledge that the family of a bruised baby contains a coagulation defect or the collagen defect of brittle bone disorder will complicate decision-making still further. No reason exists why a baby with any of these defects should not be deprived, abused or battered. The presence of such a defect will make it harder to persuade the court that the abused child is in need of care and protection. The background to suspicion has been delineated in earlier chapters. Not only the character of the injuries observed but the occurrence of sudden infant death, of poisoning and of growth failure with or without the possibility of malabsorption must be observed by clinicians with child abuse in mind.

The practical difficulty of the expenditure of time has arisen in connection with the case conference. Variations exist as to the numbers of persons to be notified of these conferences and the advantages of spreading the net wide are great in theory. In practice, the initial exploratory case conference should be limited to those immediately and personally in touch with the family and it could be sufficient for only two individuals to meet provided that they belonged to different professions and could get further information by telephone. One difficulty with social workers derives from their hierarchical system of work under which the hands of the field workers who have actually seen the clients are tied to the supervisor who has not. This relationship has not previously existed for the medical or hospital social worker and it is to be hoped that social work in connection with child abuse will in time be carried out by a worker of experience who is entrusted with the power to make decisions rather than by a sort of apprentice worker not permitted discretion[4]. The case conference must not be allowed to degenerate into a technique for shirking responsibility for decision.

The main disadvantages of the large, comprehensive case conference are that the finding of a time convenient for all is difficult and that the conference becomes a meeting, often a loquacious one, rather than an informed conversation. However in most cases, one such comprehensive conference is necessary when diagnosis is clearer and long-term treatment plans need to be settled. When plans need to be changed and at critical stages in the progress of the case, the case conference should be re-convened.

One of the main outstanding management problems concerns police participation. In England and Wales it is the police who make the decision whether to prosecute. Similar practices exist in other countries. They have the general responsibility for the protection of life and for the prevention, and the investigation as well as for the prosecutions, of crime. Police professionalism is as important to each officer as is medical professionalism to a doctor. He feels the need to make his investigation with the minimum of delay, while the scent is warm, if not hot, and before collusion can develop between parties. In the event of criminal proceedings his failure to have found evidence may be exposed in court with a consequent ill-effect upon his professional career. In ideal circumstances the police priorities would coincide with the priorities of doctors and social workers in regard both to the protection of the child and the rehabilitation of the family, and police would share with them also their mutual trust and readiness for open communication. Some families need to be handled by police but in other families the introduction of police may adversely affect the chances of rehabilitation.

An important area of difficulty is with the exploratory case conference and crises arise when, in the course of initial enquiries over suspicious injuries, the police, given the information that a family is under suspicion, are instructed to take unilateral action with a view to criminal proceedings. Improved relationships would certainly follow if the chief officer of police concerned always took seriously the views held by other members of case conferences about the need to prosecute, although everyone accepts that this decision rests by law with the police. Sharing of knowledge with the police should quickly show them that the seriousness of the case cannot always be judged by the extent or the severity of the injuries. The torn frenulum of the tongue or the finger mark bruises on the baby's face or trunk may be swiftly followed by the fatal injury. And sometimes the police have information of the greatest relevance from the past history of the family and its members. Better understanding and working co-operation between police and the other members of the team should eventually lead to the ideal arrangement under which the police are automatically kept in the picture.

The definitive case conference will often need the help of the psychiatrist. The contribution made by psychiatrically disturbed adults to child abuse is discussed in other chapters. The difficulty for the other professionals and even more for the courts is in the nature of the psychiatric information provided. Although tending to react to life's challenges by communicating through violence, the abusing parent may be entirely normal until and unless he has to function as a parent. And the only evidence of abnormality may be his failure in this respect. Whether he has himself suffered from the effects of a deprived childhood or poor or absent opportunities for bonding in his early life, he may still be able to cope with parenthood. Having killed one child, perhaps because that child failed to give the response to his parenting that he demanded or needed, he may be perfectly safe to care for other children in his family.

What to do when one child has been killed and another is born presents this problem in an acute form. Should this new baby be allowed home or should the attempt be made to take him into care on the grounds of previous parental behaviour? The only safe answer would seem to be a period of residential care for the family under observation. If the new baby is taken into care this is a serious emotional deprivation for the baby ordered by the law, unless by visiting and contributing to the baby's management, the mother and baby have the opportunity to grow together. Without this arrangement, the baby's welfare would demand placement at once with long-term foster-parents or adoption, but such plans are seldom practicable. If the child is never to return to its natural parents, their visits, especially if infrequent, may have devastating effects on both the child and the foster-parents. No general answer can be given. All too often, the child remains for many months in a nursery in which relationships are inevitably fragmented. It would be some contribution if all those implicated in making the decision, including the courts, and the solicitors, were fully aware of what was at stake.

The Department of Health and Social Security has recommended a two-tier system of management with an Area Review Committee in addition to the case conferences, suggesting in detail both membership and functions. The Department has requested Area Health Authorities to form widely based Area Review Committees including general practitioners, police and probation services as 'policy making' bodies.

This large committee has the task of modifying general policy to suit its own area needs, and many delegate their authority to districts and as occasions arise form sub-committees to review special subjects. The review committee should acquaint itself with the number and the distribution of cases but should not act in any sense as a case conference. One of the main functions in these early years should be to survey available resources of hospital facilities and of personnel so as to draw attention to any weakness in the system. Ultimately such a review committee could widen its vision to include the general surveillance of the services for all children who are deprived of a normal family life including those in long-stay hospitals. Such activities could greatly assist Social Services Departments in the discharge of their statutory duties and, of course, the closest possible co-operation should exist with these Departments as well as with the Accident and Emergency Departments. Battered children have naturally taken the limelight, but they are far from being the only deprived or damaged children in our society.

Accident and Emergency Departments, especially for urban populations, are first ports of call for a great number of battered, burnt or poisoned children. Much remains to be done to bring them up to a standard of excellence. Meanwhile the abused child is liable to be lost or at least mislaid among the multifarious clients. What is often lacking is consistency of personnel and at present there are still staff members with language problems. Some errors may be avoided by regulations about summoning paediatric staff to review the stories of all babies, infants and toddlers if not of all children, and illustrative charts on the walls of the doctor's office could show the kinds of injury which should arouse suspicion to replace these coloured posters of the rashes of what were once commonly occurring acute specific fevers with their incubation and isolation periods. It could do nothing but good if the Area Review Committee were expected to study current methods of handling children in these departments.

One function that is already 'officially' accepted is the establishment and maintenance of a register either by the Area Health Authority or the Social Services Department. The United Kingdom has at present no general reporting law, unlike the USA and Canada, but uses instead local registers which are regarded as confidential with access to information strictly limited. A minimum requirement has been outlined together with recommended methods of procedure by the Department of Health and Social Security[5]. The best methods by which families enter and leave the register have yet to be decided. As a link in the chain of communication, the register undoubtedly has an important function. The final justification for the trouble and the expense of maintaining registers comes when they can be shown to have significantly aided prevention.

All these policy-making procedures and plans are of value only to the extent in which they may be put into practice. On what data are the decisions to be made about individual patients and who is to make them? And do facilities exist for operating the decisions? Above all what help and support can the families be given? Public and professional awareness have been increased to a high degree, the index of suspicion has been raised, yet still abuse and battering, maiming and death continue. As regards the public, the movement of opinion has been away from disbelief that adults could purposely seek to destroy or damage children in their care, towards some alarm at the apparent frequency with which this does happen. Now there is a swing back of the pendulum to the feeling that the whole thing has been exaggerated. Such mass reactions do affect individual workers. Given the manipulative skills of the offenders, subjective judgement can easily be wrong. The importance of objective studies is thereby increased.

Once the suspected case has reached hospital for full assessment, he is temporarily safe and the investigation of the family, physical, social, psychological and behavioural, should lead to the correct diagnosis. The practical application of the treatment and management plans may be prevented because the parents refuse to co-operate and this refusal may be supported by the court's decision if legal action is taken. The legal framework is described in other chapters of this book. Given that co-operation by the parents or the legal decision allows the plans laid by the case conference to be put into effect, the next problem is surveillance with a crisis of decision when parents seek a change through revocation of a care order or when the conference decides to return the child to its parents. The same two difficult problems present themselves just as they did at the outset, the safety of the child and the rehabilitation of the parents.

How has the child fared, has the plan succeeded as far as the child's progress is concerned? The protection of the child from repeated battering and from physical injury is the easiest measure of success. But what also needs to be assessed is the growth of the child, firstly in physical size as measured by height and weight records over the period. Insufficient attention has in the past been paid to these measurements which are good indicators of total health. Failure to grow can point to emotional deprivation and emotional deprivation in turn can slow up or halt intellectual development. If the protection of the child is in reality the priority, these objective assessments should be made the basis on which success or failure of the management plan can be judged. Nature has provided the human body with a more efficient power to heal broken bones and bruises than to heal the effects of emotional deprivation.

The assessment of growth, of intellectual development and of emotional and social adjustment is now possible and should replace, or at least supplement at times of important decision making, the interview with the parents or guardian of the child, the 'intuitive feeling' of the worker and the look round the house for the presence of adequate clothes, bedding and toys and for evidence of satisfactory hygiene. The most deprived and miserable child can sometimes smile and play happily and can even seek, in the presence of an intruder, the safety of the abusing mother's arms or skirts. As to the mother's love for her child, everyone knows what a variety of meanings is possessed by these four letters. Certainly if love describes a wanting and a needing of another person, the immature young mother, cohabiting without security and lacking a mother to whom she herself can turn for support, may love her baby but still seek to destroy it because it cannot play the role which she has demanded.

This raises the second question of how far, in the period of surveillance, have the parents become safe for the child? Much depends on the causes of the original breakdown. Were it puerperal depression or some other critical influence the margin of safety should be greater than if it were a chronic inability to cope with life. The prospect for the parent who feels that he or she might injure the child differs greatly from that of the psychopath who is compelled to act violently and cruelly. In management decisions a knowledge of all the members of the family is essential including all sorts and conditions of consorts, legal or not, transient, occasional or more or less permanent. Men are at least as likely to damage children as women. Without such data, knowledge of the family is dangerously incomplete.

The current publicity about child abuse, inevitable as a first stage in the modern approach to management, has had its effect on the family as well as on the workers. A syndrome has been constructed, the battered child syndrome, with its diagnostic clinical, radiological, psychological and social elements. The temptation is to fill in gaps by analogy and by a trick of the mind to add to actual observations, extrapolations from general experience based on other patients. This is unjust to the client and may be dangerously misleading when the actual results or sequels of treatment programmes are being compared with some 'expected' prognosis.

From the point of view of the family, there is no battering family syndrome but the knowledge that such a label as 'the battered child' exists has its own effect on family attitudes and possibly actions. Natural feelings of exasperation common to all parents take on a sinister significance particularly for a parent not completely secure. 'Does this mean that I am a batterer?' is the question that arises and there follows, besides self-condemnation, a request for urgent re-housing or termination of pregnancy wrongly based, yet honest. Much information is being collected about the determinants of battering and of the means through which parental attitudes towards child bearing and children are engendered. While the main purpose of these insights is preventive, use can be made of them in treatment and management by illuminating the true nature of the parental dilemma. It is therefore of great importance that good research methods should be employed in gathering and collating data. In the end, each family is unique like each human being, and the problems of every family must be handled as if it were a special case.

It follows that whatever arrangements are made must be flexible. It also follows that they must be elaborate, if the safety of the abused child is to be assured within its family. The nature of the task is supportive and preventive. Since no-one can predict the timing of a family crisis, support has to be on a continuous twenty-four hours a day basis. This makes great demands on those providing the service.

The list of services now considered necessary has grown with experience, much of it based on the Denver practice developed by Kempe and his co-workers[6] and on the work of Ounstead in the Park Hospital, Oxford[7]. Local conditions, such as geography and population density, impose their own modifications.

The first essential is for the family to have some outside human being in rapport, with sympathy for and understanding of the family's real problems. Someone should be at the far end of what has come to be called the 'crisis hotline'. This part is usually to be played by a social services department, a probation officer or a specially trained NSPCC or CAS officer. For some families with insuperable difficulty in forming any true relationship with an 'official' worker, a lay worker can provide the answer. Such a person must be more than a volunteer who professes a compassionate interest. The experience of the Samaritans on selection from volunteers, the methods of their education and enlightenment as to the nature of the work and their apprenticeship could well be tapped if in any locality a volunteer lay helping agency seemed both appropriate and available. Some such preparation might well also be wise even for the trained social worker. A generic training in social work or a university degree in sociology does not necessarily produce a person with the aptitude, the attitude or the skill to provide the help which abusing families need. Whoever does take on the duty of support for the family will in turn require considerable support from and consultation with other workers. Involvement is a prerequisite for success. Judgement becomes increasingly difficult as involvement with the family deepens.

To answer the cry for help in the crisis may be enough, but for some families, or at some times, escape from the immediacy of the problem may demand respite from the unaided caring for the child. A crisis nursery may provide the answer but only if it is available on a twenty-four hours a day basis. For other families, especially with a young baby, the best prospects come from residential family treatment. Here, under supervision, the sense of isolation relieved, the responsibility for the care of the child now shared, the parents' emotional tension relaxed, the situation may come under control. For yet other families a therapeutic day centre may suffice. In such centres as these, troubled parents may find themselves able to help each other.

Apart from the case-work support, the crisis hotline, the opportunities for relief from the immediate responsibility referred to above, the parents may benefit from advice about child management and especially about what may and what may not be expected of their child's behaviour. They may also need education in what may and what may not be expected of the consort's behaviour and how to perform successfully the differing and sometimes antagonistic roles of parent and consort. Marriage guidance and parent guidance may need to be supplemented by psychotherapy and this may be on an individual or a group basis.

All of these techniques are aimed directly at the parents or the responsible adults, but the needs of the children cannot be overlooked. Some of the most serious cases concern the man who is neither husband nor consort but a transient visitor who is not the father of the child. That the child can, through its behaviour, provide a challenge to abuse from the adult is generally believed, and in these circumstances this may be relevant. There may be inordinate crying by the baby or relentless crying at inconvenient times, such as while the adults are engaged in sexual intercourse. A more subtle challenge may make the mother feel inadequate, a failure, or that the baby does not return her love. The mother expresses her frustration and anger through violent action. As the child gets older, failure to become clean and dry, or the inconvenience in the home of the child's normal exploring and occupational needs may lead to chronic or recurring battles. Play school or play therapy can provide solutions and sometimes in addition the child needs individual psychotherapy.

To provide all this, if it be accepted as necessary, makes very large demands on people and money. Add to this the expectation that some of the most serious problems arise in families that are not accessible to help, and the inevitable question is, is this the best or indeed the only way to approach the problem? The answer must at present be yes. By these means, improvement follows, the risk of re-battering diminishes and successful family life becomes once more possible. This is the immediate answer. The long term answer brings society face to face with general problems of much wider significance. These range from the nature and causes of violence and aggression, current attitudes and practices that promote or hinder stable family life, the importance attached to good parenting as an essential for the health of the child, apart from the less mysterious problems of adequate housing and income and the abuse of drugs including alcohol, which are easier to recognize but equally difficult to solve.

The identification of vulnerable families and their support is only a beginning. This constitutes secondary prevention. Primary prevention means ensuring that grand-parents provide good parenting, without which parents come into the vulnerable group. What has been undertaken in this chapter is a discussion of tertiary prevention, of how to help when circumstances have already revealed the presence of child abuse.

References

1. DHSS, LASSL (74) 13; 27; (76) 2
2. Tunbridge Wells Study Group, Report and Resolutions (1973). (Obtainable from DHSS)
3. Non-accidental injury in children (1973). *Br. Med. J.*, **4,** 656
4. Children at risk – BASW's Code of practice, *Newsletter of the British Association of Social Workers*, 4 Sept. 1975, p. 346, para 8
5. DHSS, LASSL (76) 2
6. Kempe, C. H. and Helfer, R. E. (eds) (1972). *Helping the Battered Child and his Family*, (Philadelphia: J. B. Lippincott Co.)
7. Ounsted, C., Oppenheimer, R. and Lindsay, J. (1975). The psycho-pathology and psychotherapy of the families: aspects of bonding failure. In: *Concerning Child Abuse*. A. W. Franklin (ed.) (Edinburgh: Churchill Livingstone)

5   The Epidemiology of Child Abuse

J. E. OLIVER

Part I — HISTORICAL EPISODES, CULTURAL PATTERNS, AND BIOLOGICAL PRINCIPLES, IN RELATION TO THE VARIETIES AND PREVALENCE OF CRUEL PRACTICES TO CHILDREN

The 'Ascent of Man' required group co-operation in which the young were protected. Life expectancy was so short, and sub-human and pre-human young so vulnerable that adult individuals other than the parents must have protected them. Love of the young and protection of the helpless, argues Bronowski[1] must have been essential ingredients of human evolution. Social amity and group protection of the young are older primate characteristics in pre-human evolution than the ferocity of our immediate ancestors, the man-like (group hunting) apes[2].

Nevertheless, in historical times, massacres and other outrages were accepted against children. Moral authority was inveighed in the utter destruction of Jericho (the oldest city in the world). This destruction included the children who were slain by Joshua and his nomadic warriors[3]. Later in Bethlehem, there was no difficulty in King Herod exerting his authority in the selective killing of children under 2 years old[4]. As with Joshua, so with William the Conqueror in his extermination, homestead by homestead, of the entire population between York and Durham in 1069. 'The harrying of the North was a vengeance Turkish in its atrocity, but fully in accord with the ideas and practice of the most zealously Christian warriors in mediaeval Europe'[5]. During the reign of Queen Mary (1553–1558) some children were even burned at the stake[6]. In rural areas of Ireland 'changeling babies' (usually babies with congenital defects – but sometimes ugly, screaming or hungry normal babies) were sometimes roasted alive over fires, even in the twentieth century[7]. The ultimate in horror relates to the 'Well attested ... historical fact' of the fate of the family

95

of Sawney Bean. Sawney Bean was born in East Lothian in the reign of James First of Scotland. Incest, murder, disembowelling and cannibalism by Sawney and his descendants were followed by a judicial vengeance. Inhabitants of Scotland (who 'flocked to see this cursed tribe' as they were transported from Galloway to Edinburgh, thence to be executed at Leith) considered the ensuing a 'Just punishment'. The men were dismembered and allowed to bleed slowly to death. The women and 32 grandchildren, having been forced to watch the men die (for hours) were then 'burnt to death in several fires'[8].

The style of the following extract implies widespread child neglect in the sixteenth century (the description is of hypothermia). 'Sometyme it happeneth that the lymmes are starke, and can not well come together without the greater peyne, which thyng procedeth many times of cold, as when a chylde is found in the frost, or even in the strete, cast away by a wycked mother. . . [9].'

In my lifetime, the persecution of Jews in Hungary was described by Sir Winston Churchill in July 1944, as 'The greatest and most horrible crime ever committed in the history of the world'. It is hard to disagree with this, yet thousands of officials, German, Austrian and Hungarian took active part in procedures which condemned many hundreds of thousands of Jews. Jewish children of all ages were starved, deprived of medical care, deprived of fluids, cruelly confined or exposed, subjected to cold, and to forced marches, resulting in exhaustion or death, before they were exterminated[10].

The forced march from Budapest to Austria in 1944 contained children of all ages, many of whom died en route. In Nyiregyhaza 'Children of more than one year old had to march at the same pace as the others, and this was enforced with whips'. In a Budapest ghetto, 6000 children, aged 2–14 suffered as follows: 'Their bodies were eaten by filth and scabies, their rags were infested with lice. Huddled up in fear and infinite misery, they made inarticulate sounds. They had not eaten for days . . .[10]. Many outrages by the Nazis (1940–45) involved other children (not all Jewish) in other parts of Europe[11]. Very cruel rearing practices were also reported from Soviet Russian Labour Camps in the time of Stalin, together with a classical example of baby battering[12]. It might be argued that these examples of ruthless or pathological cruelty were disastrous social aberrations. Adolf Hitler, at the peak of the chain of command of the Nazis himself had been a battered child. He was beaten 'unmercifully' by his father and was consequently once 'left for dead' as a young child[13]. This fact, combined with historical chance unleashed the ensuing savagery.

The ensuing paragraphs are intended to show the willingness of whole cultures to accept practices towards children which we would condemn as cruel[14–17]. Examples are given of flogging (Sumerian, Greek, Roman, German, French, Indian, English and American cultures); abandonment and death by exposure (Roman, Greek, East European, and Egyptian cultures).

The English public appeared to accept child slave labour (with its attendant inhumanity) for much of the 18th and 19th centuries as did Americans in the

19th and early part of the 20th centuries. The following laconic resigned statement, from 9 year old Morgan Lewis, who worked at the Ironworks in Merthyr Tydfil (1841) gives his life from the age of 7. Morgan said 'I have been working here for two years. I used to work at the squeezing machine (rolling mill), straightening bars of iron. I work for 12 hours each day for one week, then 12 hours a night for the next week. The work is very hard and I get tired, but my dinner gives me strength for I share my father's meat. Sometimes I get burned at the furnace'. Young Morgan earned 70 pence a month. He went on to say, 'When I get home from work I play about the road, and mother makes me wash myself before she lets me get into bed. Sometimes I get the stripes (beaten) for playing about'[18].

Trevelyan recognizes that exploitation of children in England did not start or finish with the Industrial Revolution, in one succinct sentence. 'The 'free labour' of children who had parents to support was also passing from the home to the mill or factory, a change that must in many cases – though not in all – have been for the worse, before the era of Factory Inspection began in 1833'[5]. Two more comments relating to the same era are worth quoting, because the author carefully considers both the industrial exploitation of children in nineteenth century England, together with the rearing practices and parental irresponsibility of the time[19]. 'An exasperated clergyman once said that in his parish the children's worst enemies were their parents. All too often this was true. We read a lot about cruelty in factories and workshops, but the cruelty that went on in some of the houses was worse, as well as being more sustained, and much harder for the children to bear since it came from their own parents. The foreman of a cotton factory said that at the end of the day he often had to drive children from behind the store and among the cotton bales. He said he could not understand why they would not go home. Had he known more about their homes he would not have been so surprised. . . . All that need be said here is that, generally, the worst employer a child could have was his own father or mother'[19].

Before 1970, certain writers in problem/advice columns of British newspapers and women's magazines condoned or even recommended the emotional exploitation of children. Doctors, probation officers and social workers often behaved likewise. Pregnancy and children were recommended to solve the emotional problems of sad or deranged women. The worthies who gave this advice were often vehemently and rightly opposed to a man or woman *marrying* and using the spouse to solve similar emotional problems. By contrast, conception and birth of a child would provide a little human who could do what no adult (husband/doctor/counsellor) could succeed in – namely treating a chronically dependent or miserable woman. Such 'treatment' rarely is successful. It does harm over two or more generations. From my child psychiatric files, I can produce recent records of more than 50 children who have endured impossible emotional demands from their parents from birth onwards, and who have been reduced to a sadder and more pitiful state than little

Morgan Lewis above.

Our culture condemns the vicious practice of the multilation of children to turn them into beggars. We also condemn mutilations and practices accepted by past cultures, such as footbinding (China), cranial deformation, facial cicatrization (e.g. African tribal scars), child castration (China, Italy[20]), slavery (deportation of slaves from Africa to Arab countries, or to America, where young children were often forcibly parted from their parents)[21]. Systematic enslavement, massacres, torture and starvation of the Guayakil Indians in Paraguay 'In the name of religion, backed by official policy' was reported in 1975. Girls of between 5 and puberty in particular were being sold as female slaves[22].

Religion has sometimes prevented, sometimes encouraged infanticide[23]. Abraham withdrew from the brink of sacrificing his son, Isaac, but the King of Moab made a burnt offering of his son. Religiously induced child killings have sometimes been amazingly cruel, as in throwing children to the Ganges crocodiles in India[23]. Cannibalism, and the use of the blood of tens of thousands of very cruelly sacrificed children during the Pre-Spanish conquest eras in Mexico and Central America was sanctioned by religion. Reports from Brazil in 1977 describe current cruel child sacrifices by religious cults. In one such Cult, members believed that throwing their live children from a precipice into the sea would ensure good harvests. The shades of Moloch, Baal and Ashtoreth are not confined to the old world of biblical times.

The politics and cultural pressures to continue the cruel practice of female 'circumcision' in Kenya (and other parts of Africa) are considered in detail by L. Bruce-Chwatt[24]. Nevertheless, we in Britain still accept or condone circumcision (of males) for non-medical reasons, this being for over 95% of permitted cases, an unnecessary operation which can cause serious complications and death. In USA and certain African and Asian countries this silly (and pointless) fashion is even more prevalent than in the UK.

Only recently in the UK have determined efforts been made in the National Health Service Hospitals and Local Authority Children's Homes, either to diminish the stress to young children suffering severance of the maternal bond, or to provide good alternative mothering. Widespread poor quality rearing in the UK can be deduced from the work of J. and E. Newson: '60% of children at 1 year of age and 97% at 4 years, are subject to physical modes of correction, 8% of them daily'[25,26]. Clearly much of this correcting is in no way cruel; the toddler is given a smack for approaching an electrical power point for the third or umpteenth time. Nevertheless, the Newson's subsequent work indicates that too high a proportion of English parents need to use weapons, such as canes on young children. Certain groups of immigrants (Irish, West Indian, African) to England seem even more inclined to use punishment by violence in rearing than the host population. Such immigrant parents frequently aggrievedly appeal to the police to support them in beating their youngsters. In Germany in the 1970s, 80% of parents beat their children, 35% using canes[17]. In all these cultures, canes can be used in cold blood – a practice which surely indicates parental incompetence, ineffectuality and weakness, as well as unkindness.

There are many social, tribal and national upheavals which put great strains on families. In countries such as Vietnam and Cambodia the disruptions of war left orphans and destitute children in extremes of material and emotional deprivation. The strength of the bonds between parents or other protective adults, and those children at risk were tested to the utmost. There must be real survival value (for a child in such war situations) in being surrounded by the more loving parents. In extremity, most citizens of Leningrad retained their honour, even during the period of prolonged starvation that occurred in the siege, which lasted nearly 2½ years. 3700 people from Leningrad died on Christmas Day 1941, mostly of starvation. Amidst courage and endurance, there were nevertheless a few individuals 'who would snatch bread from their own (starving) children'[27]. The adult or parental protective tendency also gives way to other considerations in the cases of many migrant parents and migrant-worker parents[28]. Increasing numbers of Italian parents, for instance, have been abandoning their children permanently at the Italian–Swiss frontier[29].

In the remaining sub-sections of this chapter, the figures and papers quoted are predominantly concerned with children abused by parents or individual caretakers who were performing cruel acts or cruel omissions secretly. Their destructive behaviour seemed isolated from the main social trends, and should not be necessarily compared with practices such as infanticide in primitive tribes[30,31]. This is not to say that gross child abuse does not occur in developing countries, as exemplified in papers from East Africa or Asia[32–34]. Child abuse and neglect occurs in nearly all parts of the world, although battered babies may be less often found in countries where the infant mortality is high (rejected children just do not live to be re-battered). Professor Henry Kempe has alerted the world. Further denial of the problem indicates ignorance, complacency, or arrogance. Nevertheless, cruelty to children often seems to have been so influenced by cultural patterns, and historical chance, that some writers have been inhibited over definitions of child abuse, and have implied that ascertainment of extent of the condition is an impossible task. It is necessary therefore to look at current research in human behaviour, in fields tangentially related to child abuse.

The capacity of many apparently normal human adults to be cruel or callous in certain circumstances has recently been studied in detail[35]. Stanley Milgram set out to investigate the apparent tolerence towards, or allowance of Nazi (or King Herods') persecutions[35]. His findings also explain the acceptance by whole communities and cultures of cruel practices towards children as discussed above. His experiments prove that 'It doesn't take an evil person to serve an evil system' and his work should be compulsory reading for everyone in public or professional life. Chapters 10 and 11 of his book give an analysis of the famous 'torture' experiments[35]. This analysis demonstrates how important it is to always question authority, and for people in authority to inculcate others in humane social practices (which would include rearing, the most important). Very briefly, the major headings are as follows:

Antecedent Conditions of Obedience: From babyhood, social compliance is rewarded, and there are powerful biological reasons for this. Respect for parental authority is carried into other areas of social life.

The Agentic Shift: Individuals shift (under certain social pressures) from the autonomous to the 'systemic' mode of behaviour.

Binding Factors: These include self justification, 'situational obligations' and anxiety at breaking social rules. Milgram's team used no fear, bullying, coercion or bribery in making their naive subjects 'torture' the trained subjects. However, the naive subjects often suffered terrible strain whenever they tried to resist the polite, formal, authoritative requests of the experimenter saying 'continue', or 'Go on with the experiment please'.

Milgram describes the potential of most humans, and for this reason emphasizes that his findings should not be called the 'Eichman experiments' (after Adolph Eichman, the bureaucratic Nazi persecutor). Even those subjects in his experiments who 'tortured' to extremity showed no characteristics of sadism, or any predisposition towards wanton cruelty.

Storr's essay 'Sadism and Paranoia' surveys the range of cruelty, from cultural or group induced cruel practices to tormenting of a helpless individual within the family circle. Five components are considered:

1. Aggressive psychopathy – those with this condition are impulsive individuals without concern for others.
2. 'Obedience of authority', as illustrated in the work of Milgram above.
3. Physical and/or psychological 'distance' between the aggressor and the victim.
4. The aggressors themselves having been the victims of abnormal (unkind) rearing.
5. Fear and paranoia: the aggressor projects onto the victim malign qualities[36].

All five components of human behaviour described, could, in varying proportions, be explanatory factors for battered babies, cruelly treated older children, or the persecution of a racial or cultural minority.

Following a lecture and videotape presentation on 'The Intentional Behaviour of The Young Infant', Professor John Newson was asked to pick out aspects of the parent–child interaction which would put the young child at most risk. He said that the parent must see the infant as 'a responsive individual . . . rather than an object'[31].

This corresponds with Storr's third component above. Cruel, battering or neglectful parents conceive their ill-used child as an alien; an alien, furthermore, which is disgusting, frustrating, or which tears the nerves with endless crying and screaming. This alien will not communicate at an adult level (abusive parents can have unbelievable expectations of babies and toddlers), except to register hate and ingratitude and wilfulness.

Research from Oxford emphasizes bonding failures between parent and child[38]. Cruelty by a parent, or parent substitute, towards a child may not result (entirely) from the abnormal personality of the parent, but (largely) from the failure of the process of bonding between parent and child. This helps explain why a high proportion of abusive parents are not blatantly mentally ill, psychopathic, subnormal or alcoholic. The proponents of this theory do not discount other social and biological factors. An important letter from the same department, for instance, emphasizes the dangers of the widespread use of tranquillizers in tense young mothers. The benzodiazepine tranquillizers can have an 'alcohol-like' effect in reducing higher cortical control, thereby reducing anxiety, but increasing the risk of explosions of temper[39]. Some papers emphasize defects in the attacked child, and ill-health at crucial times in the child or parent as contributing to failures of bonding and consequent child abuse. Abnormal pregnancy, abnormal labour or delivery, neonatal or early separation, illnesses in child or mother in the first year of the child's life are also factors contributing to child abuse[40].

Research from Cambridge is critical of overemphasis of 'bonding' or 'attachment' biological processes, particularly when these processes are considered in isolation[41]. In conceptualizing parental relationships '. . . their social origins outweigh the consequence of our biological evolution. . . . A mother's responses to her baby are not driven (primarily?) by any in-built biological imperatives. . . . Responses to a crying baby depend on how a mother interprets the crying and what it means to her'[41,42]. Such social sequences can be analysed in a variety of ways in terms of the Theory of Psychological Reversals. For instance, one sequence of the actual precipitation of assaults can be as follows: child tries to dominate by rages/crying/smearing faeces, etc. (paratelic behaviour) – parent attempts control (telic behaviour) . . . child gets frightened and desperate – parental guilt, fear and desperation mount until the parent also switches to the paratelic phase of irresponsible unreasoned violence[43].

A neurophysiological theory by Campbell is capable of incorporating and illuminating the other theories of child abuse[44]. The pleasure centres of the brain (septal areas, hippocampus, amygdala, etc.) must be kept activated either by sensory ('subhuman') or cortical tertiary area ('human') stimuli. Many humans function by activating their pleasure centres almost solely by sensory stimuli – a smaller number do so by a predominant use of the tertiary cortex. 'Preferred neurological pathways' are formed throughout life, especially in youth.

Battering parents have usually themselves been poorly reared youngsters. Perversion of these 'preferred pathways' leads to aberrant behaviour. Using this framework, most kindly parents live and nurture their youngsters as a consequence of their biological inheritance and their own reasonable rearing. Giving love is a delight. There are selfish parents, warm-natured but incompetent who rely almost entirely on sensory stimuli. The gurgling baby is loved, but the baulky toddler or the awkward unhappy child is rejected. Such parents may rear poorly in some respects, but not be blatantly cruel. Others, because of their own childhood deprivations and stresses may severely neglect the child, or worse, may be needing to *use* the child to activate the pleasure areas of their brains in a way the child can never live up to. The child should be dependent on the parent, but the battering parent uses the child in a situation of 'reversed emotional parasitism'.

The high IQ or intellectual parent can be equally vulnerable. A standard stereotype is of the cold upper-class English couple who employ nannies, and who toughen their child at boarding school. Nevertheless, if this same couple insist on a good loving nanny, and boarding school which fulfils all the child's essential needs, they are doing their duty as parents. The love which was given to Sir Winston Churchill by his childhood nanny (Mrs Everest) in Kent[45,46], contrasts with the failure of Adolf Hitler's biological mother to protect her little son from cruel drunken bullying in the home[13]. The facile principle 'mother = goodness'; 'no mother = irreparable harm' has often led to a belief that the *biological* mother is always better than substitute mothers. Slavish adherence to this belief is attacked in recent publications[45−48].

Many children show an unexpected biological adaptation to maltreatment. There may not be obvious expressions of fear and distress, and the children may appear to attach to the abusive or neglectful parent. This 'false-love' misleads professional people into letting the child stay in a stressful unhappy setting. The consequences of this are discussed elsewhere[48].

In summary, our children are protected by our evolutionary inheritance. Human adults tend to protect the young and helpless. Hereditary tendencies are modified during rearing by neurophysiological mechanisms, the 'preferred pathways'. Cruel, or battering or neglectful parents need to use their children to activate the 'pleasure areas' of their brains, to alleviate loneliness, inadequacy, etc., such personality traits often resulting from defects in their own rearing. The protective bonding process in humans involves biological mothers, fathers, substitute parents or others in protecting and loving the helpless. Social and cultural patterns can be superimposed, mainly in ways considered by Milgram[35] and Richards[41,42].

Children can be cruelly treated or neglected because of 'biologically abnormal' parents, (e.g. Huntington's Disease[49]), parents with lowered self-control associated with abnormal electroencephalographic patterns[50], psychosis, subnormality of intelligence, personality changes due to drugs or alcoholism, etc.) More commonly the key personality disorders are subtle, and not immediately discernible, because the parental failings of cruel parents have their origins in distorted patterns of their own rearing. If this is combined with failure in the bonding process, the child is in danger. This danger is greatly increased if society is not prepared to take action to protect its weakest citizens and if it permits cruel practices. Milgram[35] and Storr[36] show how easy it is for this to happen.

References

1. Bronowski, J. (1974). *Ascent of Man.* Ch. 1 (London: British Broadcasting Corporation Publication)
2. Ardrey, R. (1961). *African Genesis: A Personal Investigation into the Animal Origins and Nature of Man.* (London: Collins)
3. Holy Bible. Book of Joshua, Chapter 6:17–21
4. Holy Bible. Book of Matthew, Chapter 2:16
5. Trevelyan, G. M. (1959). *A Shortened History of England.* (London: Pelican)
6. Morris, C. (1967). *The Tudors,* Ch. 6 (London and Glasgow: Fontana)
7. Ward, B. (1972). *The Death of Changeling. World Med.,* **8,** 43
8. John Nicholson of Kirkcudbright (1843). Sawney Bean and his Family, Historical and traditional Tales connected with the South of Scotland.
9. Thomas Phaire (1553). *The Boke of Chyldren.* p. 31 (Edinburgh and London, 1955: E. and S. Livingstone)
10. Masters, A. (1972). *The Summer That Bled. The Biography of Hannah Senesh.* (London: Michael Joseph Ltd.)
11. Lord Russell of Liverpool (1954). *The Scourge of the Swastika. A Short History of Nazi War Crimes.* (London: Cassell and Co. Ltd.)
12. Solzhenitsyn, A. (1975). *Observer Review,* December 7. Extracted from Vol. 2 of *The Gulag Archipelago 1918–1956* (London: Collins/Harvill)
13. The Mind of Hitler. (1972). *Sunday Telegraph,* December 3
14. Radbill, S. X. (1968). A history of child abuse and infanticide. In: *The Battered Child,* R. E. Helfer and C. H. Kempe (eds.) (Chicago: University of Chicago Press)
15. Bloch, H. (1973). Dilemma of Battered Child and Battered Children. *N. Y. State J. Med.,* **73,** 799
16. Solomon, T. (1973). History and demography of child abuse. *Pediatrics,* **51,** 773
17. De Mause, L. (1976). *The History of Childhood; the Evolution of Parent-Child Relationships as a Factor in History.* Condor Press. Also summarized as *Waking from a Nightmare* by V. Sinason in *N. Psychiat.,* **3,** 18
18. Evans, R. M. (1972). *Children in the Iron Industry.* Museum Schools Service, National Museum of Wales, Cardiff
19. Speed, P. F. (1975). *Social Problems of the Industrial Revolution* (Oxford: Pergamon Press)
20. Osborn, L. (1975). Pseudohermaphrodites with the Golden Voices. *World Med.,* **11,** 55
21. Naipaul, V. S. (1975). England's Black Gold. *Radio Times.* 13th March, p. 64
22. Lewis, N. (1975). Manhunt. *Sunday Times Magazine.* January 26th, p. 26
23. Evans, P. (1968). Infanticide. *Proc. R. Soc. Med.,* **61,** 1296
24. Bruce-Chwatt, L. (1976). Female Circumcision and Politics. *World Med.,* **1,** 44
25. Royal College of Psychiatrists. Evidence for the Select Parliamentary (UK) Committee on Violence in the Family, June 1976
26. Newson, J. and Newson, E. (1965). *Patterns of Infant Care in an Urban Community.* (London: Penguin)
27. Wykes, A. (1968). The seige of Leningrad. *Purnell's History of the Second World War;* Battle Book 5. (The relevant quotations cite mainly Dmitri V. Pavlov)
28. Gelinek, I. (1974). Migrants' Children. *International Child Welfare Review,* No. 21, 45
29. Cicorela, G. and Spallino, L. (1974). Frontier Orphans. *International Child Welfare Review,* No. 21, 49
30. Noel, J. V. (1971). Lessons from a 'Primitive' People. *World Med.,* **6,** 61
31. Kiloh, L. G. (1975). Psychiatry amongst the Australian Aborigines. *Br. J. Psychiat.,* **126,** 1
32. Bwibo, N. O. (1971). Battered child syndrome. *East Afr. Med. J.,* **48,** 56
33. Bwibo, N. O. (1972). Battered child syndrome. *East Afr. Med. J.,* **49,** 934
34. Hwang, W. T., Leng, L. K. and Chin, C. (1974). Battered child syndrome in a Malaysian hospital. *Med. J. Malaysia,* **28,** 239

35. Milgram, S. (1974). *Obedience to Authority*. (London and New York: Tavistock Publications Ltd.)
36. Storr, A. (1976). Sadism and Paranoia. Paper presented at the Symposium on Child Abuse, at the Royal Society of Medicine, 2–4th June 1976
37. Newson, J. (1977). Intentional behaviour in the young infant. *Annual Scientific Meeting of the Royal College of Psychiatrists* (Child Psychiatry Section), held at The Royal College of Physicians, London, March 11th
38. Ounsted, C., Oppenheimer, R. and Lindsay, J. (1974). Aspects of bonding failure: The Psychopathology and Psychotherapeutic treatment of families of battered children. *Develop. Med. Child Neurol.*, **16**, 447
39. Lynch, M. A., Lindsay, J. and Ounsted, C. (1975). Tranquillizers causing aggression. *Br. med. J.*, **1**, 266
40. Lynch, M. A. (1975). *Lancet*, **ii**, 317
41. Richards, M. P. M. (1976). 'Parents and Children and Non-Accidental Injury'. Paper presented at the Symposium on Child Abuse, at the Royal Society of Medicine, June 2- 4th 1976
42. Richards, M. P. M. (1974). First steps in becoming social. In: *The Integration of a Child into a Social World*. (London: Cambridge University Press)
43. Apter, M. J. and Smith, K. C. P. (1977). The theory of psychological reversals and family Interaction. *International Conference on Family Interaction*. Symposium held at the University of Mexico. Mexico City. January 1977
44. Campbell, H. J. (1973). *The Pleasure Areas*. (London: Eyre Methuen Ltd.)
45. Howells, J. G. (1974). *Remember Maria*. (London: Butterworth)
46. Gathorne-Hardy, J. (1974). *The Rise and Fall of the British Nanny*. (London: Hodder and Stoughton) (Arrow edition)
47. Morgan, P. (1975). *Child Care, Sense and Fable*. (London: Temple Smith)
48. Oliver, J. E. (1976). Families in which children suffer maltreatment. Paper presented at the Symposium on Child Abuse, at the Royal Society of Medicine, June 2–4th 1976
49. Oliver, J. E. and Dewhurst, K. E. (1969). Six generations of ill-used children in a Huntington's pedigree. *Postgrad. Med. J.*, **45**, 757
50. Smith, S. M., Honigsberger, L. and Smith, C. A. (1973). EEG and Personality Factors in Baby Batterers, *Br. Med. J.*, **2**, 20

Special reference note

In this and the ensuing sub-sections there are references to evidence given to the (UK) Parliamentary Select Committee on 'Violence in the Family' in 1976. The published volumes contain as comprehensive and detailed a report on this topic as I have anywhere seen. This particularly applies to volume II.

The full reference is as follows:

The First Report from the Select Committee of Violence in the Family.

Violence to Children (Summarized report) Vol. I

Violence to Children (Minutes of Evidence) Vol. II

Violence to Children (plus Appendices) Vol. III

Printed by order of the House of Commons (H.C.329), 26.4.1977.

Part II — THE WORLD LITERATURE ON CHILD ABUSE IN THE HOME SETTING*

The extent of child abuse can be considered in two main ways. The first entails the intensive search for reasonably well defined conditions (such as battered babies). Here the researcher should have first hand clinical involvement. The second involves epidemiological projections and inferences based on official data; in this case rigid definitions and rigid methodology can give spurious results because cruel or neglectful parents are plausible, and tend to be believed. The evidence for this is seen in the extensive literature on child abuse which recognizes or emphasizes under-reporting, diagnostic failures, disbelief, incomplete information and the specialized problems of ascertainment. From the UK, the following 25 references to diverse publications illustrate the above points[1-25]. The US literature is probably even more extensive, the following examples being given from pre-1975 papers[26-44]. Publications from the European mainland, before 1975 are relatively sparse, but the ensuing make the same points[45-53]. Papers on battered babies are beginning to appear from Asian and African countries, and it is clear that certain Australians were attacking national complacency and denials over the problem of cruelty to young children in the home from 1970 onwards. Here again are listed a few pre-1975 papers from Africa, Asia and Australia which tried to heighten public awareness and sympathy in those continents and countries[54-61].

In the Appendix an attempt has been made to gather the world literature on the prevalence of child abuse, but no adequate or disciplined papers on prevalence were found from Communist Countries, or from The Third World. The estimates by Light (1973) based on a comprehensive consideration of American literature and official statistics enable the conclusion that 1 in 100 children under 18 in USA are physically abused, sexually molested or severely neglected[38]. This is the same as the number ascertained (from NSPCC statistics alone) by Chesser for England and Wales in 1951[4]. Chesser used 'cold facts' in reaching this figure; his children were under 15 and the victims of 'bad neglect or ill-treatment, or maladjustment' associated with parental ill-usage.

Chesser kept an open mind on the origins of child cruelty, considering biological, social, cultural and moral factors. He also quoted certain post-war newspaper reports, some of which seemed to illustrate how adverse social conditions could aggravate childhood suffering, and poor rearing by parents. He made the following firm, well substantiated statement in his book, about England in 1949–50. 'At some time during childhood one child in 16 is brought to the attention of the NSPCC and perhaps a majority of those involved are reported more than once'[4]. The professions and the public in England paid unforgivably little attention to Dr Chesser's cruelty to children statistics either then or since.

Whatever the effects of post-war conditions, two Yorkshire Educationalists,

---

* See also Appendix.

Alan Clegg and Barbara Megson painted a gloomy picture for the mid 1960s in their book *Children in Distress*[5]. They found that 1 in 10 of school age children 'live through extremes of wretchedness' and described the 'apprenticeship of distress' that most of this 10% suffered in their homes. This study started from the standpoint of the child's distress as observed at school, in relation to unpleasant or neglectful rearing practices. It was not based initially on 'incidents' which reached a social or medical agency.

In his evidence to the UK Parliament, Hession tries to bridge the gap of his own clinical experience of parental violence to children (at *least* 20% of his clinic cases, with a further 20% witnessing interparental [or parent figure] violence), and the more widespread poor rearing practices in London (Hession, 1976[66]). Unacceptable violence to children occurs in 1 in 10 of London families in the 1970s (closely comparable with Clegg and Megson's numbers from Yorkshire). Hession doubts that this 1 in 10 figure can be proven, as the London police were only aware of about 1% of fractures to children caused by parental violence. In his own large clinical psychiatric practice, 'about 40% of "discovered" cases of more serious injuries come from families with at least one parent with an IQ lower than 75'. In this, as in much of his evidence, his experience in London exactly matches ours in rural Wiltshire. Many psychiatrists in UK and elsewhere screen out dull problem families as 'social problems' not worthy of their expertise, thereby insulating themselves from reality. A high proportion of physically and emotionally damaged children derive from dull disintegrating problem families, but often *one, two or more* generations back[18].

Trube-Becker, from Dusseldorf states that a survey of records over a twelve month period showed that 4500 men and women in West Germany were sentenced for endangering the physical and mental well-being of 6500 children, most of whom were 3 and under[52]. This highlights another consideration; the observed rates of child abuse depend on official practices. Is the legal profession in England and Wales in a position to claim a similar knowledge of child victims and their adult aggressors?

Fairburn and Jones in the City of Bath, approach the problem from an unusual but important direction[11]. At any one time there are likely to be about 12 battering adults and 25 high-risk families (approximately 50 potentially battering adults) in Bath (population 86 000). The surveillance of these adults is exercised in order to prevent serious injury to young children. Mindlin[91], citing studies in the USA, gives estimates of child abuse ranging through Gil (6000 in 1967), Kempe[105] (60 000 in 1972), Light[38] (500 000 in 1973) and Gil[82] (circa 2.5 million, projected estimate). USA has 67 million children under 18; estimates of the rate of abuse therefore vary from less than one child in 10 000 (not a major social problem) to approaching four children in every hundred, which could be considered as an indictment of American society. These discrepancies will be discussed, and relate mainly to problems of ascertainment and definition. At all events, the public in Florida (total population 5 million) were sufficiently uneasy about child abuse to report approximately 20 000 cases of neglect and abuse via the 'hot-line' telephone system per year. Nearly half of these reports were confirmed by the agencies[93].

The variability of criteria and definitions for child abuse in general is considerably reduced when hospital based doctors publish results on a group of young victims who are perhaps at greatest risk of permanent sequelae, namely, 'battered babies'. Many hospitals have ill-defined populations in their catchment areas. Notwithstanding this, paediatricians in the United Kingdom are seeing and identifying a lot of battered babies. Table 5.1 summarizes data from six disparate localities in England with the approximate total population figures given.

Local research endeavours give higher rates of battering than even the more realistic official national returns. In Holland, for instance, in 1973, 628 'battered' children were reported to the Trust Doctors[107]. This gives a rate of approximately 50 such children (*under 20* years) per million (total population) per year in Holland, lower than the yearly rates recorded in Wiltshire, Lancashire, and Lambeth (in London) for children *under 4* years old per million (total population).

At the time of writing there were five battered babies (one also with a history of 'failure to thrive') and a sixth, a toddler, who was underfed and neglected (but not physically battered), all in the children's ward of Princess Margaret Hospital, Swindon (population of town and environs approx. 150 000).

There have been 107 references given so far. These are not mainly concerned with rough and ready beatings, or bruised youngsters 'disciplined' by simple, primitive violence. This point is reinforced by the following comments.

The importance of the Appendix is highlighted by the rate of induced brain damage resulting in degrees of mental handicap. MacKeith (1974) gives convincing projections of at least 400 new cases of chronic brain damage per year in the UK, resulting from child abuse[69]. Using the figures of Birrell and Birrell (1968), and Oliver et al. (1974), at least one quarter of the severely attacked young children are rendered intellectually damaged or subnormal as a result of battering[18,58]. Thus, if 75 (young children) per million (total population) are attacked each year, 18–19 per million (total population) suffer intellectual impairment per year, often to the extent of profound mental handicap. Projections from N.-E. Wilts. give estimates of 3000 new child victims (aged 0–3) of severe abuse in England and Wales each year. This means that 750 children in England and Wales could be rendered mentally handicapped each year as a result of attacks by their parents. A proportion of cases of microcephaly in subnormality hospitals result from the very rough shaking or battering of babies[108].

Of a series of 45 children suspected of abuse seen at the Philadelphia (USA) Children's Hospital, the neurosurgeon was involved in 20! 37 of the 45 eventually were developing reasonably normally (physically), 6 were clearly rendered mentally handicapped, and motor hyperactivity could also be a sequel to the abuse[109]. Martin (1975) found that 31% of abused children had serious

Table 5.1 The identification of battered babies in six disparate localities in England

Locality	Ref	Type of population	Ages of children	Total pop. nos.	Cases recorded in relation to the years of study	Nos. p.a. per mill. total pop.	Rate in children	Comment
Birmingham	72 106	Urban	Mostly under 2 years	1 000 000	69 cases in Birmingham in 2 years (1971 and 1972)	35	Unstated	Data predominantly from hospital sources only
Lambeth (London)	67	Urban	3 years and under	300 000	28 in 1972	93	'An incidence of 2 per 1000 in children aged 3 years and under' (per year)	Short report. Cases possibly less severe than those in the Wilts. and Birmingham studies. Data mostly from local authority sources
N.E. Wilts	18	Mixed rural and urban	Children under 4; more than 75% under 1 year	200 000	22 between Jan. 1972 and June 73	75	'1 new case per 1000 children under 4 years old per year . . .', Also 4 (very severely battered babies) per 1000 live births per annum	Very severe cases, often with repeated injuries. Data from multiple sources
Preston and environs	65	Mixed rural and urban	Unstated; mostly under 3 years	300 000	45 cases in 1969 and 1970	75	Unstated	Data from Emergency Dept. only
Leeds and Manchester Metropolitan Districts	70	Urban	Children under 4; 33% under 1 year	77 000 children under 4	89 cases in 1974	Unstated	1–1.2 New cases per 1000 children under 4 years old per year	1. Discussion on the value of registers 2. Repetitions and rebatterings considered

neurological dysfunction $4\frac{1}{2}$ years after the abusive episodes. Less than half of the originally abused children had suffered fractures or subdural haemorrhages, yet approaching one third had developed seriously impaired neurological function associated with a mean IQ of 78[110]. At each stage, these are all cautious statements of the minimum extent of mental handicap induced by battering, and other forms of child abuse (such as shaking babies).

Vagueness creeps in when 'failure to thrive' (starved) babies are included in baby battering studies, where such babies have not been shown to be physically battered. The Melbourne Study,[58] breaks the cases down into physical violence (battered babies) only 25; physical violence *and* gross neglect 10; gross neglect only, 7. The overwhelming assumption of nearly all investigators is that degrees of neglect are far more common than active abuse. The relative proportions in such studies therefore indicate artefacts of identification and selection. It is easier to identify and demarcate classical battered babies (though still hard enough!) than to identify and demarcate children who are being deprived of adequate food, fluids, warmth, love or protection by their parents.

The extent of child abuse is also measured on the basis of the numbers and percentages of abused children in hospital admissions or by paediatric, emergency or casualty referrals. These disturbing figures are given in Table 5.2. Smith and Noble in 1973 estimated that 4400 children each year are treated in hospital casualty departments in the UK, with injuries of an inadequately explained nature[111]. Sceptics who might accuse the investigators of soft criteria over the definitions of the child abuse considered ('everyone knocks their children around in the East End – it doesn't mean anything'!) should look at columns D (and J in certain rows) of the Appendix dealing with the death rates. The lowest estimates come from legal and official sources. Derivations from the Department of Health and Social Services (1970) figures for England and Wales only reveal 40 infant deaths per year known to be the result of wilful violence[64]. Nevertheless, for a number of reasons, it would be very naive to accept official or national death rates for children 'known to be the result of wilful violence' as anything but the barest minimum estimates, representing the most blatantly obvious killings. No pathologist could risk his reputation by pinning the blame on parents in six examples of killings (most falling within common categories, which categories also encompass innocent or purely medical causes of death in some or most cases) given in a letter to the *British Medical Journal* in 1975[112]. Extrapolation from our data (Oliver *et al.*, 1974)[18], would give a minimum figure of 300 deaths of children aged 0–3 by parental violence for the same population (50 million approx.). The Tunbridge Wells Study Group[74], estimates 700 deaths of children by parental violence per year for the UK. Trube Becker[104], found that 6.4% of deaths of newborn infants and children under 6 in and around Dusseldorf in West Germany were due to neglect and/or maltreatment. In 1973, Trube Becker stated that 100 young children per year die of maltreatment in W. Germany (pop. 62 million)[52].

In Canada (pop. 21 million), Rodenberg (1971)[103], gave a figure of 74 legally

Table 5.2 Proportions of children seen in routine medical practice who are the victims of violence or ill-usage at the hands of their parents or guardians

References		Subject	% Abused children
89 Lauer et al. (1974)	USA	Admissions to San Francisco General Hospital.	3% of total admissions are due to child abuse.
35 Kempe (1969)	USA	Children under 5 seen in Emergency Room.	15% of the children seen are the victims of child abuse.
36 Kempe (1971)	USA	Children under 2 seen with fractures.	25% of the children seen are the victims of child abuse.
84 Green F. C. (1975)	USA	Children under 3 seen in the Emergency Room at the Washington Children's Hospital.	10% of trauma is inflicted rather than accidental.
84 Green F. C. (1975)	USA	Children under 2 years with fractures.	30% of these fractures have been inflicted, rather than being accidental.
84 Green F. C. (1975)	USA	Children who are 'established abuse cases'.	50% of such children have been victims previously.
101 Fried (1973)	CANADA (Citing USA sources)	Young children and babies with fractures.	15% of the children seen are the victims of child abuse. (See also Dawe[99])
101 Fried (1973)	CANADA (Citing USA sources)	Young children and babies seen with trauma in the Hospital Emergency Room.	25% of the children seen are the victims of child abuse. (See also Dawe[99])
15 Okell C. (1971)	UK	Children under 3 attending the Casualty Department.	6.7% of total children are victims of physical abuse. 8.9% are victims of obvious neglect.
66 Hession M. (1976)	UK	Children attending the assessment diagnostic and treatment services for certain London Social Services Departments.	'At least 20% of such children have been at the receiving end of parental violence of a degree greater than society considers normal or reasonable.'
1 British Medical Journal (1973)	UK	Casualties in children under 2 years.	10% of total children are victims of physical abuse.
1 British Medical Journal (1973)	UK	Fractures in children under 2 years.	25% of total children are victims of physical abuse.
14 Jackson (1972)	UK	London children seen with physical injury at Kings College Hospital, London.	18% of total children are victims of physical abuse.
19 Ounsted C. et al. (1975)	UK	Paediatric Referrals to Park Hospital, Oxford.	11% of total children are victims of physical abuse.

ascertained child murders by depressed parents in 5 years. These small numbers compare with the DHSS estimate in the UK[64]. Here again, ascertainment depended on formal legal methods. Smith and Hanson in 1974 comment on five babies on whom the Birmingham coroner reached an open verdict; the authors relate[72] that '... none (of these battered children killed by their parents) appeared in the Registrar General's figures for "homicides and injuries purposely inflicted" in 1971'.

Weston (1969) found that in 5 years there were 60 children killed by abuse and neglect in Philadelphia for 212 394 births, or at least one child killed for every 3500 born[97]. However, many of the suspicious deaths evaded autopsy, or there was not sufficient data to form a definite conclusion. The cases that Weston illustrates are again examples of the most blatant abuse leading to death[97]. Weston's cases, like those in other pathological series, do not incorporate the (probably larger) numbers of children killed by suffocation, inhalation of gastric contents in an abusive situation and other modes of death alluded to above[112]. This point, together with the obvious diversity of the selections of series of cases and the varied methodology in the different papers, should be borne in mind in considering the implications of the ensuing paragraph.

The percentages of total attacked children who are killed by their parents varies according to different publications as follows: 1–5% (UK)[23], (USA)[28,82,83,89]; 5–10% (after excluding cases where parents had gone to prison[72]) (UK)[69], (USA)[37*,44,86]; 10–33%, (Australia)[59], (UK)[6,18,65,72], (USA)[29,34,79,83,94,95,98,113]. With some exceptions, the series with the youngest children tend to have the highest death rates.

Unkind, neglectful, or incompetent rearing cannot be measured solely by consideration of the most blatant, or most easily identified cases of child abuse. One country in Europe, Holland, has methods of collecting statistics which are a gradual move towards a system by which society can know how many children are victims in the home setting. Parents may fail their children by ill-will, indifference, or incompetence. Parental guilt or blame may therefore be irrelevant to the child who is suffering. Child care in the Netherlands would seem to take account of this[114,115]. The categories of children requiring child care and protection are as follows:

(1) Children under guardianship:
   (a) Deprivation of parental rights occurs *in cases where very serious facts have come to light.*
   (b) Release from parental rights. Here the intention is to assist families where parents are unable or unfit to carry out parental duties properly.
   (c) Compulsory release from the parental power, which may be decreed against the parents' will; or in cases where parents cannot express their will because of insanity.

* 'Initial mortality' only, of 70 000 children battered annually in USA.

(2) Children under family guardianship:

Supervision (by the Judiciary) of children who are in an unfavourable situation in the home setting, or who are threatened with moral or physical danger.

(3) Juvenile Offenders:

The third category does not imply direct child abuse or neglect, but many (or most) antisocial children become as they are, as a consequence of defective rearing. Juvenile offenders who have been punished only account for less than one in 8 of the 45 000 who require care and protection out of a population of 4.5 million Dutch children.

Child care and protection therefore involves one Dutch child in every hundred[114]. It is tempting to compare this 'one child in 100' with the actual findings of Chesser[4] in England and the projections by Light[38] in USA (see Appendix), which gave the same proportion. It should be noted that Chesser's data are entirely derived from NSPCC sources, whereas the Dutch data are derived from official sources in which 'serious' facts have come to light, such facts having been also processed by judicial procedures. Underascertainment is likely in both.

There are pitfalls in interpreting the official statistics for England and Wales, which are not easy to compare with the Dutch numbers. On 31st March 1973, there were 93 188 children in care in England and Wales. For England, this represents 6.8 per 1000 of the estimated population under the age of 18 (DHSS and Welsh Office, 1973)[116]. The circumstances listed in which children came into care may be misleading. Thus, 15 532 children are listed as coming into care at the time of a short-term illness of parent or guardian. A total of 8863 were admitted following a Care Order, under the Children's and Young Person's Act (1969). Some 4596 were deserted by their mother, and 956 were abandoned or lost. A further 4206 were listed as having unsatisfactory home conditions. There are 17 different designations, each with varying social implications. Some designations imply parental incompetence or callousness – some imply unhappy and uncontrollable circumstances. For any one family, the designation given for the national statistics could be arbitrary. At the time of writing, I know of a nearby large family of children, of a borderline intellectually subnormal mother who is also a prostitute. The mother has a 'short term illness' which is given as the reason why her children go into care (yet again). These children have been reared roughly and incompetently, and have suffered degrees of unnecessary violence and intellectual, social and emotional deprivation. The real reason for their reception into care is that their parents are incompetent rearers of children, and Society cannot, or will not intrude or cares too little to intrude effectively into parental rights on behalf of child victims. Conversely, if I visit a local reception centre or children's home, I can pick out children from only too many known problem families, such children having suffered unmeasurable degrees of neglect and/or ill-usage.

Mia Kellmer Pringle in 1971 stated that over 70 000 children were in care in England and Wales[117]. However, she estimated[117] that the combined totals of children technically in care, plus children unloved and rejected by parents, or children understimulated and culturally deprived in their own home amounted each year to three times 70 000 or at least 210 000. The point is that national statistics on children in care are influenced by the poor rearing abilities of their parents, as well as by more obvious policies or other social factors. Indeed in the UK, there have for years been consistent efforts and much propaganda to *resist* children going into care. To examine the implications of the Home Office and DHSS command papers on 'Children in Care in England and Wales' from 1969–1973 one must not only consider, say, the effects of the provisions of the 1969 Children's and Young Person's Act (implemented in January 1971). It is also necessary to look behind some of the convenient labels, the 17 designated 'circumstances in which children came into care'. Many, or most children in care have been victims of unkind, neglectful or incompetent rearing[116,118–121]. Other indirect indices of parental incompetence could include (a) maladjusted children, (b) children in schools for the maladjusted, (c) uncontrollable children (between 14 and 16 years) in jails or remand centres, and (d) a proportion of the pupils attending for Child Guidance. In 1973 the respective figures for these four groups were (a) 10 494 (b) 5713 (c) nearly 4000 and (d) 79 093 (provisional).[112]

At first sight, it would seem that the current National Society for the Prevention of Cruelty to Children statistics should give a direct index of the rate of ascertained child abuse in England and Wales, but the NSPCC numbers are also influenced by many factors unrelated to parental cruelty. Reorganization of Local Authority Social Services Departments has resulted in changing proportions of child welfare cases being taken on by Local Authority social workers rather than by NSPCC Inspectors. NSPCC propaganda is aimed at helping parents *before* they harm their children, rather than taking action after the damage is done. This increased the heterogeneity of the NSPCC new cases. Thus, there were 21 143 new cases in 1972 involving 62 227 children, but 47 352 of this total were labelled 'at risk', whereas only 792 (children of all ages) were unequivocally stated to be physically injured[123]. Yet from Table 5.1 it can be seen that there cannot be less than 2000–4000 newly battered babies (mostly children under 3) in England and Wales each year! As an index of parental cruelty and incompetence, another NSPCC total should be considered: Of the 62 227 children helped by the NSPCC in 1972, only 2347 were reported to be 'well cared for – no case'[123].

In 1973 the equivalent NSPCC figures for the 12 months January–December were 20 273 new cases opened, involving 60 076 children[124], and a further 43 160 were considered at risk. Although 1070 were unequivocally stated to be victims of physical injury, only 3048 of the 60 076 were reported to be 'well cared for – no case'[124]. In both years, the NSPCC were worried by the increasing numbers of young children being left on their own by parents who were opting out of rearing responsibilities. Taking all these considerations into account, 'Child Care and Protection' is probably involved in about one English child in every 100, as in Holland.

At the start of this sub-section, I referred to the statement by the two educationalists Alan Clegg and Barbara Megson[5], that one in 10 of school age children 'live through extremes of wretchedness', most suffering in their own homes. It is significant that this estimate, which is ten times greater than either the Dutch figure[114,115], or the UK and USA numbers and estimates discussed above, is derived by direct observations of distressed schoolchildren, picked out from the entire school population. This contrasts with the medical, medico-legal, social work, NSPCC and other estimates on child abuse, for these are all based on incidents and injuries which *by chance* have come to light, have *not* been overlooked, have been acted on *and confirmed* by professional people, who are *not* in the home, and who usually spend far less time with the children than the abusive parent or the child's teacher. In his memorandum containing evidence for the British Parliamentary Select Committee in May 1976, Hession estimated that 'physical violence beyond a generally accepted norm occurs in about 10% of families'. He also estimated that 'at least 20% of new children seen each year at the psychiatric assessment diagnostic and treatment service for the Social Services Departments (of certain London Boroughs) had been at the receiving end of parental violence of a degree greater than society considers normal or reasonable. A further 20% have witnessed an exceptional amount or intensity of inter-parental (or parental figure) violence'. Hession made a special point of focusing on certain vulnerable groups of parents prone to violence 'about 40% of all the discovered cases of serious injuries come from families with at least one partner with an IQ lower than 75'[66].

Those who estimate that 10% of children receive violence and maltreatment in their own homes must be taken seriously even though their claims, they admit, are hard to prove. It does not mean that they are not right. The '1 in 100' figures for child victims represent the proven apparent cases, the maggot in the core of society that cannot be ignored. The '1 child in 10' usually just suffers, and his plight is only apparent to conscientious people who spend an appreciable part of the day with him. His situation represents the rotting from the core of society and he is the likely parent of the blatantly battered baby in the next generation.

References (to Part II and Appendix)

1. *British Medical Journal* (1973). Deliberate injury of children. **4,** 61
2. Cameron, J. M. (1972). The battered baby syndrome. *Practitioner,* **109,** 302
3. Castle, R. L. and Kerr, A. M. (1972). A study of suspected child abuse. National Society for the Prevention of Cruelty to Children publication, September, 1972
4. Chesser, E. (1951). *Cruelty to Children.* (London: Victor Gollancz Ltd.)
5. Clegg, A. and Megson, B. (1968). *Children in Distress.* (London: Penguin)
6. Cooper, C. (1975). The Doctors Dilemma. In: *Concerning Child Abuse,* A. W. Franklin (ed.) (Edinburgh: Churchill-Livingstone)

7. Court, D., Lister, J. and Franklin, A. W. (1974). Experts and child abuse. *Br. Med. J.*, 3, 801

8. Court, J. (1969). An historical review of the american child abuse laws. *Child Care News*, 92

9. Court, J. (1971). The battered child syndrome: 1. The need for a multi-disciplinary approach. *Nursing Times*, 67, 659

10. Diggle, G. and Jackson, G. (1973). Child injury intensive monitoring system. *Br. Med. J.*, 3, 334

11. Fairburn, A. C. and Jones, S. (1975). Beta 5 and battering (child abuse – a scheme of interdisciplinary linkage and co-ordination). *New Society*, 31.7.75

12. Franklin, A. W. (1975). *Concerning Child Abuse*. (Edinburgh: Churchill Livingstone)

13. Howells, J. G. (1974). *Remember Maria*. (London: Butterworth)

14. Jackson, G. (1972). Child abuse syndrome: the cases we miss. *Br. Med. J.*, 2, 756

15. Okell, C. (1971). Childhood accidents and child abuse. *Community Med.*, 126, 124

16. Okell, C. (1972). The battered baby syndrome: (a) recent research and implications for treatment. Royal Society of Health Congress held at Eastbourne, 24–28th April 1972

17. Oliver, J. E. and Cox, J. (1973). A family kindred with ill-used children: the burden on the community. *Br. J. Psychiat.*, 123, 81

18. Oliver, J. E., Cox, J., Taylor, A. and Baldwin, J. A. (1974). Severely ill-treated young children in North-East Wiltshire. Unit of Clinical Epidemiology. Oxford Record Linkage Study. Oxford Regional Health Authority. Research Report No. 4. August 1974.

19. Ounsted, C., Oppenhimer, R. and Lindsay, J. (1974). Aspects of bonding failure: The psychopathology and psychotherapeutic treatment of families of battered children. *Devel. Med. Chld Neurol.*, 16, 447

20. Parker, G. E. (1965). The battered child syndrome. *Med. Sci. Law*, 8, 160

21. Powis, D. (1974). Violence to children. *Police Review*, November 15th, p. 1473

22. Renvoize, J. (1974). *Children in Danger*. (London: Routledge and Kegan Paul)

23. Skinner, A. E. and Castle, R. L. (1969). 78 Battered children: A retrospective study. (London: NSPCC)

24. Smith, S. and Noble, N. (1973). Battered children and their parents. *New Society*, 26, 393

25. Stark, J. (1969). The battered child: does Britain need a reporting law? *Public Law*, 48

26. Avery, J. C. (1973). The battered child. *Mental Hyg.*, 57, 40

27. Dodge, P. R. (1962). Medical implications of physical abuse of children. In: *Protecting the Battered Child*. American Humane Association Publication, p. 23

28. Ebbin, A. J., Gollub, M. H., Stein, A. M. and Wilson, M. G. (1969). Battered child syndrome at the Los Angeles County General Hospital. *Am. J. Dis. Chld.*, 118, 660

29. Fontana, V. J. (1971). *The Maltreated Child*. (Illinois: Charles C. Thomas)

30. Fontana, V. J. (1971). The diagnosis of the maltreatment syndrome in children. Symposium on Child Abuse. New York University Medical Centre. June 15th 1971. Published in *Pediatrics*, 51, April 1973

31. Gregg, G. S. and Elmer, E. (1969). Infant injuries: accident or abuse? *Pediatrics*, 44, 434

32. Helfer, R. E. and Kempe, C. H. (1968). *The Battered Child*. (Chicago: University of Chicago Press)

33. Holter, J. C. and Friedman, S. B. (1968). Child abuse: early case-finding in the emergency department. *Pediatrics*, 42, 128

34. Kempe, C. H., Silverman, F. N., Steele, B. F., Droegemueller, W. and Silver, H. K. (1962). The battered child syndrome. *J. Am. Med. Assoc.*, 181, 17

35. Kempe, C. H. (1969). The battered child and the hospital. *Hosp. Pract.*, 4, 44

36. Kempe, C. H. (1971) Paediatric implications of the battered baby syndrome. *Arch. Dis. Chld.*, 46, 28

37. Kempe, C. H. (1974). Duty to report child abuse. Editorial in the *W. J. Med.*, 121, 224

38. Light, R. J. (1973). Abused and neglected children in America: a study of alternative policies. *Harvard Educational Review*, 43, 556

39. Murdock, C. G. (1970). The abused child and the school system. *Am. J. Pub. Hlth*, **60,** 105
40. Pickett, L. K. (1972). The role of the surgeon in the detection of child abuse. *Connecticut Med.*, **36,** 513
41. Reeb, K. G., Melli, M. S., Wald, M. and Wesenberg, R. (1972). A conference on child abuse. *Wisconsin Med. J.*, **71,** 226
42. Silver, L. B., Barton, W. and Dublin, C. C. (1967). Child abuse laws: are they enough? *J. Am. Med. Assoc.*, **199,** 101
43. Silver, L. B., Dublin, C. C. and Lourie, R. S. (1969). Child abuse syndrome: the 'gray areas' in establishing a diagnosis. *Pediatrics*, **44,** 594
44. Simons, B., Downs, E. F., Hurster, M. M. and Archer, M. (1966). Child abuse: epidemiologic study of medically reported cases. *N. Y. State J. Med.*, **66,** 2783.
45. Verbeeck, J. (1971). The physician confronted by unloved children. *Med. Hyg.*, **29,** 362
46. Vesterdal, J. (1972). The battered child syndrome. *Ann. Nestle*, 27, 5
47. Moszer, M. and Bach, C. (1969). The battered child syndrome. 'Le syndrome des enfants maltraités'. *Prog. Méd.*, **97,** 303
48. Neimann, N. and Rabouille, D. (1969). Maltreated children. *Rev. Prat.*, **19,** 3879
49. Straus, P. and Wolf, A. (1970). A topical question: maltreated children. *Psychiatrie de L'Enfant*, **12,** 577
50. Köttgen, U., Greinacher, I., and Hofmann, S. (1968). Radiological diagnosis of maltreatment of children (Battered Child Syndrome), *z.Kinderheilkde*, **6,** 384
51. Nau, E. (1967). Maltreated children. *Monatsschr.Kinderheilkde*, **115,** 192
52. Trube-Becker, E. (1973). Child abuse and its consequences. *Paediat. Prax.*, 12/3, 389 (English Summary in *Psychiatric Briefs*, **7,** 70)
53. Underhill, E. (1974). The child and his surroundings. The strange silence of teachers, doctors and social workers in the face of cruelty to children: *International Child Welfare Review* (Geneva), No. 21, p. 16 (In English)
54. Bwibo, N. O. (1972). Battered child syndrome. *E. Afr. Med. J.*, **49,** 934
55. Hwang, W. T., Leng, L. K. and Chin, C. (1974). Battered child syndrome in a Malaysian hospital. *Med. J. Malaysia*, **28,** 239
56. Irwin, C. (1974). Specialists on child battering. Golden jubilee of the South African National Council for Child Welfare. Pretoria, 21–25, October 1974. Reported in *Child Welfare* (Kindersorg) December 1974
57. Bialestock, D. (1973). Custody of children. *Med. J. Aust.*, **2,** 1128
58. Birrell, R. G. and Birrell, J. H. W. (1968). The maltreatment syndrome in children: a hospital survey. *Med. J. Aust.*, **2,** 1023
59. Colclough, I. R. (1972). Victorian Government's report on child abuse: a reinvestigation. *Med. J. Aust.*, **2,** 1491
60. Editorial Article (1974). *Med. J. Aust.*, **2,** 231
61. Gibson, G. H. and Watson, J. V. (1973). Battered baby syndrome. *Med. J. Aust.*, **2,** 1073
62. British Paediatric Association and British Association of Paediatric Surgeons. (1976). Evidence Presented to the Select Parliamentary Committee, 8.6.76
63. Beswick, K., Lynch, M. A. and Roberts, J. (1976). Child abuse and general practice. *Br. Med. J.*, **2,** 800
64. The Battered Baby (1970). Prepared by The Standing Medical Advisory Committee for the Central Health Services Council, England and Wales. Dept. of Health and Social Security. (London: HMSO)
65. Hall, M. H. (1972). The battered baby syndrome: (b) non-accidental injuries in children. Royal Society of Health Congress, held at Eastbourne 24th–28th April, 1972
66. Hession, M. (1976). Evidence for the select parliamentary (UK) Committee on violence in the family, from the Institute of Child Psychology. May 1976
67. Holman, R. R. and Kanwar, S. (1975). Early life of the battered child. *Arch. Dis. Chld.*, 78
68. Editorial (1971). Violent Parents. *Lancet.*, **ii,** 1017

69. MacKeith, R. (1974). Speculations on non-accidental injury as a cause of chronic brain disorder. *Devel. Med. Chld Neurol.*, **16**, 216
70. Rose, N., Owtram, P., Pickett, J., Marran, B. and Maton, A. (1975). Registers of suspected non-accidental injury. (London: NSPCC)
71. Scott, P. D. (1973). Parents who kill their children. *Med. Sci. Law.*, **13**, 120
72. Smith, S. M. and Hanson, R. (1974). 134 battered children: a medical and psychological study. *Br. Med. J.*, **3**, 666
73. Sills, J. A., Thomas, L. J. and Rosenbloom, L. (1977). Non-accidental injury; a two year study in central Liverpool. *Devel. Med. Chld Neurol.*, **19**, 26
74. The Tunbridge Wells Study Group. (1973). Non-accidental injury to children. Compiled by Alfred White Franklin, sponsored by the Spastics Society
75. Adelson, L. (1961). Slaughter of the innocents. *N. Engl. J. Med.*, **264**, 1345
76. Akbarnia, B., Torg, J. S., Kirkpatrick, J. and Sussman, S. (1975). Manifestations of the battered-child syndrome. *J. Bone Joint Surg.*, **56-A**, 1159
77. Blumberg, M. L. (1974). Psychopathology of the abusing parent. *Am. J. Psychother.*, **28**, 21
78. Bryant, H. D., Billingsley, A., Kerry, G. A., Leefman, W. V., Merrill, E. J., Senecal, G. R. and Walsh, B. G. (1963). Physical Abuse of Children. An Agency Study. *Child Welfare*, **42**, 125
79. Elmer, E. (1967). *Children in Jeopardy*. (University of Pittsburgh Press)
80. Furst, W. D. (1975). The medical profession and child abuse in Texas. *Texas Med.*, **71**, 87
81. George, J. E. (1973). Spare the rod. A survey of the battered child syndrome. *Forensic Sci.*, **2**, 129
82. Gil, D. G. (1970). *Violence Against Children* (Cambridge, Mass: Harvard University Press)
83. Gil, D. G. (1968). Incidence of child abuse and demographic characteristics of person involved. In: *The Battered Child* (R. E. Helfer and C. H. Kempe, (eds.)). (University of Chicago Press)
84. Green, F. C. (1975). Child abuse and neglect. *Pediatr. Clin. N. Am.*, **22**, 329
85. Hall, D. A. (1974). Protecting the abused child in Maine. *J. Maine Med. Assoc.*, 148
86. Helfer, R. E. and Pollock, C. B. (1968). The Battered Child Syndrome. *Adv. Pediatr.*, **15**, 9
87. Hudson, P., Bagdon, L., Haroutunian, A. and Winters, H. (1975). The health professions and child abuse and neglect. *J. Med. Soc. New Jersey*, **72**, 605
88. Jaffe, A. C. Dynneson, L. and ten Bensel, R. W. (1975). Sexual abuse of children. *Am. J. Dis. Chid.*, **129**, 689
89. Lauer, B., Broeck, E. T. and Grossman, M. (1974). Battered child syndrome: review of 130 patients with controls. From the Dept. of Pediatrics, San Francisco General Hospital and University of California, *Pediatrics*, **54**, 67
90. Merrill, E. J. (1962). Protecting the battered child: Part I. Physical abuse of children. American Humane Association, Children's Division report for the 89th Annual Forum of the National Conference on Social Welfare, New York City, May 31st 1962
91. Mindlin, R. L. (1974). Child abuse and neglect; The role of the pediatrician and the academy. *Pediatrics*, **54**, 393
92. Morse, C. W., Sahler, O. J. Z. and Friedman, S. B. (1970). A three year follow-up study of abused and neglected children. *Am. J. Dis. Chld.*, **120**, 439
93. Nazzaro, J. (1974). Child abuse and neglect. *Exceptional Children*, **40**, 351
94. Schloesser, P. T. (1964). The abused child. *Bull. Menninger Clin.*, **28**, 260
95. Silver, L. B. (1968). Child abuse syndrome: a review. *Med. Times*, **96**, 803
96. Solomon, T. (1971). History and demography of child abuse. Symposium on child abuse. New York University Medical Centre, 15.6.71. Published in *Pediatrics*, **51**, April 1973
97. Weston, J. T. (1968). The pathology of child abuse. In: *The Battered Child*, R. E. Helfer, and C. H. Kempe (eds.). (Chicago: University of Chicago Press)
98. Zalba, S. R. (1966). The abused child. A survey of the problem. *Social Work*, **2**, 3

99. Dawe, K. E. (1973). Maltreated children at home and overseas. Royal Children's Hospital, Melbourne Australia. *Aust. Paediat. J.*, **9**, 177

100. Dawe, K. E. (1973). Child abuse in Nova Scotia. *Aust. Paediatric J.*, **9**, 294

101. Fried, C. T. (1973). Child Abuse is a Family Social Disease. *Can. Family Phys.*, Aug. 1973, 53

102. McRae, K. N., Ferguson, C. A. and Lederman, R. S. (1973). The battered child syndrome. *Med. Assoc. J.*, **108**, 859

103. Rodenburg, M. (1971). Child murder by depressed parents. *Can. Psychiatr. Assoc. J.*, **16**, 41

104. Trube-Becker, E. (1971). Autopsy of children who have died suddenly. *Medizinische Klinik*, **66**, 58 (English Summary in the Journal *Ann. Nestle*, **27**, 67, 1972)

105. Kempe, C. H. (1972). Paper Presented to Harvard interfaculty Seminar on Child Rearing in Urban America.

106. Smith, S. M. (1975). Personal communication

107. Bonjer, A. J. (Director, Vereniging tegen kindermischandeling) Personal communication

108. Oliver, J. E. (1975). Microcephaly following baby battering and shaking. *Br. Med. J.*, **2**, 262

109. James, H. E. and Schut, L. (1974). The neurosurgeon and the battered child. *Surg. Neurol.*, **2**, 415

110. Martin, H. P. (1975). The effect of child abuse on the neurologic and personality development of children. *Developmental and Child Neurology*, p. 389. (Paper given during annual meeting of the American Academy for Cerebral Palsy, 1974)

111. Smith, S. and Noble, S. (1973). Battered children and their parents. *New Society*, **26**, No. 580, 393

112. Oliver, J. E. (1975). Statistics of child abuse. *Br. Med. J.*, **3**, 99

113. Brown, R. H. (1973). The battered child. *Chicago Med. Soc. Bull.*, March 1973

114. Rood-de-Boer, M. (1971). Child care in the Netherlands. National Federation for Child Welfare. The Hague

115. Directie Kinderbescherming-Ministerie Van Justitie. (1973). Verslag over de jaren, 1969–70. Staatsuitgeverij's-Gravenhage (English summaries and English notes explaining the tables)

116. Children in Care in England and Wales, (1973). Dept. of Health and Social Services and the Welsh Office, Command Paper, 5815, HMSO

117. Pringle, M. L. K. (1971). *Deprivation and Education*. Studies in Child Development; National Bureau for Co-operation in Child Care. (London: Longmans)

118. Children in Care in England and Wales (1969). Home Office Command Paper 4263, reprinted 1972, HMSO

119. Children in Care in England and Wales (1970). Home Office Command Paper 4559; HMSO

120. Children in Care in England and Wales (1971). DHSS and the Welsh Office, Command Paper 5100, HMSO

121. Children in Care in England and Wales (1973). Dept. Health and Social Security and the Welsh Office, Command Paper 5434, HMSO

122. Montagu, N. L. J. (1975). Personal communication

123. Annual Report (1972). National Society for the Prevention of Cruelty to Children

124. Annual Report (1973). National Society for the Prevention of Cruelty to Children

125. Gil, D. G. (1969). Physical abuse of children. Findings and implications of a nationwide survey. *Pediatrics*, **44**, 857

126. De Francis, V. (1966). *Child Abuse Legislation*. (Denver: American Humane Association, Children's Division)

127. Kempe, C. H. (1972). Paper presented to Harvard Inter-Faculty Seminar on Child Rearing in Urban America

128. Jacobziner, J. (1964). Rescuing the Battered Child. *Am. J. Nursing*, **64**, 92

129. *Planning for the Protection and Care of Neglected Children in California* (1964). (Sacramento: National Study Service)

130. American Public Welfare Association (1958). Preventive and Protective Services to Children. A responsibility of the Public Welfare Agency. Chicago

131. Newcombe, H. B. (1966). Familial tendencies in diseases of children. *Brit. J. Prevent. Soc. Med.*, **20**, 49

132. Kempe, C. H. and Helfer, R. E. (1972). *Helping the Battered Child and his Family.* (Philadelphia: Lippincott)

133. Scott, P. D. (1973). Fatal battered baby cases. *Med. Sci. Law*, **13**, 197

134. Smith, S. M., Hanson, R. and Noble S. (1974). Social aspects of the Battered Baby Syndrome. *Br. J. Psychiat.*, **125**, 568

6 The Extent of Child Abuse

J. E. OLIVER, JANE COX AND ANNE BUCHANAN

Part I – SEVERELY ILL-TREATED YOUNG CHILDREN IN NORTH-EAST WILTSHIRE (J. E. Oliver, Jane Cox and Ann Buchanan)

INTRODUCTION AND ACKNOWLEDGEMENTS

This clinical and epidemiological study appears to be the first to attempt intensive assessment of the extent of severe child abuse in a defined population. The methods of case detection which had to be adopted were those of person and family record linkage[1]. The clinical part of this study of child abuse was carried out by a psychiatrist (J. E. Oliver), a sociologist (Jane Cox), and a social worker (Audrey Taylor) with the support of clinical research funds from the Oxford Regional Hospital Board. Other aspects of the study were completed and analysed with the help of the Director of the Oxford University Unit of Clinical Epidemiology, J. A. Baldwin (also a psychiatrist).

Part I contains much of the epidemiological data from the published report of 1974, but does not include most of the clinical detail from that report, nor the 33 pages of family histories, nor the appendices on classification or 'Points of Suspicion'[1]. The parts of that report which classify the reasons for absence of information on cases of cruelty to children ('submerged data') are also not included here. The Results and Discussion headings closely follow a more recent publication, which combines the epidemiological findings of the 1974 report with additional data on the 1972–73 families[2]. Our gratitude is expressed to our colleague Dr John Baldwin, who undertook a major part both of the data analysis, and of the assessment of the implications of the data for this study; also to the very large number of doctors, social workers, probation officers, police, and charitable society workers, who gave freely of their time and made great efforts to help and collaborate with us.

Certain children referred to the child psychiatry services and to subnormality hospitals in north-east Wiltshire were seen to have been ill-treated or neglected by their parents or guardians. Careful documentation showed that some mentally handicapped children had been normal at birth, and that subnormality associated with brain damage was a consequence of assaults by parents[3]. A systematic survey was started in January 1971 with a primary aim of identifying all young children known to have been actively ill-treated in a given geographical area, and so yield an estimate of the extent of the condition. Secondary aims of the study were to assess the types and severity of injury, and the duration over which assaults occurred in the presenting families; and to describe features of the families which might justify a reappraisal of our existing organization of records and services if our society seriously wishes to limit cruelty to young children in an effective way. North-east Wiltshire had a population of 200 000 with 18 500 children under 5 years old and 3600 live births annually. The period 1965–1970 was studied retrospectively. The year 1971 was used to alert professional people to the extent and complexities of the problem, and the numbers of children ascertained from January 1972 to June 1973 were obtained for comparison with the earlier period. It soon became apparent that the initial project was too ambitious because of the unexpected extent of child abuse, and the very great difficulties in obtaining reliable information[4–16]. Selection of families for detailed study therefore was narrowed to those in which the presenting child was aged under 5 years, and had been subjected to very severe active physical ill-treatment, the 'severe abuse' category.

Criteria for severe abuse

Satisfaction of any one or more of the following six criteria merited inclusion of the family of a child under 5 years old:

(1) Prolonged assaults of such severity that death ensued[17–20]. Infanticides and murderers were not included automatically[21–23].
(2) Skull or facial bone fractures[24].
(3) Bleeding into or around the brain[11,24–29]; brain damage with consequent impairment of either intellect or functioning of one of the senses, or proper functioning of the central nervous system; direct damage to the vision[30,31].
(4) Two or more instances of mutilation requiring medical attention such as bites, burns, crushes or cuts[32,33].
(5) Three or more separate instances of fracture and/or severe bruising requiring medical attention[7,17,34–40].
(6) Multiple fractures and/or severe internal injuries[17,25,35,40].

We were not able to consider as a criterion for severe abuse temporary impairment of oxygenation of the brain caused by assault. Reports of unconsciousness, resulting from the intentional placing of polythene bags over the child's head, obstruction of breathing (including one instance of holding the child's head so that vomit was inhaled), obstruction of neck vessels, and holding the child's head under water were frequent in certain families.

Moderate abuse

Degrees of assault or injury which approached but did not entirely meet the criteria for severe abuse were classified as 'moderate abuse', and episodes of suffocation were included here. Sibs of severely abused children frequently met the criteria for moderate abuse and data on them are presented briefly. Families were referred with children who could be placed only in the 'moderate abuse' category, but these were underestimated, and are considered further in Part II.

Neglect

Many of the presenting children and their sibilings had undergone other forms of ill-treatment in addition to the essential criteria for selection. These included deprivation of food, fluids, freedom, warmth, medical treatment, etc.[41-45], prolonged unnecessary psychological stress, and various mental assaults[46-49]. This group of ill-treatments was classified as 'neglect' and further subdivided into 'severe' and 'moderate' according to the severity and duration of the deprivation, and age of the child. Abandonment was classified as a form of neglect.

Criteria for inclusion in study

If a child was ascertained as having been injured in such a way as to satisfy one or more of the criteria for severe abuse, the family was included in the study if the severe abuse occurred:

(1) When the child was under 5 years old.

and (2) In the period January 1965 to June 1973.

and (3) While the family were resident in north-east Wiltshire.

Certain of the brothers and sisters had been assaulted in similar or more severe ways than the presenting children. These sibs were not counted as index children if the injuries were not inflicted during the relevant period, or if the child was over 5 years old at the time of the injury, or if the family was not in the demarcated area of north-east Wiltshire at that time. The figures for severely physically abused young children in 1972 and the first half year of 1973 are given separately from the figures for the years 1965–1971 because increased awareness amongst the professional people concerned indicated widespread under-reporting in the whole area before 1971.

Ascertainment of the numbers of young children fulfilling the 'severe abuse' criteria, and selection of families for intensive study

One of us (JEO) was in an almost unique situation in which to obtain access to confidential data. Our responsibilities encompassed most of the departments directly or indirectly concerned with child welfare in the area. Three of us (JEO, JC, and AT) personally saw most of the officials and professional people concerned with the health and welfare of young children in north-east Wiltshire, explaining our criteria and listening to comments, reservations and other points of issue. The individuals and agencies which identified severely and actively ill-treated young children over the period January 1965 to June 1973 are shown in Table 6.1. The total number of such children was 60. Nomadic and certain army families posed special problems. Families on the Tidworth Military and Lyneham RAF camps were excluded unless their children were referred to local services. We investigated as far as possible other families in the area whose children were assaulted in north-east Wiltshire but taken elsewhere for treatment, and a few nomads on the fringe of the area whose children were treated in our hospitals.

By June 1973 there were altogether 34 families with 38 presenting children firmly ascertained for the seven year period 1965–1971 who were studied in detail. A further 22 children were ascertained in the 18 months January 1972 to June 1973.

SUBMERGED DATA: INVESTIGATION IN DEPTH OF THE 34 FAMILIES WITH 38 YOUNG CHILDREN WHO HAD BEEN SEVERELY ABUSED IN THE SEVEN YEARS 1965–1971

Two of us, personally and separately, saw half the total parents, and more than half the presenting children. Three of us saw children, parents, relatives and professional people concerned with the families and were involved in the treatment of some families. For 4 out of 34 families the information was gleaned entirely from other professional people and written notes. For the other 30 the information was both first hand and from professional people and from files. The sources of information and methods of substantiating data have been discussed elsewhere[50,51].

Obtaining reliable and relatively complete data on the 34 families was a complex task, making heavy demands on time, energy and imagination. Information was kept in coded confidential files to which we alone had access. Nevertheless, considerations of confidentiality often limited availability of data. This aspect, combined with episodes of professional incredulity ('I know she's an inadequate Mum, but never a batterer'), made the work emotionally very demanding.

Parents also misrepresented themselves without necessarily consciously lying, omitting information or deceiving. They frequently presented an ideal or facade which bore little relation to reality (cf. Abrahamson[52]). Sentimentality could conceal irresponsibility in essentials. Sentimental or idealized versions of the parents' own upbringing often had led professional people to record accounts of neutral or innocuous family histories which were misleading. Parents commonly made global statements which indicated a belief in the normality of

Table 6.1 Severely abused young children in north-east Wiltshire, 1965–1973. Numbers of notifications[1] and confirmations by agencies and professional or other groups of individuals

Agency and group	Notifications	Confirmations	Agency and group	Notifications	Confirmations
Doctors and Nurses			*The Family*		
Paediatricians	20	18	Parent (or parent substitute)	3	10
Paediatrician or Neurologist at Special Care Baby Unit	—	4	Other relative (not a child)	1	2
Casualty Officer	3	—	The attacked child or a sibling	—	1
Orthopaedic Surgeon	3	—	TOTAL	4	13
Family Doctor	5	9			
Medical Officer of Health	4	5	*The Public*		
Health Visitors	6	6	Local newspaper	3	—
Infant Welfare Clinic	1	3	Neighbours	3	1
Other Nurse	1	—	Anonymous	—	1
Adult Psychiatrist	1	5	Police	6	1
Child Psychiatrist	2	10	TOTAL	12	3
Subnormality Psychiatrist	1	2			
Ophthalmologist	—	1	Study Team[2]	10	6
Prison Medical Officer	—	2	GRAND TOTAL[3]	94	120
Military Hospital Doctor	2	1			
Pathologist	4	2			
TOTAL	53	68			
Social Welfare Organizations					
NSPCC	6	7			
Dept. of Social Services	7	8			
Hospital Social Workers	1	13			
Probation Officers	1	2			
TOTAL	15	30			

1. Notification here means either that the professional or agency informed us, or that the Wiltshire Medical Officer of Health was informed, or that the diagnosis of baby battering was claimed in newspaper articles.
2. Information obtained by us while following up other children in the family suspected of having been ill-treated.
3. The totals are greater than the number of severely abused young children (60) because notifications and confirmations could come from more than one source.

their own upbringing in general terms, which contrasted dramatically with contradictory and unpleasant specific accounts couched in detailed terms (cf. Abrahamson[52]). Such parents usually appeared unaware of these discrepancies, and became bewildered when their previous statements were compared. In this respect, old records sometimes proved more reliable than direct interviews. Much of the evidence involved memorizing and promptly recording verbatim statements. Experience had taught us to be sceptical about negative information and vague generalizations. Facts were collected from as many sources as possible, and data from each source checked against those from other sources.

The general method of investigation is schematized in Table 6.2. The following are examples of problems encountered in compiling a family history, illustrating the points to check which are listed in Table 6.2:

(i) In 8 families the presenting child was known by two or more different surnames. In 5 families two or more first christian names were used.

(ii) The presenting child in one family had notes filed under three surnames: his mother's birth surname (spelt four different ways) because he was illegitimate, his first step-father's name (spelt two different ways), and his second step-father's name. There were six variations in spelling of the family surname in another family as well as three aliases in the grandparents' generation.

(iii) In one kindred the child did not live in Wiltshire at the time of the investigation in 1971, but was treated in north-east Wiltshire because he was in the local hospital's catchment area. He thus had local medical notes, medical social work notes, NSPCC notes, and a file with a local child psychiatrist. He had social service department notes, not only for his current area, but also a separate file in another part of Wiltshire where he used to live. In addition, there was a variety of files in an adjacent county.

(iv) In the master index of the local general hospital, a system of putting cards for psychiatric patients next to those for general patients had been started about two years previously, so that in theory it could be established quickly if a person was receiving or had received psychiatric treatment. In one case, great-grandmother did not have such a card, but was found to have been a psychiatric inpatient in the past. The maternal uncle did not have a card because his treatment started very recently and the record had not reached the master index.

(v) Only 10 out of the 34 families had apparently straightforward structures (2 parents + legitimate children). In one family there had been six children up to 1973. All were illegitimate, with three fathers involved. One died of pneumonia at nine months. The second was adopted by grandmother, the third (the presenting child) and fourth were in care, and the fifth and sixth were with mother and cohabitee.

(vi) This check revealed that the eldest child in two families was no longer alive. In direct interviews, parents often fail to reveal dead, damaged or aban-

Facts required	Sources of information	Points to check
A. The presenting child	(a) Files, notes and personal knowledge of child and his family by referring agency	(i) If the child has changed his name in full or part, or a past or present alias
1. Present surname and all forenames		
2. Date and place of birth	(b) All other medical, legal and social work depts. which might know the family either locally or in another area	(ii) A child's notes may be filed under one of his parents' names, a family name, the name of a cohabitee, foster parent, etc. There may be various spellings of each surname
3. Present and past addresses		
4. Details and dates of injuries		
5. Physical, intellectual and social progress from birth onwards	(c) Direct interview with families and relatives of the child	(iii) The catchment areas of hospitals, medical practitioners, social work offices etc., vary. They may also be altered by new legislation
		(iv) Changes in office procedure
B. Sibs of the presenting child	(a) (b) (c) plus:	(i) (ii) (iii) (iv) plus:
6. Total number of full, half and step sibs. Their surnames and previous surnames	(d) Birth and death records in register offices and churches	(v) Sibs may be missed who have died, been adopted, are living with a relative, friend or foster parent
7. Their relationships to the presenting child	(e) Pathologists' records	(vi) Compare dates of birth records of mother's confinements
8. Their dates and places of birth		
9. Addresses, past and present		
10. Their medical and social histories		
11. Number and identity of ill-treated and poorly cared for sibs		
12. Surnames of cohabitees of the parent (past or present) caring for any of the children in the family		
C. Relatives of the presenting child*	(a) (b) (c) (d) (e) plus:	(vii) Name changes, aliases and variations
13. Family membership and relationships. Forenames, birth surnames of mothers and grandmothers	(f) Marriage records in register offices and churches	(viii) Notes may be filed under a variety of names
	(g) Street directories and voters' lists in reference libraries locally and in any other area where a relative is known to have lived	(ix) Cross-check all known names with known addresses, in street directories, voters' lists and indexes of names in medical and social work offices. Look at all people of the given surname plus variations and check if there are relatives
14. All addresses, present and past. Dates and places of birth		
15. Medical and social histories of all family members	(h) Housing lists	(x) Ask all departments, both local and out of the area, if old records exist and if so, from what date and where they are kept
16. Number of ill-treated and poorly cared-for children in previous generations	(i) Newspaper cuttings	

---

* Gibbens and Walker[33] commented that 'nearly half (of the battering fathers in their series) were either ignorant of their siblings' whereabouts, indifferent, or actively hostile to them'. Here early files on uncles and aunts of battered children often furnished detail for the case histories which were given in appendix I of our main study'. Certain of the abusive parents in this series did not even know of the existence of their sibs, let alone their whereabouts!

doned previous children.

(vii) (viii) (ix) Many family members were established by this 'detective-work' method of investigation, who were not revealed by the parents in family histories given to doctors or social workers[51].

(x) Ill-treatment and/or neglect by the present abusing parents in the 1940s in 4 families was still on record at the local NSPCC office. Records of children in care since the 1948 Act are kept in central county archives until the individual is aged 21. Psychiatric notes from the mid-nineteenth century were found for some elderly relatives in the survey families. Records were lost by authorized destructions, damp, a bulldozer accidentally pushing the wrong wall, changes of sitings of hospitals and departments, unauthorized destruction, and for many other reasons. Known records of hospital admissions, etc., often were not found from areas outside the county, even when much detail was given to help in tracing. Nevertheless, it was surprising how much information was retrieved, considering the variety of reasons for non-availability of earlier records.

It is necessary to discuss family fact-finding in detail because the process of the submerging of relevant factual data in the known *severely* abusive families, occurred even more insidiously in the much more numerous abuse and neglect families discussed in Part II.

RESULTS

A total of 38 children were ascertained as having been assaulted in the seven years 1965–1971 in north-east Wiltshire to such an extent as to meet the criteria for severe abuse. These presenting children came from 34 families, 4 families each contributing two children, and these families were the subjects for detailed study. A further 22 children were ascertained as meeting the same criteria in the 18 months January 1972 to June 1973, but detailed consideration of the children and their families is mainly concentrated on the retrospective series.

The presenting children

The sex and age distributions of children in the two series are shown in Table 6.3. In the retrospective series four fifths were under 1 year old at the onset of severe abuse and none were in the second year, while in the prospective series about the same proportion were fairly evenly divided between the first and second years of life. It was thought that in the earlier period 1 year old children, having passed from the responsibility of the paediatric services, were not under such close surveillance until they reached pre-school age. This suggestion is supported by the annual sex/age specific rates per thousand population (Table 6.4). Of children under 1 year 83% of the retrospective series and 89% of the prospective series were under 6 months. Very few children were ascertained over the age of 2 in either series. A possible explanation of the small numbers of

Table 6.3 Severely abused children in north-east Wiltshire, 1965–mid-1973. Numbers and percentage distribution by sex and age at commencement of abuse

Age in completed years	Males 1965–1971		Males 1972–mid-1973		Females 1965–1971		Females 1972–mid-1973		Total 1965–1971		Total 1972–mid-1973	
	No.	%	No.	%	No.	%	No.	%	No.	%	No.	%
0	16	72.7	3	37.5	15	93.7	6	42.8	31	81.6	9	40.9
1	0	—	2	25.0	0	—	6	42.8	0	—	8	36.4
2	4	18.2	2	25.0	1	6.3	2	14.3	5	13.2	4	18.2
3	2	9.1	0	—	0	—	0	—	2	5.2	0	—
4	0	—	1	12.5	0	—	0	—	0	—	1	4.5
TOTAL 0–4	22	100.0	8	100.0	16	100.0	14	99.9	38	100.0	22	100.0

χ^2 for females aged 0 and $> 0 = 6.95$; $p = < 0.01$ (with Yates' correction)
No significant differences in males, or between males and females aged 0 or > 0

Table 6.4 Severely abused children in north-east Wiltshire, 1965–mid-1973. Annual sex/age specific rates per thousand population, 1965–1971, 1972–mid-1973.

Age in completed years	Males 1965–1971	Males 1972–mid-1973	Females 1965–1971	Females 1972–mid-1973	Total 1965–1971	Total 1972–mid-1973
0	1.22	1.07	1.20	2.25	1.21	1.64
1	—	0.72	—	2.26	—	1.47
2	0.31	0.73	0.08	0.73	0.20	0.73
3	0.15	—	—	—	0.08	—
TOTAL 0–3	0.42	0.62	0.32	1.31	0.37	0.96

3 and 4 year olds is that by this age they are more robust and so less easily damaged to such an extent as to meet the criteria for severe abuse. Either their injuries are less severe because they are stronger or because they are more successful in avoiding the most serious assaults. Less severely injured children in this age group were ascertained. Furthermore, proof that injury is not accidental is more difficult. Fractures, for example, may occur during play and it may be impossible to determine the precise cause.

Males outnumbered females in the retrospective series in the ratio 1.4:1. In contrast, males were fewer than females in the prospective series in the ratio 1:1.7.

Rate of severe abuse

The single case aged 4 years has been omitted from rate calculations so that, unless otherwise specified, total rates are for the age group 0–3 years. Table 6.4 shows that the annual rate for children under 4 in the prospective series (1972–mid-1973) was 2.6 times that in the retrospective series (1965–1971) and was almost 1 per thousand. The increase affected both sexes and each age group but was most marked in girls and those aged 1 year.

There were 4 deaths from abuse in the retrospective series, giving an annual rate of 0.04 per thousand under 4 years old. There were 2 deaths from abuse in the prospective series, an annual rate of 0.09 per thousand under 4, an increase of 2.55 times.

Features of the retrospective series of children

The children were much more frequently abnormal at birth than in the population as a whole. Eight (21%) were premature compared with 6.7% in the Perinatal Mortality Survey[54]. Four children (10%) had congenital defects compared with about 3% in most surveys. Three had heart defects, one of whom was a mongol. One of these three had a squint, and the fourth had abnormally long second toes which required surgical correction. Nine (23%) of the children were illegitimate compared with 7.6% in the local population. The mothers of eight of the children had originally requested termination of the pregnancy or sterilization, but had been refused.

Prominent clinical features of the presenting children were closely similar to those reported by Galdston[55]. They included fear of parents or other adults (42%), withdrawal, listlessness or drowsiness (42%), hyperactivity or repetitive motor activity (29%), persistent crying or irritability (45%), and marked pallor (34%). All these figures are exclusive of severely subnormal children. Fear of adults was often extreme and sometimes associated with situations in which abuse had occurred such as toilet training, bathing or play. Unresponsive, apathetic children sometimes showed no reaction to their injuries, and often were characterized by their parents as 'useless' or 'lazy'.

Withdrawal, irritability, and crying or screaming apparently brought on by neglect or abuse, often precipitated further attacks which reinforced the behaviour.

Injuries

A total of 225 separate incidents consisting of one or more injuries were ascertained among the 38 children, a mean of 5.9 incidents per child with a range of 1 to 23. The main classes of injury and numbers of children affected are shown in Table 6.5. As might be expected, nearly all the children had soft tissue injuries and were judged to have been emotionally affected by the assaults, but the high proportions of children severely physically damaged in several ways is outstanding. A total of 517 separate physical injuries and illnesses, including healed or partially healed fractures, was ascertained, a mean of 13.6 per child. This is almost certainly a considerable underestimate because healed superficial injuries which were not medically treated were missed. There were 40 instances of brain damage, speech and locomotor defects probably caused by injury, most of the affected children exhibiting more than one defect. The specific injuries and defects are enumerated, together with the numbers of children affected, in Tables 6.6 and 6.7. Fractures, bruising of the head, face, body and limbs, and lacerations about the head and face were most common, but episodes of unconsciousness were also outstandingly frequent. Malnutrition, dehydration, and infections associated with these insults were common. Severe and irreparable damage to the brain and central nervous system caused by fractures of the skull and bleeding into or around the brain were disturbingly frequent. The mean annual rate for skull fracture over the 7 year period of the study was 0.12 per thousand under 4 and that for intracranial haemorrhage was 0.16 per thousand. Since these rates are likely to be underestimates of similar order to the overall rate for the retrospective series, it is probable that abuse

Table 6.5 Type of injury

Type of injury	No. at risk*	No. affected	Proportion affected (%)
Skull fracture	38	12	31.6
Intra-cranial haemorrhage and other brain injury	37	16	43.2
Fractures other than skull	38	22	57.9
Soft tissue injuries	38	36	94.7
Severe neglect reported	36	18	47.4
Starvation, deprivation of fluids, failure to thrive for non-medical reasons, medically confirmed	36	10	27.8
Persistent or severe emotional trauma	28	25	89.3

* Includes only children known to have been at risk.
Some types of damage such as 'failure to thrive' and emotional trauma were not applicable to some children, as when the child was not with the relevant parent for a long enough period.

Table 6.6 **All ascertained injuries and disabilities of the 38 index children**

Injury	Children	Instances
Skull fracture	12	≮17
Subdural haematoma	12	15
Subarachnoid haemorrhage	10	14
Retinal haemorrhage	7	8
Other intra-cranial bleeding	8	9
?Brain damage due to injury	9	—
Temporary obstruction of breathing*	9	14
Fits, loss of consciousness	15	31
Speech defects	16	—
Locomotor defects	15	—
Fractures other than skull	22	≮52
Bruising of head	22	55
Bruising of face and ears	14	37
Bruising of neck	9	12
Bruising of mouth	3	4
Bruising of nose	7	10
Bruising of eyes	9	18
Bruising of body and limbs	21	47
Lacerations of head	8	14
Lacerations of face	9	21
Lacerations of lip	3	5
Lacerations of body and limbs	9	15
Crushed fingers and nails	2	6
Finger-grip bruises of face	3	14
Finger-grip bruises of body and limbs	5	12
Scratched neck	1	1
Mutilation of penis	1	≮3
Bites	2	3
Burns and scalds	7	14
Failure to thrive, malnutrition	14	28
Dehydration	5	5
Anaemia	7	12
Bronchitis/pneumonia during periods of neglect	11	23

* Reports by parents, relatives or neighbours. Includes holding head under water (5 instances), head in polythene bag (2 instances), hands round throat (1 instance), hands or pillow over face (6 instances).

Table 6.7 **Fractures of the 38 index children**

	Children	Instances
Skull	12	<17
Femur	7	8
Tibia	2	2
Fibula	2	2
Clavicle	2	2
Humerus	3	3
Radius	3	3
Ulna	4	4
Pelvis	2	2
Ribs	7	26
3 or more fractures at once	7	7

contributes substantially to the total rates for these injuries in this age group. Multiple injuries and multiple incidents are well known features of these assaults, and it has been observed that injuries to the head and face are often experienced repeatedly by the same child[5,56]. This was found also in some of our series of children. Although multiple fractures were common, it appears that, apart from the skull and ribs, the same fracture rarely recurs in the same child.

Duration of severe abuse

The total periods (regardless of age at ascertainment) over which severe abuse extended varied widely. In 3 cases severe battering took place only in the space of 1 to 4 hours, and in 2 others over 1 to 3 days. Four children were severely abused over 1 to 2 weeks. The most common history was of severe abuse extending over 1 to 10 months (17 children), while the remaining 12 children were subjected to repeated episodes covering from 1 to over 8 years. When lesser degrees of abuse were taken into account the distribution shifted toward the very long periods with 16 children affected from 1 to over 8 years.

An example can be given of the chronological pattern of injuries and disorders seen in one little girl over 4 years. The cauliflower ears are still apparent at the age of 8, together with many residual scars to the fingers. The child looks, in some respects, like a professional boxer, this being largely the consequence of her experiences in the first 4 years of life.

It is important to emphasize that, of the five children who were assaulted over a period of hours or days, only one escaped permanent damage. One was killed, two were rendered severely subnormal and one of these became blind and deaf as well, while the fifth became epileptic with an abnormal EEG and probably was made educationally subnormal.

OUTCOME FOR THE 38 (1965–1971) CHILDREN

By mid-1973, four children (10%) had been killed by parents or had died in suspicious circumstances, two (0.02/1000/annum) from brain haemorrhage following skull fracture, and two (0.02/1000/annum) from asphyxia caused by inhalation of vomit (cf. Gormsen and Vesterdal[57]; Vesterdal[58]). Of those remaining alive on whom an assessment was possible 8 out of 30 (27%) were intellectually impaired due to induced brain damage, 10 out of 30 (33%) had fits or abnormal EEG patterns, and 17 out of 31 (55%) had permanent scarring or disablement caused by their injuries. Social, educational or emotional disturbance, or probable intellectual impairment was noted in 22 out of 29 (76%) children (cf. Part III; also[24,25,59–64]).

Of the 34 survivors, 14 (41%) remained with the parent or parents responsible for the injuries, and only 3 (9%) were with parents or relatives who had not injured them, by the end of the study. A further three had been adopted, 13

(38%) were permanently or intermittently in foster homes, and 10 (29%) had been in hospitals or institutions for long periods.

Structure and features of the retrospective* series of 34 families

Marital condition

In 26 (76%) of the families, the married natural parents were responsible for the children when the principal injuries occurred. Four families consisted of a natural parent and a step-parent or cohabitee, 2 were adoptive families, while 2 had unmarried mothers. In 8 (24%) families at least one of the natural parents had been divorced, compared with 0.58 expected in a sample of married and divorced persons of the same sex and age structure in north-east Wiltshire, 9 (27%) had been separated, and 2 had been widowed. Six (18%) of the men were away for long periods in the armed forces or in prison. (The proportion of natural parents in the prospective series of 22 families who were divorced, separated or parted by, for instance, imprisonment or hospitalization, was 36%.) Four men and three women were in their second marriages. The mean age at marriage or cohabitation of the responsible parents was 21 for women (ranging from 16 to 39) and 23 for men (ranging from 16 to 37). Sixteen women and six men were under age 20 at marriage or start of cohabitation.

Origin

The place of birth distribution of the parents or guardians in the 34 families is shown in Table 6.8. It can be seen that, while the majority of parents of each sex came from England, there was a larger proportion of the males than of the females who 'belonged' to north-east Wiltshire.

Occupation and social position

It was difficult to construct reliable occupational histories of the male parents or guardians. Most of the men had unstable work records with frequent changes of job and periods of unemployment. Table 6.9 gives the best distribution which could be compiled, though its reliability is not high. A number of the unskilled labourers did occasional spells as lorry or van drivers, and there was a tendency for the women to accord their partners higher occupational attainments than the facts warranted. Nevertheless, at least two out of three were social class V families in the retrospective series and a similar proportion of the prospective series were also of the same class. Of the 33 families with

---

* Some information (in Tables 6.9 and 6.11, as well as in the text) is also given on the prospective series, for comparison with the earlier group.

fathers or father surrogates, 16 (48%) of the men were unemployed at the time of the principal injuries. (The comparable figure in the prospective series was 27%.)

Place of residence

The addresses of the index children at birth and during the most severe assaults are set out in Table 6.10. These do not reflect the high level of residen-

Table 6.8 Place of birth distribution of the parents or guardians of the 34 (1965–1971) families

	Males	*Females*
Swindon	11	7
N.E. Wilts.	2	2
London	8	4
Other England	6	14
Scotland	1	1
N. Ireland	1	1
S. Ireland	1	1
Foreign	2	1
Unknown	2	3
TOTAL	34*	34

* Includes one father of the child of an unmarried mother, who had little or no contact with his child.

Table 6.9 Designated occupation of fathers or male guardians (when not unemployed – see text)

1965–1971 series		*1972–mid-1973 series*	
Unskilled labourers or drivers	24	Unskilled labourers or driver	13
Machine operators	2	Machine operator	1
Railway signalman	1	Mechanic	1
Clerical	1	Plasterer's assistant	1
Draughtsman	1	Policeman	1
Electronics engineer	1	Bookbinder	1
Armed Forces	4	Armed Forces	3
		None (blind)	1
TOTAL	34	TOTAL	22

Table 6.10 Place of residence of index children

	At birth	*During most severe assaults**
Swindon	22	23
N.E. Wilts.	4	8
London	3	2*
Other Britain	7	5*
Foreign	2	—
Total	38	38

* Other assaults precipitated the intervention in N.E. Wilts.

tial mobility of the families, many of whom moved house abruptly, unexpectedly and frequently. Some families appeared to try to conceal their movements, which evidently were made in response to pressures such as creditors, health or social service staff seeking access, or hostile neighbours. The types of accommodation often were of poor quality, but half the families were living in relatively good conditions at the time of the main assaults, such as council houses, some privately rented properties and owner occupied homes (Table 6.11). It is noteworthy that two of the children were assaulted while in mother and baby homes. The proportion sharing accommodation was lower in the retrospective series (13%) than in the prospective series (45%).

Table 6.11   Accommodation at time of main assaults

	1965–1971 series	1972–mid-1973 series
Private rented	13	0
Council rented	10	8
Shared (including 'squatting')	5	10
Caravan	2	0
Motorway construction hut	1	0
Own home	2	1
L.A. mother and baby home	2	0
Army accom. (not camps)	3	3
Total	38	22

Adults in loco parentis

A characteristic of these families was frequent changes of adults in charge of the children as spouses, cohabitees, and relatives came and went. The distribution of the 129 parents and step-parents or cohabitees (not including grandparents and foster parents), reponsible at various times for the presenting children and their siblings is shown in Table 6.12. Only 12 (35%) families had but two parents. The larger families tended to have more adults involved in care of the children, a mean of 4.7 in families with 4 children and 5.6 in families with 5 or 6 children.

Sibling structure

The sibling structures of the 34 (1965–1971) families are summarized in Table 6.13. There was a total of 116 children in the 34 families, a mean of over three children per family. Over half the families had four or more children, two had six and only two were single child families. Over half the 38 severely abused children came from families with four or more children, and nearly three quarters from families with three or more children. The large size of these

Table 6.12 Parents and parent surrogates responsible for children in the 34 (1965–1971) families

No. of parents or parent surrogates	No. of children in family						Total families	Total parents or parent surrogates
	1	2	3	4	5	6		
2	2*	4	4	2	—	—	12	24
3	—	1	3	4	—	—	8	24
4	—	2	—	3	—	—	5	20
5	—	—	—	1	1	1	3	15
6	—	—	—	—	2	1	3	18
7	—	—	—	1	—	—	1	7
8	—	—	—	—	—	—	0	—
9	—	—	—	1	—	—	1	9
10	—	—	—	—	—	—	0	—
11	—	—	—	—	—	—	0	—
12	—	—	—	1	—	—	1	12
Total families	2	7	7	13	3	2	34	—
Total parents or parent surrogates	4	19	17	61	17	11	—	129

* Cells show number of families.
Note: Foster-parents and grand-parents are not included.

Table 6.13 Sibling structure of the 34 families

	No. of children in family						Total families	Total children
	1	2	3	4	5	6		
No. presenting children								
1	2*	6	6	13	2	1	30	30
2	—	1	1	—	1	1	4	8
Sub-total children	2	8	8	13	4	3	34	38
No. full sibs								
1	—	5	4	1	1	1	12	12
2	—	—	3	2	—	—	5	10
3	—	—	—	5	—	—	5	15
4	—	—	—	—	—	1	1	4
Sub-total children	—	5	10	20	1	5	23	41
No. step or half sibs								
1	—	1	3	2	—	—	6	6
2	—	—	—	1	1	—	2	4
3	—	—	—	5	—	—	5	15
4	—	—	—	—	2	1	3	12
Sub-total children	—	1	3	19	10	4	16	37
TOTAL families	2	7	7	13	3	2	34	
TOTAL children	2	14	21	52	15	12		116

* Cells show numbers of families.

families compared with the country as a whole is shown in Table 6.14 and would be even more marked if account were taken of the youthfulness of the parents. The siblings of the presenting children were nearly as likely to be step or half sibs as they were to be full sibs. Thirty (26%) of the 116 children were illegitimate, and these 30 came from half the 34 families.

Table 6.14   Distribution by family size N. E. Wilts. of child abuse families and of all families in Great Britain*

Number of children	N.E. Wilts. child abuse families		Great Britain 1966*	
	No.	%	No. (thousands)	%
1	2	5.9	2572	41.4
2	7	20.6	2177	35.0
3	7	20.6	914	14.7
4	13	38.2	348	5.6
5 or more	5	14.7	208	3.3
Total	34	100.0	6219	100.0

* Source: Social Trends, 1972.

Features of sibs of the presenting children in the retrospective series

Child abuse

Of the 78 full and step or half siblings of the presenting children, 65 (83%) were considered to be at risk of abuse by reason of their age, and presence in the family in the care of adults responsible for attacks on the presenting children. Of these 65 children, severe or moderate active physical abuse was ascertained in 41 (63%) and suspected in a further 6 (9%), though the abuse did not meet one or more of the criteria of severity, time, place or age necessary for inclusion in the group of presenting children. Much smaller numbers of injuries were identified in the siblings than in the presenting children. There were recorded 10 fractures including 1 of skull, 5 instances of suffocation, 14 of fits or loss of consciousness caused by assault in 7 children, 73 instances of bruising, 16 of lacerations, 4 of crushed fingers or nails, 2 of bites and 9 of burns. No instances of bleeding into or around the brain or retinal haemorrhages were recorded. In view of the severe damage ascertained in many of the siblings, it seems likely that injuries such as these were not looked for, particularly those which are easy to conceal, or those such as retinal haemorrhages which can be detected only by special examination. Others, such as fractures of the ribs, would have been discovered only on X-ray. Five (8%) of the siblings were brain damaged, 12 (18%) had speech defects and 6 (9%) had locomotor defects, all caused by injury or other abuse or neglect. Severe neglect (starvation of deprivation of essentials or failure to thrive for non-medical reasons) was found in 28 (43%) of these children, and repeated or severe emotional trauma in the same number. Four of the siblings had been killed by a parent or guardian, two having died from suffocation and two from brain injury. Intellectual, social, educational or emotional damage caused by abuse was judged present in 28 (43%) of the siblings.

An even higher proportion (57%) than of the presenting children remained with the parents or guardians responsible for the assaults. Seventeen children (26%) were with relatives who had not injured them, two had been adopted, six were in foster homes, and four were in a hospital or institution.

The clinical features noted in the index children were reported in the siblings in the following frequencies: fear 11 (17%), withdrawal 13 (20%), hyperactivity 13 (20%), irritability and excessive crying 22 (34%), and pallor 12 (18%).

Other pathology

In addition to the four deaths from injury, five siblings had died from other causes (prematurity, inhalation of vomit following bronchitis aggravated by hypothermia, broncho-pneumonia following bronchitis, mongolism and congenital defects, and neuroblastoma). The last two of these deaths occurred in the same family, there were three siblings with congenital conditions in another family (one heart disease and talipes, one heart murmur and dislocation of hips, one cyanotic heart disease), and one child in another family had a squint and a benign systolic murmur.

Beyond the immediate sibs there were more extensive histories in several families. Five families had histories of asthma and eczema in several members over two or more generations. One family had a number of members in three generations afflicted with a form of ataxia which may have had a genetic origin or may have been a consequence of poor rearing. One family was reported as having 'puny' neonates over three generations. There were cases of albinism, ovarian dysgenesis, and subnormality in another family.

The detailed family histories given previously, often covering 3 or more generations, are suffused with dullness or subnormality of intelligence, personality disorder, and mental illness in the direct lines[1]. Such disorders, the meat of psychiatric practice, were conspicuous in the antecedents of the battered children[1].

EXTENT OF CHILD ABUSE IN THE RETROSPECTIVE SERIES OF FAMILIES (1965–1971)

It was evident from the data on siblings of the index children that the stringent criteria by which they were identified erected artificial boundaries around the problem of child abuse which did not accord with reality. It appeared to be partly a matter of chance whether injury was inflicted of such severity as to meet the criteria. For instance, blows to the head or shaking might cause intracranial or retinal haemorrhage in one child but not in another of similar age. In order to obtain a fuller picture of the extent of child abuse by the parents or guardians in these families, the data on both severe and moderate physical abuse were combined and coupled with cases of neglect for both index children and siblings. Of the 116 children in these families, 15 were not at risk, either because they had died from natural causes, or were not living in the family (two children in this group had been abused by relatives while in the family but were not included in the following analyses). Of the 101 children at risk only 14 (14%) were well cared for. A further six (6%) had been subject to neglect but not active abuse. Thus in all, 81 (80%) had been abused. Eight (8%) had been killed, 40 (40%) had been severely abused, and the remaining 33 (33%) moderately abused.

An important aspect of the pattern of child abuse in these families was the tendency noted in an earlier study for assaults to be propagated from one child to the next as family size increases[56]. In our series, 79% of first born children were attacked, the proportion rising to 93% of second born, then falling to 70% of third born, and 88% of fourth born. A more precise calculation can be made on the basis of eldest to youngest at risk, eliminating vicarious absences which distort the birth order pattern of risk. Of eldest children at risk, 82% had been attacked. If the eldest had been assaulted, the likelihood of the second eldest being abused was 78%. If the two oldest children were abused, 64% of third oldest children were also. The proportion of fourth children abused if their three older siblings had been was 50%.

CHARACTERISTICS OF THE PARENTS (1965–1971 FAMILIES)

The abusing behaviour

Although there was a multiplicity of parent figures at various times in most of the 34 families, it was possible to identify a man and a woman in all but one case who were responsible for the presenting children at the time of the injuries, one or both of whom were implicated in the attacks in varying degrees. The exception was a family with an unmarried mother and no father figure present at the time. The sex and ascertained degree of involvement of the parents or guardians present at the time of the assaults is shown in Table 6.15. There was a significant excess of females responsible or thought to have complied actively in the assaults (χ^2 with Yates' correction = 6.66, d.f. = 1, $p < 0.01$). There were 16 (47%) families in which the female parent or guardian alone was responsible for the assaults, and four (12%) in which the male alone was responsible. In the remaining 14 (41%) both partners attacked the children or one actively complied in assaults by the other (seven families).

There was a tendency for the main assaults to take place soon after marriage or the start of cohabitation, the mean age of female parents being 24 years and that of males 25 years. The mean time elapsing between marriage or commencing cohabitation and the start of severe child abuse was, for abusing females 2

Table 6.15 Sex and ascertained degree of involvement of parents or guardians in abuse of presenting children

| | Males | | Females | |
	No.	%	No.	%
Responsible	12	40.0	27	81.8
Active complicity	6	20.0	3	9.1
Not involved	12	40.0	3	9.1
Total*	30	100.0	33	100.0

* There were 4 families in which no male and one in which no female could have been responsible for the severe assaults because they were away at the time.

years 9 months, and for abusing males 1 year 8 months. Seven women and 5 men severely assaulted the children less than a year following legal or common law marriage. Sixteen women and five men severely assaulted the children less than a year after the birth of their first child. There was evidence that lesser degrees of abuse occurred still earlier.

Characteristic behaviour patterns were noted in many of the parents or guardians. Gross neglect of the children was common, usually by deprivation of food and fluids, but also of warmth, light, treatment or protection, or simply leaving babies or toddlers alone for several days or nights. Eighteen (47%) of the index children were affected in this way on 49 occasions, and 37 (57%) of the siblings on 68 occasions. Abandonment or leaving children in the care of unwilling relatives or strangers occurred less frequently [8 (21%) index children in 14 episodes, and five (8%) siblings in six episodes]. Non-attendance at clinics for inadequate reasons and refusal of access in the home by professional people were very common [29 (76%) index children on 86 occasions, 39 (60%) siblings on 64 occasions]. It is noteworthy that this deliberately manipulative behaviour often gave rise to friction between the different professional people concerned, such as hospital service staff, social workers, and staff of the local health authority.

Pathological histories (1965–1971 families)

Confirming earlier work perhaps the most impressive feature of the parents and parent substitutes was the constellation of pathologies and of their own unsatisfactory childhoods which they exhibited[1*,50,51,65]. Table 6.16 shows the frequency of 19 characteristics in the 67 parents or guardians responsible for the index children at the time of the principal assaults. The high rates of

* Appendix 1 of the 1974 Report[1] contains 33 pages of short clinical descriptions relating to family and personal histories, up to 3 or more generations back.

Table 6.16 Frequency of certain characteristics in 67 parent figures of the severely abused children

Characteristic	Present No.	Present %	Absent No.	Absent %	Not applicable No.	Not applicable %	Not known No.	Not known %	Total No.	Total %
Childhood										
1. Severe or moderate physical abuse	28*	41.8	17	25.4	—	—	22	32.8	67	100
2. Severe or moderate neglect	28	41.8	16	23.9	—	—	23	34.3	67	100
3. Severe or prolonged mental abuse	39	58.2	4	6.0	1	1.5	23	34.3	67	100
4. Illegitimate or pre-marital conception	10	14.9	47	70.2	—	—	10	14.9	67	100
5. Abandoned, institutionalized or fostered	18	26.9	33	49.3	—	—	16	23.8	67	100
6. Prolonged separation (over 1 mth) from one or both parents	28	41.8	21	31.3	—	—	18	26.9	67	100
7. History of ESN or special schooling	11	16.4	37	55.2	6	9.0	13	19.4	67	100
8. Conduct, learning or emotional disorder	33	49.2	11	16.4	6	9.0	17	25.4	67	100
9. Extensive agency support[50]	26	38.8	14	20.9	6	9.0	21	31.3	67	100
Adulthood										
10. History of stealing, violence, sex offences or other criminal behaviour	31	46.3	34	50.7	—	—	2	3.0	67	100
11. Extensive agency support[50]	45	67.2	21	31.3	—	—	1	1.5	67	100
12. Chronic physical ill-health or disability	17	25.4	50	74.6	—	—	—	—	67	100
13. Episodes of unconsciousness	19	28.4	48	71.6	—	—	—	—	67	100
14. History of uncontrolled drug or alcohol use	8	11.9	54	80.6	—	—	5	7.5	67	100
15. Borderline or moderate mental subnormality	20	29.8	45	67.2	—	—	2	3.0	67	100
16. Personality or neurotic disorder	51	76.1	10	14.9	—	—	6	9.0	67	100
17. History of suicidal attempts or gestures	20	29.8	43	64.2	—	—	4	6.0	67	100
18. History of psychiatric treatment	39	58.2	24	35.8	—	—	4	6.0	67	100
19. History of psychiatric inpatient treatment	23	34.3	38	56.7	—	—	6	9.0	67	100

* Includes 10 cases in whom severe or moderate physical abuse was probable but evidence was not complete.

Table 6.17 Proportion of parents or guardians with various characteristics by sex and implication in assaults

	Directly implicated						Indirectly implicated					
	Males		Females		Total		Males		Females		Total	
	No.	%	No.	%	No.	%	No.	%	No.	%	No.	%
Childhood												
1. Severe or moderate physical abuse	9	81.8	15	68.2	24	72.7	3	33.3	1	33.3	4	33.3
2. Severe or moderate neglect	9	90.0	13	59.1	22	68.7	4	44.4	2	66.7	6	50.0
3. Severe or prolonged mental abuse	12	100.0	22	100.0	34	100.0	3	42.9	2	66.7	5	50.0
4. Illegitimate or pre-marital conception	2	14.3	6	21.4	8	19.0	—	0	2	66.7	2	13.3
5. Abandoned, institutionalized or fostered	5	38.5	11	42.3	16	41.0	1	11.1	1	33.3	2	16.7
6. Prolonged separation (over 1 mth) from one or both parents	7	50.0	17	68.0	24	61.5	2	28.6	2	66.7	4	40.0
7. History of ESN or special schooling	5	38.5	2	9.1	7	20.0	3	30.0	1	33.3	4	30.8
8. Conduct, learning or emotional disorder	10	90.9	17	77.3	27	81.8	4	50.0	2	66.7	6	54.5
9. Extensive agency support[50]	9	81.8	11	57.9	20	66.7	4	57.1	2	66.7	6	60.0
Adulthood												
10. History of stealing, violence, sex offences or other criminal behaviour	11	64.7	14	48.3	25	54.3	6	40.0	—	—	6	31.6
11. Extensive agency support[50]	14	82.4	22	73.3	36	76.6	6	40.0	3	75.0	9	47.4
12. Chronic physical ill-health or disability	5	27.8	8	26.7	13	27.1	4	26.7	—	—	4	21.1
13. Episodes of unconsciousness	5	27.8	10	33.3	15	31.3	4	26.7	—	—	4	21.1
14. History of uncontrolled drug or alcohol use	4	25.0	1	3.6	5	11.4	3	21.4	—	—	3	16.7
15. Borderline or moderate mental subnormality	4	23.5	12	40.0	16	34.0	4	28.6	—	—	4	22.2
16. Personality or neurotic disorder	15	88.2	27	93.1	42	91.3	7	63.9	2	50.0	9	60.0
17. History of suicidal attempts or gestures	8	47.1	9	32.1	17	37.8	3	21.4	—	—	3	16.7
18. History of psychiatric treatment	10	62.5	21	72.4	31	68.9	6	42.9	2	50.0	8	44.4
19. History of psychiatric inpatient treatment	8	47.1	11	39.3	19	42.2	3	25.0	1	25.0	4	25.0

physical and mental abuse and neglect in their childhoods were outstanding. The proportions of illegitimacies, abandonment and fostering, special schooling, behaviour disorder, and agency support were all extremely high (cf. Sayre *et al.*[66]). The pathological behaviour and ill-health was equally striking in adulthood. Bearing in mind the youthfulness of these parents, there were gross excesses of psychiatric disturbance, physical illness and disability, and criminality. Even in the absence of controls it may be assumed that these characteristics together mark off this group of inadequate and unhealthy individuals from the general population.

In order to assess the importance of these characteristics in relation to actual abuse of the index children, parents and guardians who were directly or indirectly implicated were compared with those who were not (Table 6.17). The small numbers and the high proportion of cases in which data were not available made precise evaluation difficult. There were no significant differences between males and females, but taking both sexes together, where there were more than trivial numbers of cases, implicated parents or guardians were more likely to exhibit these features than those who were not. Implicated males were more likely to have each of the characteristics except subnormality than unimplicated males, though the difference reached significance only with respect to social agency support as an adult (χ^2 with Yates' correction $= 4.43$, d.f. $= 1$, $p < 0.05$). There were no statistically significant differences among the mothers or female guardians. With respect to neglect as a child, illegitimacy or premarital conception, history of educational subnormality or special schooling, and extensive agency support as a child and as an adult, those not implicated in the assaults were more likely to be affected than those who were. Although these results suggest that those exhibiting assaultative behaviour were not readily distinguishable from their unimplicated partners in these terms, significant differences were obtained when the characteristics were grouped. Implicated parent figures were more likely to have been subjected to physical or mental abuse or neglect in their own childhoods (Table 6.18) and they were more likely to have one or more features of an unhealthy or unsatisfactory childhood (Table 6.19).

DISCUSSION (Part I)

Extent of severe child abuse

The rate of about 1 new case referred per thousand children under 4 years old per year followed intensive educative activity with the medical and social welfare professions. For England and Wales as a whole this rate would entail referral of over 3000 children aged 0–3 each year. Although this rate was an increase of over two and half times the ascertainment rate in the previous 7 years, there were clinical indications of residual under-reporting and the true rate is almost certainly higher. Though we have detailed data only on the retrospective series, it seems likely that the proportion with brain damage is similar in the prospective series.

From the text ('Outcome' subheading) and Table 6.5, it can be seen that 27% of the 1965–1971 children were rendered intellectually impaired from in-

Table 6.18 Comparison of implicated and unimplicated parents or guardians with definite or probable physical or mental abuse or neglect in childhood

	Implicated		Not implicated		Total	
	No.	%	No.	%	No.	%
Abuse or neglect	34	91.9	7	50.0	41	80.4
No abuse or neglect	3	8.1	7	50.0	10	19.6
Total	37	100.0	14	100.0	51	100.0

Exact probability = 2.93% (two-tailed)

Table 6.19 Comparison of implicated and unimplicated parents or guardians with one or more features of an unsatisfactory childhood*

	Implicated		Not implicated		Total	
	No.	%	No.	%	No.	%
Unsatisfactory	40	85.1	8	50.0	48	76.2
Normal	7	14.9	8	50.0	15	23.8
Total	47	100.0	16	100.0	63	100.0

Exact probability = 1.28% (two-tailed)
* Based on items 1–9 of Table 6.16.

duced brain damage, but 43% suffered intracranial haemorrhage or other brain injury. Projecting these figures to England and Wales, this means that at least 750 children per year in the country could suffer gross reduction in their intelligence as a result of parental attacks, and up to 1200 children per year could suffer blunting of their intellect as a direct result of brain damage induced by parental assaults.

These figures may be taken as a reasonable estimate of the extent of severe abuse in this age group using the criteria and methods of ascertainment of the study, yet they are by no means an indication of the extent of child abuse as a whole. Three principal qualifications must be taken into account. First, almost no children over age 3 were ascertained because this group appears to escape injury of such severity, though it frequently is subject to less damaging assaults. Our figures for brain damage may therefore be fairly firm. Indeed, all but 2 of the 38 children in the retrospective series and 1 of the 22 in the prospective series were under 3 years, so that it may be held that severe physical abuse as here defined and identified is virtually confined to the age group 0 to 2 years. In the prospective series the total annual rate for this group was about 1.3 per thousand. Second, the criteria for severe abuse were very stringent. Lesser degrees of abuse were ascertained in over half the sibs of index cases at risk in addition to the 16% of sibs who were severely abused. Families in which the children were not known to have been injured seriously enough to meet the criteria were excluded altogether. Third, nearly all the families were in social classes IV and V and it must be questionable whether this is at least partially a consequence of the methods of ascertainment rather than a reflection of the real situation. Kempe[67] for instance believes that child abuse occurs more or less equally in all social classes. It can be argued that concealment of child abuse would be more effective in the higher social classes and there were indications from interview material with medical and other professionals that this was so. Higher social class parents rarely seek the help of social service agencies, confining themselves to contact with the medical profession. Nevertheless, it is unlikely that abuse of the severity necessary to meet our criteria would have escaped ascertainment to any great extent in the climate of opinion of the prospective study in 1972 and 1973. It may well be that severity is class related.

It is difficult to make useful comparisons with other studies since definitions have been less precise and usually all grades of abuse, and sometimes neglect, have been included. Our total rate for severe abuse is not incompatible with the results from the Tunbridge Wells Study Group[68], but the extent of brain damage is considerably higher in our study. If moderate abuse had been included our total rate also might have exceeded the Tunbridge Wells figures. Light[69] made a 'best estimate' of 3 per thousand United States children under 18 for all grades of physical abuse, and a further 7 per thousand for severe neglect and sexual abuse to reach his total of 1%. Kempe[67] gave a figure of 6 per thousand live births for all types of abuse from severe assaults to passive rejection in the United States. The rate for severe abuse only in the present study is 4 per thousand live births per annum. Judging from clinical experience, application of the rates for all types of abuse given by these American authors to the United Kingdom would not be unrealistic.

The death rate in the prospective series was about 0.1 per thousand under 4 years old per year. This rate is between one third and two thirds of the rate for traumatic causes in the Oxford Record Linkage Study area, and represents between 2% and 2.5% of all deaths in children aged 0–3. Extrapolated to England and Wales as a whole, this death rate would account for over 300 deaths a year with a range within one standard error (70% of samples) of 31 to 526. This contrasts with, on the one hand the Tunbridge Wells Study Group figure of 700 a year[68], and on the other with the official figure of 80 in 1972[70]. Although deaths were included only if the abuse had been prolonged sufficiently to meet the criteria, so that not all infanticides or murders necessarily were counted, it seems unlikely that additional deaths of this type occurred in the north-east Wiltshire population in the 18 months period of the prospective study. It is possible that rates may be higher in other, perhaps more heavily urbanized, parts of the country.

It is of some interest to examine possible reasons for the apparent marked under-reporting of deaths from abuse in the official figures. In the retrospective series there were four deaths of index cases and four deaths of their sibs, and in the prospective series a further two index deaths were ascertained. Of these ten deaths, inquests were held in nine, and convictions for infanticide or manslaughter obtained in three. In one other case the mother was acquitted of causing the death but convicted of cruelty to a person under 16. In only four of the nine cases investigated by inquest, therefore, was there considered to be evidence of assault. Coroner's verdicts in the other five were either accidental death (three cases) or open (two cases). The diagnosis in all the accidental deaths was some variant of asphyxia caused by inhalation of gastric contents. The diagnosis in one of the open verdicts was cerebral haemorrhage following fracture of skull and in the other cerebral haemorrhage following a tentorial tear. The diagnoses in the cases associated with convictions were (1) bronchopneumonia and cerebral haemorrhage following fracture of skull and ribs, (2) subdural haemorrhage following fracture of skull, and (3) asphyxia. In the case associated with a conviction for cruelty the diagnosis was asphyxia caused by inhalation of vomit. The tenth case, without inquest, was diagnosed after post mortem as acute bronchitis and certified by the coroner. Multiple bruising and episodes of deliberate exposure to cold had been noted by medical, nursing and social work staff at different times. Two of the deaths occurred in hospital, and two other babies were dead on arrival at hospital, none of these being associated with conviction for infanticide or manslaughter.

These records suggest that where the cause of death is not overt violence there is less chance of allegation of assault leading to trial, and not all cases of overt violence such as fracture of skull have this outcome. Adequate evidence clearly is difficult to obtain, but it may, be useful to note that eight out of the ten deaths occurred at ages less than 1 year. Death from intra-cranial haemorrhage associated with injury not clearly caused in situations precluding assault, or asphyxia (whether or not caused by inhalation of vomit) occurring under 1 year of age should be investigated most thoroughly. It would be useful if the external cause (corresponding to the E code of the International Classification of Diseases) were noted on the death certificate wherever applicable, so that the frequency of supposed accidental causes which stretch credibility (such as being dropped, falling down stairs, etc.) might be obtained.

Family characteristics

Large size, youthfulness, instability, and gross excesses of psychiatric and physical illness and disability and criminality characterized the retrospective series of child abuse families. Clinically, families in the prospective series, though referred at the much higher rate, were similar. So marked were these features that, even in the absence of controls, it is likely that they identify a group of inadequate and unhealthy families to whom severe physical abuse is largely confined. These results are generally in accord with those of Smith and his colleagues in the Birmingham area[59,71-74]. They also reinforce the main finding of the New York City Epidemiological Study, in which a very high proportion of the abusing families were 'multiproblem families' (Simons *et al.*[75]).

The frequency of pathologies in these families is suggestive of clustering of disorders and is reminiscent of Newcombe's finding of greatly increased relative risk in siblings of handicapped and stillborn children for a wide range of conditions, including accidents, poisonings and violence[76]. This is clearly a subject for detailed study for which a system of linked medical records depicting the primary and intergenerational family relationships would be necessary. If disease clustering in such families were confirmed and its nature and extent specified, there could be important implications for both medical knowledge and the organization of health and social care. Child abuse appears to be but a manifestation of widespread, heterogeneous, and often severe, medical and social pathology affecting virtually the whole family. Multiple pathology and the consequent disability may become so overwhelming that the means of coping with the difficulties of living are no longer available to the adult members. Violent impulsive aggression, shifting dependence on acquaintances and relatives, and deep ambivalence towards health, social welfare and social control agencies on which extraordinary demands are made, become a characteristic way of life. We have discussed elsewhere some implications for ascertainment, secondary and primary prevention, and organization of services[1].

POSTSCRIPT, 1973–1977

From 1973 onwards, attitudes changed amongst professional people. Doctors, social workers, lawyers and others in N.E. Wilts. and elsewhere, more efficiently identified and alleviated the plight of child victims of severe abuse. Individuals who had taken action on their own were increasingly supported, paediatricians usually taking the key role where children had been admitted to hospital.

During the 4 year period July 1973–July 1977, 'severe abuse' cases as defined have diminished. There have been about a quarter as many as hitherto. There has almost been a complete cessation of the saddest cases of children suffering repetitive, severe physical cruelty. The *proportion* of battered children *based* in the locality, as opposed to children identified from families transiently in N.E. Wilts. seems also to have diminished. Throughout this time interval, there has been little evidence of improved rearing practices. There has been a continued flow of marginal and/or less severe cases reported, together with early or partial baby batterings.

'Supportive case work' with cruel families has been much less favoured since 1973. On the social work side, there had often been much triviality in the pre-1972 case work, the notes often running to dozens or even hundreds of pages: ('... called again, this time successful. Discussed the rent arrears but did not want to pursue this ... did not see the children but hear they had a nice day in the park on Wednesday. ... Mrs. X is doing quite well considering her limited abilities etc.'). This contrasted with the stark reality of sufferings to the children recorded over the same time intervals; mutilations, terror, and scarring of body and mind. Young children could enter an era of suffering whilst the psychiatric notes confidently recorded successful treatments of depressions or derangements in their mothers. As the adult was invariably the presenting patient or client, the adult had become hedged about with the confidential treatment considerations at the expense of child victims, who could not speak for themselves. The professional taboo in psychiatric and social work circles against value judgements had been confined to *adverse* criticism. Frequent accounts by social workers, probation officers or others had appeared in the files noting 'loving' or 'caring' of children by plausible parents who had put on a convincing front. Sometimes these facile opinions had been used (and believed) in court reports to get a lighter sentence for parents convicted of other offences! In cruel families there had usually not been any evidence of protective, useful love to the child. By contrast there had frequently been records in the same or separate files of extremely damaging behaviour by the parent, who was needing love from, not giving love to, the child victims.

After 1973 there was a more general acceptance of the rights of children as individuals, rather than them being seen as chattels. There was a recognition that there was not necessarily a magic natural biological bond. 'Family therapy' was not always the right treatment. A proportion of children, whether 10% or 0.1%, were being damaged by their parents to such an extent that they would be better being reared, partly or wholly, by someone else (cf. Howells[77]). Medical, social work, legal and other agencies in N.E. Wilts. co-operated in applications for full Care Orders to assume the parental rights on behalf of child victims, with consequent better control exercised on behalf of the child. The feebler Supervision Orders were viewed with distaste by most of us. On occasion, court applications were made to remove a newborn baby from mothers who had been severely and/or persistently cruel to their other babies and toddlers. Such severe (albeit uncommon) measures were supported by the courts providing witnesses were firm, clear, conscientious and honest. The same process was occurring in the adjacent area of Bath City and Avon[78].

Reasons for the improved situations with respect to the severe abuse, or repetitive cruelty cases, could be as follows:

1. Generally improved rearing practices: an unlikely reason, because of the continuing flow of less severe cases of cruelty, neglect and unkind or irresponsible behaviour towards young children.

2. Improved local and national awareness, a swing in public attitudes coinciding with improved local organization, and more efficient local and national efforts to co-ordinate proper care for the battered babies and toddlers[79].

3. Realization that even severely cruelly treated children could cling to, and appear to attach to, the parent responsible for their plight: older children could defend, and collude in the stories of their parents[80,81].

4. Decline in birth rate. Family planning is also starting to reach the more helpless and feckless problem families in N.E. Wilts. (and England as a whole) over the past few years (cf. Light[69]).

5. Awakened public conscience, with less hypocrisy and evasion. People no longer look away pretending that cruelty to young children does not occur, or only occurs with parents or guardians who are clearly and obviously mad and bad[82].

6. Heightened authority and increased group pressure, acting against the tolerance of parental cruelty to children, and in particular towards babies and pre-school children (cf. Milgram[83], and Part I).

None of the foregoing considers punitiveness or its obverse, compassion to the cruel parent for her own suffering and inadequacy. These aspects can be appropriate to the treatment of individual families, and have been the theme of many papers and much propaganda since Kempe's 1962 paper. Nevertheless we contend that the six points above have the greatest relevance to the figures and findings given in Parts of Chapters 5 and 6 and in Appendix I, subsection III, for our part of England and probably for communities in any part of the world. The last 5 points account for the striking decline in known cases of repetitive or severe cruelty to young children (despite increased vigilance), in N.E. Wilts. since June 1973.

References

1. Oliver, J. E., Cox, J., Taylor, A. and Baldwin, J. A. (1974). Severely ill-treated young children in North-East Wiltshire. Oxford Unit of Clinical Epidemiology, University Research Report No. 4

2. Baldwin, J. A. and Oliver J. E. (1975). Epidemiology and Family Characteristics of Severely Abused Children. *Br. J. Prevent. Soc. Med.*, **29**, 205

3. Oliver, J. E. (1975). Microcephaly following Battering and Shaking. *Br. Med. J.*, **2**, 262

4. British Medical Journal (1973). Deliberate injury of children. *Br. Med. J.*, **4**, 61

5. Castle, R. L. and Kerr, A. M. (1972). *A Study of Suspected Child Abuse.* National Society for the Prevention of Cruelty to Children

6. Colclough, I. R. (1972). Victorian government's report on child abuse. *Med. J. Aust.*, **2**, 1491

7. Ebbin, A. J., Gollub, M. H., Stein, A. M. and Wilson, M. G. (1969). Battered child syndrome at the Los Angeles County General Hospital. *Am. J. Dis. Child.*, **118**, 660

8. Fontana, V. J. (1971). *The Maltreated Child.* 2nd Edition. (Illinois: Charles C. Thomas)

9. Jackson, G. (1972). Child abuse syndrome: the cases we miss. *Br. Med. J.*, **2**, 756

10. Nau, E. (1967). Maltreated children. *Monatsschr. Kinderheilkunde*, **115,** 192
11. Neimann, N. and Rabouille, D. (1969). Maltreated children. *Rev. Prat.*, **19,** 3879
12. Okell, C. (1971). Childhood accidents and child abuse. *Community Med.*, **126,** 124
13. Okell, C. (1972). The battered baby syndrome: (a) recent research and implications for treatment. Royal Society of Health Congress
14. Parker, G. E. (1965). The battered child syndrome. *Med. Sci. Law*, **8,** 160
15. Silver, L. B., Barton, W. and Dublin, C. C. (1967). Child abuse laws: are they enough? *J. Am. Med. Assoc.*, **199,** 101
16. Silver, L. B., Dublin, C. C. and Lourie, R. S. (1969). Child abuse syndrome: the 'grey areas' in establishing a diagnosis. *Pediatrics*, **44,** 594
17. Cameron, J. M., Johnson, H. R. M. and Camps, F. E. (1966). The battered child syndrome. *Med. Sci. Law*, **6,** 2
18. Scott, P. D. (1973). Fatal battered baby cases. *Med. Sci. Law*, **13,** 197
19. Trube-Becker, E. (1971). Autopsy of children who have died suddenly. *Medizin. Klin.*, **66,** 58
20. Weston, J. T. (1968). The pathology of child abuse. In: *The Battered Child*. R. E. Helfer and C. H. Kempe (eds.) (Chicago: University of Chicago Press)
21. Lukianowicz, N. (1971). Infanticide. *Psychiat. Clin.*, **4,** 145
22. Rodenberg, M. (1971). Child murder by depressed parents. *Can. Psychiat. Assoc. J.*, **16,** 41
23. Scott, P. D. (1973). Parents who kill their children. *Med. Sci. Law*, **13,** 120
24. O'Neill, J. A., Meacham, W. F., Griffin, D. P. and Sawyers, J. L. (1973). Patterns of injury in the battered child syndrome. *J. Traum.*, **13,** 332
25. Birrell, A. G. and Birrel, J. H. W. (1968). The maltreatment syndrome in children: a hospital survey. *Med. J. Aust.*, **2,** 1023
26. Guthkelch, A. N. (1971). Infantile subdural haematoma and its relationship to whiplash injuries. *Br. Med. J.*, **2,** 430
27. Kottgen, U. (1967). Maltreatment of children. *Monatsschr. Kinderheilkunde*, **115,** 186
28. Straus, P. and Wolf, A. (1970). A topical question: maltreated children. *La Psychiatrie de L'Enfant*, **12,** 577
29. Caffey, J. (1974). The Whiplash Shaken Infant Syndrome: Manual Shaking by the Extremities with Whiplash-Induced Intracranial and Intraocular Bleedings, Linked with Residual Permanent Brain Damage and Mental Retardation. *Pediatrics*, **54,** 396
30. Harcourt, B. and Hopkins, D. (1971). Ophthalmic manifestations of the battered baby syndrome. *Br. Med. J.*, **3,** 398
31. Mushin, A. S. (1971). Ocular damage in the battered baby syndrome. *Br. Med. J.*, **3,** 402
32. Cameron, J. M. (1972). The battered baby syndrome. *Practitioner*, **209,** 302
33. Sims, B. G., Grant, J. H. and Cameron, J. M. (1973). Bite-marks in the battered baby syndrome. *Med. Sci. Law*, **13,** 207
34. Caffey, J. (1972). The parent-infant traumatic stress syndrome. *Am. J. Roent.*, **114,** 218
35. Cameron, J. M. (1970). The battered baby. *Br. J. Hos. Med.*, **4,** 769
36. Grantymyre, E. B. (1973). Trauma X – Wednesday's Child. *Nova Scotia Med. Bull.*, **52,** 29
37. Griffiths, D. L. and Moynihan, E. J. (1963). Multiple epiphyseal injuries in babies ('battered baby' syndrome). *Br. Med. J.*, **2,** 1558
38. Maroteaux, P. and Fessard, C. (1969). The battered child syndrome: Silverman's syndrome. *Concours Medical*, **91,** 6704
39. Roeb, K. G., Melli, M. S., Wald, M. and Wesenberg, R. (1972). A conference on child abuse. *Wisconsin Med. J.*, **71,** 226
40. Silverman, F. C. (1968). Radiologic aspects of the battered child syndrome. In: *The Battered Child*. R. E. Helfer and C. H. Kempe (eds.) (Chicago: University of Chicago Press)
41. Elmer, F. (1960). Failure to thrive: role of the mother. *Pediatrics*, **25,** 717
42. Leonard, M. F., Rhymes, J. P. and Solnitt, A. J. (1966). Failure to thrive in infants – a family problem. *Am. J. Dis. Child.*, **111,** 600
43. Maginnis, E., Pivchik, E. and Smith, N. (1967). A social worker looks at failure to thrive. *Child Welfare*, 335

44. Smith, S. M. and Hanson, R. (1972). Failure to thrive and anorexia nervosa. *Postgrad. Med. J.*, **48**, 382

45. Young, L. (1964). *Wednesday's Children*. (New York: McGraw-Hill)

46. Chesser, E. (1951). *Cruelty to Children*. (London: Victor Gollancz Ltd)

47. Cherry, B. J. and Kuby, A. M. (1971). Obstacles to the delivery of medical care to children of neglecting parents. *Am. J. Publ. Hlth.*, **61**, 568

48. Clegg, A. and Megson, B. (1968). *Children in Distress*. (London: Penguin)

49. Pavenstedt, E. and Bernard, V. W. (1971). *Crises of Family Disorganization*. (New York: Behavioral Publications)

50. Oliver, J. E. and Cox, J. (1973). A family kindred with ill-used chilren: the burden on the community. *Br. J. Psychiat.*, **123**, 81

51. Oliver, J. E. and Taylor, A. (1971). Five generations of ill-treated children in one family pedigree. *Br. J. Psychiat.*, **119**, 473

52. Abrahamson, D. (1974). Procedure re-examined. *Lancet*, **i**, 1153

53. Gibbens, T. C. N. and Walker, A. (1956). *Cruel Parents*. (London: Institute for the Study and Treatment of Delinquency)

54. Butler, N. R. and Bonham, D. G. (1963). *Perinatal Mortality*: the first report of the 1958 British Perinatal Mortality Survey. (London: Livingstone)

55. Galdston, R. (1965). Observations on children who have been physically abused and their parents. *Am. J. Psychiat.*, **122**, 440

56. Skinner, A. E. and Castle, R. L. (1969). *78 Battered Children: A Retrospective Study*. National Society for the Prevention of Cruelty to Children

57. Gormsen, H. and Vesterdal, J. (1968). *Ugeskr Laegar*, **130**, 1203.

58. Vesterdal, J. (1972). The Battered Child Syndrome. *Annales Nestlé*, No. 27, p. 5

59. Smith, S. M. and Hanson, R. (1974). 134 Battered Children: A Medical and Psychological Study. *Br. Med. J.*, **3**, 666

60. Silver, L. B. (1968). Child Abuse Syndrome: A Review. *Med. Times*, **96**, 803

61. Elmer, E. (1967). *Children in Jeopardy. A Study of Abused Minors and their Families*. (University of Pittsburgh Press)

62. Martin, H. P. (1975). The Effect of Child Abuse on the Neurologic and Personality Development of Children. (Paper given during the Annual Meeting for Cerebral Palsy, 1974). *Develop. Med. Child Neurol.*, June 1975, p. 389

63. Cooper, C. (1975). The Doctors Dilemma. In: *Concerning Child Abuse*. A. W. Franklin (ed.) (Edinburgh: Churchill-Livingstone)

64. Kempe, C. H. (1974). Duty to Report Child Abuse. *Western J. Med.*, **121**, 224

65. Oliver, J. E. and Dewhurst, K. E. (1969). Six generations of ill-used children in a Huntington's pedigree. *Postgrad. Med. J.*, **45**, 757

66. Sayre, J. W., Foley, F. W., Zingarella, L. S. and Kristal, H. F. (1973). Community Committee on Child Abuse. *N.Y. State J. Med.*, p. 2071

67. Kempe, C. H. (1971). Paediatric implications of the battered baby syndrome. *Arch. Dis. Child.*, **46**, 28

68. Franklin, A. W. (1973). *Tunbridge Wells Study Group on Non-Accidental Injury to Children*. Spastics Society

69. Light, R. J. (1973). Abused and neglected children in America: a study of alternative policies. *Harv. Educ. Rev.*, **43**, 556

70. Peckham, C. S. and Jobling, M. (1975). Deaths from non-accidental injuries in childhood. *Br. Med. J.*, **2**, 686

71. Smith, S. M., Hanson, R. and Noble, S. (1973). Parents of battered babies: a controlled study. *Br. Med. J.*, **4**, 388

72. Smith, S. M. and Noble, S. (1973). Battered children and their parents. *New Soc.*, **26**, 393

73. Smith, S. M., Honigsberger, L. and Smith, C. A. (1973). EEG and personality factors in baby batterers. *Br. Med. J.*, **2**, 20

74. Smith, S. M., Hanson, R. and Noble, S. (1974). Social Aspects of the Battered Baby Syn-

drome. *Br. J. Psychiat.*, **125**, 568

75. Simons, B., Downs, E. F., Hurster, M. M. and Archer, M. (1966). Child Abuse: Epidemiologic Study of Medically Reported Cases. *N.Y. State J. Med.*, **66**, 2783

76. Newcombe, H. B. (1966). Familial tendencies in diseases of children. *Br. J. Prev. Soc. Med.*, **20**, 49

77. Howells, J. G. (1974). *Remember Maria*. (London: Butterworths)

78. Fairburn, A. C. and Jones, S. (1975). Beta 5 and battering (child abuse – a scheme of interdisciplinary linkage and co-ordination). *New Soc.*, 31.7.75.

79. Department of Health and Social Security. (1970). *The Battered Baby*. HMSO

80. Oliver, J. E. (1978). Families in which Children Suffer Maltreatment. In: *The Challenge of Child Abuse*. A. W. Franklin. (ed.) (London: Academic Press)

81. Rogers, D., Tripp, J., Bentovim, A., Robinson, A., Berry, D. and Goulding, R. (1976). Non-accidental poisoning; an extended syndrome of child abuse. *Br. Med. J.*, **1**, 793

82. Ounsted, C. (1975). Gaze aversion and child abuse. *World Med.*, **10**, 27

83. Milgram, S. (1974). *Obedience to Authority*. (London: Tavistock Publications Ltd.)

Part II – ILL-TREATED CHILDREN IDENTIFIED IN N. E. WILTS (J. E. Oliver and Jane Cox)

Blatantly battered babies, including the dead and brain-damaged young children identified in Chapter 5, Part II, and Chapter 6, Part I and Part III, form a small proportion of the total children born and reared – a minimum of 3000 children aged 0–3 in England and Wales per year. Battered babies do not just appear from seed-beds of severely abusive families. Their parents often come from large families of distressed, dull, incompetent, ill, chaotic, cruel, intermittently cruel, or neglectful rearers[1]. The parents of big, poorly reared families provide most of the battered babies for the ensuing third or fourth generations.

A confidential comparison was made between the earliest (incomplete) hospital research team lists of names of ill-treated children in N.E. Wilts. and an independently made check on the roll list of names of children at 3 special (ESN) Schools in N.E. Wilts.[2]. 7% of the children on the roll of the 3 special schools had a record of ill-treatment. There is no saying how much cruel or incompetent rearing had contributed to the mental handicap of the children concerned (see Part III of this chapter). There are publications to the effect that the dual deficit of food deprivation and understimulation synergistically impairs the intellect[3]. If this dual deficit occurs throughout the period of the human baby's maximum brain growth spurt period, that baby will become a dull or mentally subnormal citizen. Many problem families in N.E. Wilts. have unloved, understimulated, intermittently underfed babies and toddlers.

In this Part, an attempt is made to give a more complete picture of the extent of ill-treatment of children in N.E. Wilts. than was given in Part I. The average population for the locality for the 1965–1973 time interval was 45 000 children under 12 years old. The numbers are prepared in two groups.

1. Assault cases (see Table 6.20 A-D inclusive; Table 6.21, A, B1, C1)

These range from blatant and/or prolonged battering to irate or unjustified damaging blows to a baby, toddler or young child, which caused professional involvement. Included are some previously unidentified severe battering cases and a few fatal cases, which have not been recorded in the numbers in Part I.

Table 6.20   Children under 5 suffering maltreatment in the home (pre-school children)

(A) *Infanticide or murder victims.*
(B) 1. *Classical battered babies.*
    2. *Babies or children with facial bruising, one fracture, or other injury as a result of parental assault.* Such pre-battering, or partial battering, situations were much commoner than the full 'battered baby' picture.
(C) 1. *Severely shaken babies,* who may suffer intracranial damage, or damage to the retinae, with little evidence of external injury.
    2. *Babies or toddlers subjected to suffocatory techniques,* such as holding under bath water, hand (or pillow) over face to the point of unconsciousness etc. As with shaken babies, there may be few surface injuries, but the parent may eventually complain of the baby having inexplicable 'fits' or 'turns'. Respiratory infections may be frequent, or the baby may inhale gastric contents. Toddlers fear reminders of the suffocatory situation (see also D below), for instance by being terrified of water.
    3. *Children intentionally poisoned, victims of concealed cruel or bizarre practices[10,11].*
(D) *Young children who have suffered the effects of frequent pain, fear, mental cruelty or other prolonged or frequent stress, in the home setting.* One or more of the following disturbances were seen: Unnatural fearfulness of parents, or other adults, or of certain situations; withdrawal or listlessness or drowsiness; hyperactive or repetitive motor activity; persistent crying or irritability; pallor; unresponsiveness.
    There can be other reasons to account for any one of these disturbances (such as ill health in the child) but in this group one or more of such features were associated with parental maltreatment.
(E) *Babies who have failed to thrive* as a result of their mother's failure to feed or love them. Young children who are wasted and neglected, victims of malnutrition resulting from parental neglect are included here. The combined effects of underfeeding and understimulation are markedly synergistic in impairing the intellectual function of the child.
(F) *Babies of young children with disorganized social behaviour, with poor abilities or poor performance, or with low scores as measured by developmental quotients.* In this group the child's disabilities were not the result of ill health or inherent intellectual defects, but were attributable to degrees of stress, or psycho-social deprivation related to inadequate or chaotic rearing.
    The unsatisfactory early environment in which the child is reared can permanently affect the mental abilities of that child. There are crucial times such as the period of maximum post-natal brain growth spurts, but the total length of time over which the child suffers inadequate or stressful rearing is also important. The effects of the maltreatment are generally recognized in the designation 'mental retardation associated with psycho-social (environmental) deprivation' which appears in the International Classification of Diseases.

Note: Not all pre-school children showed clearly the effects of intermittent cruelty. Babies sometimes smiled at abusive parents. Two to five years olds (as well as older children) could defend abusive or neglectful parents with apparent loyalty.

Table 6.21   Children under 12 suffering maltreatment in the home

(A) *Child victims of murder or sudden serious assaults.* Publications often emphasize that the assaulting parent frequently has a psychotic depression but most of the (few) cases of this sort in N.E. Wilts. resulted from explosive behaviour in a parent who had a serious personality disturbance rather than a psychosis.

(B) 1. *Child victims of consistent activity cruelty; deliberate physical cruelty occurring over a period of time.*

　2. *Children intentionally poisoned or subject to other (semi) concealed cruel or bizarre practices*[10,11].

　3. *Child victims of passive cruelty, rejection or blatant physical neglect.* Included here also are children who suffered mental cruelty over long periods of time.

　4. *Children suffering as a result of chronic chaotic disorganization in their rearing.* Parents who are chronically incompetent and/or irresponsible are sometimes not viewed by professional people as being cruel to their children.

　　The children here were expected to rear themselves, and there were varying degrees of psycho-social or emotional deprivation. There tended to be frequent placement of children in care, and frequent arbitrary removals from care. Intervals of unnecessary neglect of the children's needs could be followed by assaults during periods of social upheaval, particularly when the problem family in question increased in size as a result of a rapid sequence of unplanned births.

　　Episodes of stress to the children could be interpreted as being due to social pressures (bad housing, debts, father in prison, etc.) but when all incidents were collected, collated and subjected to close scrutiny it could be seen that the children were suffering maltreatment. Multi-agency support was often used by such parents to the detriment of everyone concerned, and the parents seemed to out-manoeuvre the attempts to help both the children and themselves. The capacity of such parents to form useful protective (as opposed to shallow sentimental) bonds with their children was very limited.

　　Chronically unhappy children, children working below capacity, children with conduct disorders, antisocial youngsters, 'latch-key kids', truants, vandals – these are usually the victims of poor rearing, although in some such cases there are sometimes factors other than parental incompetence or irresponsibility contributing.

　5. *Child victims of exploitation* by their parents for emotional/neurotic reasons, or for material reasons. The child may have been conceived as a cure for parental depression, loneliness, or inadequacy, or 'to hold the marriage together'. Sometimes the parental emotional needs were so overwhelming that no child or adult could ever fulfil them. A special feature of emotional exploitation was the use of children by a husband and wife in conflict as 'marital footballs'[13], a common situation much discussed by the NSPCC workers. A special example of exploitation of children by inadequate unrestrained parents was seen in the cases of incest.

　　There were, in N.E. Wilts, examples of direct material exploitation of the children, the parents using conceptions to get points for a council house, or using the allowances for the children as financial crutches for themselves. A famous international example was the English train robber Ronald Biggs who was said to have planned the conception of his child as a means of avoiding extradition from Brazil. Nevertheless, material exploitation of the child was generally much less damaging than emotional exploitation. Child victims of the latter could suffer a great variety of conduct and neurotic disturbances.

(C) *As for (B) 1–5 but here the child victims only suffered episodic maltreatment.* In these families, supportive treatment by social workers or others had much more chance of success than in group B. External social stresses or illnesses were important in impairing the parental capacities, and were related closely to the episodes of maltreatment. If the stresses were alleviated, the children were properly cared for. Reopened cases, and multi-agency support were not prevalent features in this group.

　　The above 2 classifications are crude divisions of the types of child victims seen in our survey of N.E. Wilts. They should not be considered in isolation, but in the context of the considerations discussed in Chapter 5, Part I.

2. Neglect/ill-usage cases (See Table 6.20, D-F inclusive; Table 6.21, B2 and 3 and some cases of B4, and some cases from categories C2-4)

The neglect cases ranged from starved, or repeatedly dehydrated or abandoned young children, to young children irresponsibly left on their own for varying periods. Examples of blatant irresponsibility in failing to provide minimum essentials of parental care for young children came from a variety of agencies. The criterion for inclusion in the maltreatment (neglect/ill-usage) numbers was a situation caused by the parents which necessitated professional involvement on behalf of the children.

Abandonments, and receptions into care with repeated capricious removals, were often considered forms of parental neglect. The world of transient adults, evanescent relationships, unpredictable 'Uncles' and 'Daddies' appearing in the home and taking over, ensuing strife, children's homes, failed visits, sudden appearances by a sobbing mother with 'conscience gifts' followed by months or years of absence, are indicative of a failure* of biological parenting. Sometimes a child even had his name taken away – a new cohabitee arrives, and if his children happen to be called 'Wayne', 'Gary' and 'Darren', the existing 'Wayne', 'Gary' or 'Darren' is arbitrarily told he must be called another name.

COLLECTION OF INFORMATION ON MALTREATED CHILDREN (SEE ALSO PART I AND TABLE 6.1)

The numbers given at the end of this Part relate to numbers of children under 12, irrespective of the number of incidents, repetitions, or cases in a particular department. The age of 12 was chosen as a maximum because of biological considerations, and because teenagers are less vulnerable than the younger children. Those papers discussed in the Appendix had two peaks of interest – children under 3 (16 papers) and children under school age (38 papers). There were only about 15 papers[18] clearly concerned with the whole range of ages 0–16. It is pointless considering children over 16, because some 16 and 17 year olds were already maltreating their own children!

There was a dichotomy between abbreviated short periods or one or two lines on an isolated family of 3 or 4 total individuals, and other families with a huge network of socially incompetent people. Often these latter families extended their social (and medical) pathology over several generations, with multiple files on sibs and uncles and aunts, step and half sibs, and cohabitees[4,5]. Abusive, neglectful and problem families were remarkably often linked with each other by transient association, cohabitation, brief marriages or unsuspected kinships[5]. Multi-agency involvement often resulted in 'paper depots' of uncollated and unstandardized files in which items of 'hard' information on abuse and neglect of children were buried in sheaves of socio-psychological observations on adults, and bureaucratic administrative correspondence on in-

---

* Feeble, faulty or non-existent parental *protective bonding capacity*.

dividuals within the families who had created a problem to society. A practical difficulty resulting from the above considerations was that it was difficult to cross-check new items of incomplete or abbreviated information on individuals with common or commonly given names such as Smith, Jones, or Singh.

Social workers and allied professions vary greatly in their attitudes to parents in families with suffering dependants. Carter[6] neatly categorizes the main viewpoints. The words 'cruel' or 'neglectful' imply the penal/punitive attitude. The phrase 'parent behaviour problem' implies the traditional 'compassionate' attitude. Words such as 'subnormal intelligence', or 'hysterical psychopath' are indications of an attempt at the medical (scientific) sympathetic/neutral attitude. A phrase applied to the Children's Bill, that it could be 'anti the working-class parent' seems to have been made within the framework of the radical (social liberation via reorganization) approach, which blames the organization of society for rearing failures. The wilder expressions of the last are considered and criticized in a letter by Stroh[7].

The collecting of the ensuing numbers was influenced from all four of these standpoints, but parental motivation was not a major factor in defining the cases[8]. A child can suffer fear, pain, stress and ill-treatment whether his parent is a dull, deprived, exploited teenager with no home, or a selfish sadist. The approach of Clegg and Megson[9] is therefore preferred to that of Gil[8], and maltreated children in N.E. Wilts. were identified from the viewpoint of the children in their homes. The geographical boundaries, populations (N.E. Wilts.), years considered, and other aspects of methodology are the same as considered in Part I, except that collecting and collating of data continued until September 1975, and included children up to the age of 12.

Information was derived by:

1. Personal contact with the agencies and professionals listed in Table 6.1. Unfortunately, ascertainment from many of these agencies and individuals was unsystematic and incomplete.
2. Systematic examination of NSPCC cases. These included neglect and assault cases of 1965–1970. The NSPCC categories changed in 1971 from designations such as 'neglect' to those such as 'parent behaviour problem' or 'lacks proper care'. Superficially innocent designations such as 'housing problem' or 'child behaviour problem' or 'advice sought' could conceal cases of blatant cruelty, as evidenced from other medical or other social files. Less than half of the total official NSPCC new cases recorded for the circumscribed area of N.E. Wilts. were included in either the physical abuse or the neglect/ill-usage numbers.
3. Systematic re-examination of confidential files kept at Burderop Hospital since 1969, which in turn were derived from (1) immediately above, from child psychiatry and subnormality sources (mainly J. E. Oliver), and from research work associated with Part I.

Information on less than half the maltreated children emanated from NSPCC sources. Information on the most severely attacked children derived predominantly from hospital sources.

NUMBERS OF MALTREATED CHILDREN ASCERTAINED IN NORTH-EAST WILTSHIRE

Over an $8\frac{1}{2}$ year period 1921 children under 12 were ascertained from an average population of 45 000* children under 12 years old. A minimum of 4.2% of children under 12 are therefore victims of maltreatment by their parents. It can be seen from Table 6.22 that the ascertainment improved in 1972/73 as compared with the 1965/71 interval. In 1972/73 period there was a rate of 8.1 children under 12 maltreated, per thousand children under 12 per annum. The ratios of assault to neglect/ill-usage cases were 1:4.24 for the 1965/71 interval, but 1:2.36 in the 1972/73 interval. These numbers represent minimum estimates for under 12's because only $8\frac{1}{2}$ years were considered, and ascertainment was known to be incomplete. We found that certain families were 'repeating' as we scanned new agencies, but each new source invariably revealed some new families.

An accurate estimate of the amount of maltreatment in a community would require teams from the different agencies working in unison, for a total population of about 1/5–1/4 million. This could not be done on a larger scale, *as personal contacts are essential*. Formal reporting procedures will never reveal the true extent of child maltreatment. The teams would have to contain representatives from most of the agencies listed in Table 6.23.

It could be said that the 4% of English children so maltreated represents an indictment of our culture. There are other communities which simply do not provide welfare agencies corresponding to those in N.E. Wilts., and thus conceal the facts about bad rearing practices. For such cultures it is impossible to know the extent of maltreatment of children.

POSTSCRIPT

Since completing the collecting and collating of the 1921 cases, *routine* clinical work in child guidance and subnormality has revealed another 140–150 cases which would have fulfilled the criteria for inclusion in the 1965–1971, or 1972–1973 numbers. This reinforces our contention that the numbers given are minimum estimates, and that one maltreatment case (requiring professional intervention) per 100 children per year, for the 1972–1973 period, is closely approached. Light's (1973) estimates from Harvard University, and Chesser's post-

---

* The extra children born over the $8\frac{1}{2}$ year period, plus immigrants to the locality, swell the total population of under 12's, but this is balanced by those potential victims who were still babies at the end of the $8\frac{1}{2}$ year interval, plus emigrants who may have suffered abuse elsewhere.

Table 6.22   Results. Maltreated children under 12 years in N.E. Wilts. Population of 44 846 children under 12 in the areas considered (1971 Census)

Time interval (years inclusive)	Type of care (all children under 12)	Numbers of affected children over the time interval (repeat cases not counted)	Numbers of affected children under 12 (per thousand children under 12 per annum) for the relevant time interval	Rate per thousand per annum
1965–1972, with first half of 1973 (8½ yrs)	Maltreatment (all types)	1921	(42.8)	(5.0)
,, ,,	Assaults	425	(9.5)	(1.1)
,, ,,	Neglect/ill-usage	1496	(33.4)	(3.9)
1965–1971 (7 years)	Maltreatment (all types)	1374	(30.5)	(4.4)
,, ,,	Assaults	262	(5.8)	(0.8)
,, ,,	Neglect/ill-usage	1112	(24.7)	(3.5)
1972 with first half of 1973	Maltreatment (all types)	547	(12.2)	(8.1)
,, ,,	Assaults	163	(3.6)	(2.4)
,, ,,	Neglect/ill-usage	384	(8.5)	(5.7)

* The ratios of Assault to Neglect/Ill-Usage children were as follows:
1965/71 = 1:4·24
1972/73 = 1:2·36
1965/73 = 1:3·52

war statistics from England and Wales, as discussed in Chapter 5, Part II, are therefore supported here.

EXAMPLES FROM MEDICAL PRACTICE AND SOURCES OTHER THAN THE NSPCC (1–33)

1. *Baby girl 3 months*: Baby abandoned by mother who was sleeping rough and taking illicit drugs.

2. *Baby boy, 3 months*: Admitted to hospital with swollen left upper arm, bruising on left cheek and left leg, and swelling of right lower tibia. X-ray showed skull fractures and fractures of left humerus, fractured right lower tibia and healed fractures left 7th, 8th, and 9th ribs.

3. *Baby girl aged 13 weeks and girl aged 3*: The mother of these two children had an hysterical personality. Numerous suicidal attempts and gestures caused the involvement of many doctors and social workers. Suicidal threats as a manipulative technique had given way to homicidal threats towards the children, who had been mildly attacked and severely neglected on occasion. This mother had also threatened to inflict pain on the children, or cause permanent harm to them if her husband and others did not do as she asked. This mother complained that her 13 week old 'never smiles at me, she just doesn't care about me'. She also complained revealingly 'The only one who has come out of this (the psychiatric and social attention given) with anything worth while is M (the 3 year old)'.

4. *Baby girl, 6 months*: Admitted to hospital with failure to thrive and semi-starvation. The baby was rejected by the mother, who was dull of intelligence. This mother and her sister had been both severely ill-treated themselves as children, her sister ending up in a subnormality hospital. The baby's mother had married into another family with ill-treated children and multiple social problems.

5. *Baby boy, 7 months*: Put into care following episodes in which he was found with bloodshot eye, bruising to the face, severe bruising to the arm, scratches to the cheek and neck, and other episodes of bruising on different occasions. The mother felt she was too young when she had the baby and she could not stand his crying.

6. *Baby boy, 7 months*: Fractured femur and other traumata attributed to battering.

7. *Baby boy, 14 months*: 'So emaciated and his buttocks so infected that his life was in danger. . . . Considered calling in the police for this gross neglect.'

8. *Baby boy, 15 months*: Child repeatedly attacked. His arm was broken by his father, who insisted on looking after him, and threatened his wife with violence if she tried to intervene. The baby received more bruising and facial bleeding. The father eventually admitted being jealous because the child went to his mother rather than to him. The father had said that he had 'devils' inside him, as an explanation for the attacks.

Note: The excuse of 'devils' and like malign influences to explain and excuse aberrant behaviour resulting in cruelty to children and other family members is uncommon amongst English abusive parents. These types of beliefs recall mediaeval culture. They are dangerous because they preclude attempts to redress cruel acts towards more defenceless members within the family. An individual (who may not be psychotic) should not be encouraged in such beliefs because he can be reached neither by scientific psychiatry nor by moral exhortation. Somebody 'with devils' can do what he likes.

9. *Boy aged 2 years*: Child found with an unexplained fractured femur. Initially, the mother claimed that the child had jumped off a chair. Then she admitted breaking his leg, then retracted. This family depended on multiple agency support and had done so ever since the birth of the eldest of the 5 children. The 5 children had at least 3 different fathers. 'Uncles' came and went from the household, which had also been a haven for petty criminals on the run.

   Severe congenital defects were present in 4 out of 5 sibs and in 6 out of 9 uncles and aunts on the maternal side. There were large numbers of cousins on the maternal side with congenital defects. The sibs of the attacked child, plus cousins on the maternal side, had a range of psychiatric/social problems including prolonged school refusal. The legal father of the child and the cohabitee, who may have fathered the boy, both had criminal records. Two of the fathers' brothers had criminal records, and cousins on the paternal side were recorded as having been ill-treated and neglected in NSPCC and other files.

10. *Boy aged 2 years*: This boy was not changed or fed from morning to night by his mother, 'a simple fat, slow woman, who was in care herself as a child, and who does not like children and would rather work'.

11. *Girl aged 2½ years*: Bruising of child's face inflicted by this mother.

12. *Girl aged 2½ years*: Died 'as a result of falling over flex'. The child had a split liver, bruised heart, finger-grip bruises and fractured ribs.

13. *Boy aged 2¾ years*: '(The father) will not let M use his hands or touch anything, and requires him to sit motionless for long spells (hours). He has behaved like this since M was 1½. He hits him continuously, with heavy blows to the face, although these are openhanded slaps and not the clenched fist. There is no logical discipline. If M touches the staircase or wall, or anything else, he shouts "Hands off you little rat" and hits him. If M moves when he (the father) is at home, he says "Sit still, you little rat". M flinches whenever Mr D. moves. If M makes a noise, Mr D. says "Don't make a noise you little rat".' The mother left the father on account of his behaviour. The parents later reunited in another locality where M and his brother were both assaulted more severely than hitherto.

14. *Boy aged 3 years*: From babyhood, until the age of 4, this boy was 'Always being beaten up excessively – but his parents are so dull that they do not

know what they are doing'.

15. *Boy aged 3 years*: Repeated unjustified slapping, facial bruising, face held under water.

16. *Boy aged 3¼ years*: This little boy was anaemic, apathetic, withdrawn, had developed no speech even though of potentially average intelligence. He was vacant, drooling, and isolated. He had suffered minor (?finger-grip) bruising. His mother suffered very florid schizophrenia and she had incorporated her son into her delusional system. Her thought disorder was such that he was quite unable to cope with her vagaries, capriciousness and paranoid pre-occupations.

17. *Boy aged 4 years*: This little boy was hyperactive, with very limited attention and concentration. His mother never spoke to him, except to abuse him verbally. He was sometimes allowed to go to the lavatory and sometimes not allowed, depending on her mood. Despite this, he was repeatedly attacked for wetting himself, his mother shouting 'You dirty little sod', or 'You damned nuisance'. Her threshold of frustration was so low that she tolerated hardly anything from him. The mother then turned her husband against his son. This boy had a continual fear of violence, and lived in an atmosphere of hostility and verbal abuse. He was not accepted as a person, just as a permanent menace. He was subjected at times to primitive deconditioning but his mother's capriciousness, unpredictability and moodiness was such that he was in a permanently distressed state. If he moved in any direction he was shouted at 'Get out of the way ... Don't you break that bloody iron ... F ... off'. The boy was potentially of near average intelligence, but had been reduced to a dull, distractible, hyperactive state, with a vocabulary of oaths and threats and little else.

Observation of this state of affairs was exceptional. The facade presented by the family to naive observers was convincing – the mother seemed a bit inadequate; her son seemed unmanageable; she obtained sympathy. However, the observer found that the mother's laziness and lack of self control which had continued for years had worsened in the child's third and fourth year of life. 'It (the mental and physical cruelty, mainly the former) starts first thing in the morning, and goes on and on. There is no end to it. It is really bad. The pressure is constant, except when she knows she is being watched.'

18. *Boy aged 4 years*: From 4 until after the child started school, this boy was burnt several times by his father because of father's anger, at his (?feigned) deafness.

19. *Girl aged 4½ years*: Episodic bruising to face and buttocks. Head held under water. Held down and 'worked over' by mother and elder sibs. A 12 year old brother was given the duty of beating her by his mother.
   Note: There were several examples of parents permitting or encouraging sibs to attack a younger victim in the family. Professional staff tend to be naive in accepting explanations that injuries inflicted on ill-treated young

children were caused by sibs in innocent circumstances.

20. *Girl aged 5 years*: Referred by the school, following the finding of marks on her legs. Her twin brother then revealed that she had suffered by having her head banged against the wall by her mother. Bruises and bumps were found under the hair on this occasion, and on other occasions.

21. *Boy aged 5 years*: Paediatrician felt that this child had suffered delayed growth and delayed or stunted intellectual development, following severe emotional and material deprivation from birth onwards.

22. *Boy aged 6 years*: Found with marks on his throat, believed to have been inflicted by one or both parents.

23. *Boy aged 7 years*: D. 'very hit about . . . she drags him about by the wrists . . . marks on all the other children'. Neighbours asked for help (of the NSPCC and Social Services) saying that his mother 'really goes to town on D.'.

24. *Boy aged 8 years*: Rejected as a baby, and subsequently dressed as a girl by his neurotic mother, who never cuddled him. At 8 he was stealing and lying and soiling; his mother repeatedly listed his failures in front of him, and he was blamed for his sister's and mother's ill health, and the various marital difficulties. For years his mother had been saying 'You will go into a home . . . You are hateful. . .'. Apart from times in which the boy and his sister had been left for periods on their own by their mother, and the times that his mother had not wished to feed him or care for him as a baby, there were no recorded episodes of severe physical violence or gross neglect.

25. *Boy aged 9 years:* This boy had been used as ammunition in the marital conflicts of the two parents preceding their divorce, and following their re-marriages (ref. NSPCC[13]). His mother, an hysterical psychopath, alternated between telling him that she hated him, with telling him that she loved him but his father hated him. There was no violence and no gross neglect in the sense of having refused the boy material essentials of life. He had, however, suffered episodes of abandonment and had been used as a pawn. Reports of neglect were limited to the boy being left on his own, being unsupervised, or just being forgotten when he should have been picked up by a parent. He also suffered by having to cope from a young age with his mother's bouts of hysteria.

26. *Boy of 10 years*: Repeatedly beaten with belt for enuresis. Sent to school in torn, baggy canvas clothes as a reproach to him for wetting, so that other boys would know. He suffered multiple tics, poor progress and excessive anxiety symptoms. But his parents claimed 'he is just lazy'.

27. Father often in jail. Mother copulating with several men, whilst elder daughter had to control the younger children, who had been given beer to keep them quiet during the proceedings. The eldest daughter remonstrated and was subsequently attacked by another male in the household, a sadist, who had not taken part in the multiple sexual intercourse. This man having beaten the elder daughter (with the mother's approval) pursued her by car

out into the streets, until she was taken to someone's home. He himself had been reared in an environment of cruelty and sexual perversion, an individual from a described Huntington's disease kindred[14].

28. It took 10 weeks, with 8 hours concentrated work, for one doctor to collect and collate data on one neglected and ill-treated child of 4 years old in this large problem family. The result of this was an overflowing box file with 5″ depth of paper and files on this child and his family. This quantity of information was only obtained from medical sources before a start had been made on Probation, Social Services, NSPCC, Official Archives, Children's Home notes and many other sources.

No one professional person considered the child to come from a severe abuse family. Health visitors, doctors, social workers, probation officers alike all considered that the family represented a classical neglect/problem family. Different branches of the family had been encouraged not to co-operate in giving names and addresses of either themselves or their cohabitees, in an attempt to get extra money, extra accommodation, etc., as some were squatters. This family was linked by marriage, kinship or episodic cohabitation with 5 severely abusive (battering) families which had been independently studied.

The professional people trying to give family support had tended to consider isolated items of neglect or abuse from the standpoint of the motivation of adults caring for the abusive or neglected child at any one particular time. The impression was given in reports that the professionals could influence the course of events. Collecting and collating of information revealed, however, that the children had received much unnecessary violence as well as neglect. Their development had been impaired by the poor quality rearing.

From the child standpoint, their dull, damaged mothers or stepmothers had attracted unpredictable and untrustworthy cohabitees or husbands. Name changes, address changes, swapping of sexual partners and rapid mobility, meant that the children lived in a chaotic world where known adults were unkind, incapable or unreliable, and new adults might inflict pain or fear, even if they were called 'Uncle' or 'Daddy'. Whatever the circumstances described in reports of varying lengths on the social difficulties of the adults, many children in this family received severe ill-usage over long periods of time, often amounting to years or even decades.

The injuries and neglect episodes to the originally considered child, his half and step-sibs and his cousins, involved multiple bruising of different ages, head injuries, episodes of failure to thrive, burns, scalds, bites and lacerations. More frequent, however, were references to non-co-operation in clinic attendances, children hyperactive, apathetic, infested, infected, ill-cared for, and suffering repeated chest infections. The children appeared miserable. In some, impaired intellectual development and severe emotional disturbance was noted.

29. Three children under the age of 8 repeatedly left on their own in the dark in filthy surroundings. Electricity disconnected. Both parents out drinking at nights, sometimes not returning home, or returning home staggering and partly conscious. Family seen by NSPCC Inspectors on previous occasions.

30. Three children abandoned on two or more occasions by their mother. Four year old girl, the eldest, admitted to hospital with dehydration. Two year old boy hit and shaken hard by his mother for insufficient reason. 'The mother has a violent temper.' The mother was in care herself, as was her mother. 'She is used to welfare.' Her brothers and sisters were also in care, etc. Bruising to children reported on other occasions.

32. The eldest of four sibs had at the age of 10 become an experienced shoplifter, leading his younger brothers in antisocial acts. This boy, whose mother had been a juvenile delinquent, was rejected from birth onwards, and had many hospital admissions in another part of the country as a baby and toddler. Irrational hatred had been expressed so often towards him that he had ceased to respond to normal human social pressures. He and his younger sibs were unsupervised, 'latch key' children, fending for themselves in a criminal subculture.

33. Young children not fed adequately and not cared for. Indications of prolonged failure of social adjustment by their mother, and adult members of the family, including rent arrears, attacks on the police, different unstable cohabitees, etc.

EXAMPLES FROM THE NSPCC 34–42

The NSPCC reports did not specify very much detail about individual acts of cruelty or gross neglect towards children, as did many of the medical reports. They deal more with the world of social chaos, with wives out at Bingo, or leaving home for a variety of reasons. Chaotic disorganization within the family was the main recurring feature. Children were left on their own, or with unspecified, unknown or underaged babysitters. Husbands and wives used their children as marital footballs[13].

Unemployment was a recurring theme, but many of the fathers and cohabitees made no determined effort to stick at any jobs they achieved. Likewise, the children did not persist in school attendance. Mothers could not persist either in keeping babies and toddlers happy, or in effective contraception. Rent arrears, debts, lack of money for children's food, and maintenance problems arose. Problems involved the home, emergency accommodation, evictions, overcrowded caravans, and living illegally in other people's council houses. There were episodic family rows, sometimes with violence, or frustrated vandalism, or fights. The police, prison authorities and the probation service featured with regular monotony.

Health problems were associated with deprivation – father threw things at the children when he was depressed; mother was too depressed to cope, or she was nervous or neurotic, or had spells in mental hospital; both parents 'went sick' when they could not manage. Parents seemed to find refuge in hospitals, or in the houses of friends or neighbours, but the children ended up from time to time in children's homes, or temporarily fostered. The parents also tended to let the children rear themselves. The transient nature of the social bonds between the individuals in these disorganized families was often demonstrated by family complexity, with step and half and full sibs in different places in different permutations at different times.

34. Designation: Parent behaviour problem.

Family disorganized, with fighting and children out of control. Police involvement on account of mother's shoplifting. Violence in the home. Financial difficulties culminating in mother's nervous breakdown. Father away. Five children all eventually taken into care.

35. Designation: Parent behaviour problems.

Mother previously divorced. Second husband a gambler who severely beat up his wife when he lost money. Mother frequented Bingo halls. Family well known to the police and probation departments. Children suffering as a result of the assaults, and the parental pre-occupation with their own problems. Of the 5 children, 4 returned to the custody of mother's first husband.

36. Designation: Lack proper care.

Two children aged 6 and 9, left to their own devices day and night. Parents were separating, and mother was waiting for a divorce. Warnings from NSPCC, police and housing manager.

37. Designation: Leaving children on their own.

Two children aged 1 and 2, left on their own for long periods at nights. Doubtful paternities. New baby expected shortly, again paternity doubtful.

38. Designation: Parent behaviour problem.

Reopened case. 8 year old boy disturbed in behaviour as a result of parental mismanagement. Repeatedly beaten. Mother disinterested in children, except to beat the boy. Neighbours repeatedly reported beatings of the elder child and ill-treatment of the 1 year old and the baby of 3 months. Multi-agency involvement, repeated rent arrears, chaotic disorganization in the household. Both parents evaded family responsibilities. The 8 year old was subsquently taken into care.

39. Designation: Lacks proper care.

$1\frac{1}{2}$ year old left in dirty disorganized house with 4 men. Police noticed the child when called to deal with disturbance amongst the men. Mother found with another young girl aged 4 from another household. Empty milk bottles and empty beer bottles lying around. Baby's father in prison. Subsequent telephone call from neighbour saying the toddler was being neglected, when 6 men, some known to the police, were in the house. The child was removed to the care of the maternal grandmother.

40. Designation: Child behaviour problem.

Four children, aged 12, 9, 6 and 3 often alone on their own. Eldest boy stealing, and entering houses illegally. 'This is another case where parents are out working and do not know what their children are up to.'

41. Designation: Lack proper care.

Four children aged 1–7. Accusations from passer-by and neighbours that children had been hit excessively. Borderline subnormal mother with many relatives of similar ilk. History of child neglect in several branches of this family. Fighting between mother and her husband, mother walking out of the home and leaving children. Social disorganization, marital discord, involvement with the police and other agencies.

42. Designation: Advice sought.

No beds or bedding for two children, aged $2\frac{1}{2}$ and 18 months. Mother requested help with food and clothing. Two months later, the two children were taken to hospital following the ingestion of illicit (hallucinogenic) drugs used by the mother and her cohabitee. Subsequent gaol sentence on cohabitee, and probation for the mother.

References

1. Oliver, J. E., Cox, J., Taylor, A. and Baldwin, J. A. (1974). Appendix 1 of Severely Ill-Treated Young Children in North-East Wilts. Oxford University Unit of Clinical Epidemiology, Oxford Regional Health Authority

2. Myers, P. A., (1975). 'Can Education help break the pattern in families where there is cruel, neglectful or incompetent rearing?' Thesis submitted to University of Oxford Department of Educational Studies (A.C.E. special educational course)

3. Lewin, R. (1974). Malnutrition and the Human Brain. *World Med.*, **10,** 19

4. Oliver, J. E. and Taylor, A. (1971). Five generations of ill-treated children in one family pedigree. *Br. J. Psychiat.*, **119,** 473

5. Oliver, J. E. and Cox, J. M. (1973). A family kindred with ill-used children; the burden on the community. *Br. J. Psychiat.*, **123,** 81

6. Carter, J. (1974). In: *The Maltreated Child.* (London: Priory Press)

7. Stroh, G. (1975). Children at Risk. In: *Mind Out,* p. 11. June, 1975.

8. Gil, D. G. (1970). *Violence Against Children.* (Cambridge, Mass.: Harvard University Press)

9. Clegg, A. and Megson, B. (1968). *Children in Distress.* (London: Penguin)

10. Meadow, R. (1977). Munchausen Syndrome by Proxy. The Hinterland of Child Abuse. *Lancet,* **ii,** 343

11. Rogers, D. *et al.* (1976). Non-accidental injury – an extended syndrome of child abuse. *Br. Med. J.*, **1,** 793

12. Registrar General's Advisory Committee on Medical Nomenclature and Statistics (1968). *A Glossary of Mental Disorders,* Studies on Medical Poulation Subjects No. 22. (London: HMSO)

13. National Society for Prevention of Cruelty to Children (1974). Children as Marital Footballs. *The Child's Guardian,* Issue 6, 6

14. Dewhurst, K. (1970). Personality Disorder in Huntington's Disease. *Psychiat. Clin.*, **3,** 221

Part III – MALTREATMENT OF CHILDREN AS A CAUSE OF IMPAIRED INTELLIGENCE (J. E. Oliver and Ann Buchanan)

Child maltreatment as a cause of impaired intelligence can be considered as follows. The brain may have been damaged by direct violence to such an extent that the intellect has been obviously impaired. There would be concomitant neurological features, although in *some* cases these might diminish with time. A number of papers on battered babies include such cases (five of many possible examples are given from the UK, the USA and Australia[1-5]). Nevertheless, few papers so far have considered the problem from the point of view 'How much mental handicap is caused by baby battering?' A second, and probably numerically more important, group encompasses children whose brains have been damaged by secret and severe shaking[6-8]. Not only can subdural haematoma form as a result of the shearing of vessels between the dura and the brain surface, but punctate haemorrhages may form in the substance of the brain. Such haemorrhages should be compared with the retinal haemorrhages often seen in battered babies.

Children, such as the shaken babies with damaged brains, or children with brains damaged by other forms of indirect violence (such as repeatedly holding the baby or toddler under water[9], or intentional poisoning), may develop mental handicap without a history of skull fractures or even any evidence of bruising. Mentally subnormal children in both these first two groups (mental handicap following direct violence to the head, or following violence or active maltreatment which indirectly adversely involves the brain) are seldom given adequate diagnostic labels. The standard text books on subnormality do not consider this topic. The children tend to become classified as having their mental handicap caused by other factors – birth injury, prematurity, congenital abnormalities, etc. Evidence which may be minimal at first (e.g. retinal haemorrhages) soon disappears. Fractures resolve within weeks or months. In time, histories of possible parental involvement as a cause of a child's mental handicap become attenuated in the ensuing and subsequent notes. Doctors and social workers are reluctant to attribute mental handicap to parental violence whenever alternative explanations are possible, even if the idea enters their mind[1,2,30].

The third group contains children with intellects stunted by malnutrition, especially during the period of the maximum postnatal brain growth spurt (0–2 years, and to a lesser extent 2–4 years). Famine can affect whole populations in this way[10-17]. Publications on babies and toddlers with 'failure to thrive' due to neglect/deprivation of food, generally depict groups of children whose intellects are certainly temporarily retarded, with probable permanent effects. From these groups there are a proportion of babies who seem to have suffered permanent reduction in intelligence as a consequence of their mothers starving them at crucial intervals in their development[18-20].

Psycho-social deprivation, or 'experiential' deprivation, has long been recognized as a cause of subnormal intelligence[21-24]. Children in this fourth group usually would fall in the IQ ranges of 60–85, for experiential deprivation on its own is seldom held to be the cause of permanent, severe or profound mental retardation (IQ below 50). Psycho-social deprivation as a cause of mental handicap, is also recognized by all the international classification systems (for instance General Register Office[25], and Grossman[26]).

For completeness, a fifth group must be considered. Here the children have suffered such emotional trauma at the hands of their parents that they are unlikely ever to reach the full intellectual potential that they had inherited. This aspect is considered by Jones[27] in follow-up studies on battered babies, many of whom may *not* have suffered actual brain damage.

The sixth group is undoubtedly the most important numerically. Here are included children who have suffered intellectual impairment from combinations of the 5 (preceding) adverse influences discussed above. Attempts have been made to demarcate the 'neglect' families from the 'active abuse' families[28]. Despite such attempts there are consistent threads running through the literature that battered babies are often neglected (sometimes starved, sometimes deprived of stimulation). Likewise, neglected children have often suffered episodes of inappropriate violence. The neglected 'problem family' child may well have been severely shaken as a baby, to the extent of suffering punctate brain haemorrhages either during, or between, episodes of ill-health, infections, etc. associated with neglectful early rearing. It has been strongly emphasized by Dobbing and others that malnutrition and under-stimulation (experiential deprivation) are mutually synergistic influences[11-13,17,22-24,29]. We also believe that the concept of 'vulnerable' brains should be recognized. Impairments of intellect from abuse and neglect, especially in those children with vulnerable brains due to pre-existing abnormality or latent weakness, may be much commoner than generally realized[30]. Conversely, certain deprived children from poor backgrounds are sufficiently resilient to overcome handicapping events, and can become successful people.

During the past six years, several authors have drawn attention to the consequences of child abuse in relation to brain damage and mental function[6,7,27,30-36]. The British Paediatric Association Survey reported to the Parliamentary Select Committee on Violence in the Family that 92 out of 869 'non-accidental injury' cases reported by paediatricians in the United Kingdom were left with brain damage, and 48 with visual defects[37]. The Royal College of Psychiatrists, reporting to the same Committee, estimated '... if 75 young children per million of total population (UK) are severely attacked each year, then 18–19 per million could suffer intellectual impairment each year, often of a profound degree'[38]. Baldwin, projecting from the N.E. Wilts. data, gives a crude minimum estimate of 240 new cases of severe subnormality (IQ below 50) in England and Wales per year resulting directly from parental assaults on babies and toddlers[39].

To our knowledge, there have been two systematic surveys concerned with evaluating child abuse/maltreatment as a cause of subnormality of intelligence from reasonably large populations of mentally handicapped people. The first of these is from Alaska, and involves a retrospective case study analysis of 436 cases of mental retardation diagnosed in Anchorage between 1957 and 1973 (Eppler and Brown[40]). Eppler and Brown found that 65 of 436 (15%) of their cases had evidence of abuse and neglect prior to identification of their retardation. They discuss the paucity of reported studies of abuse and neglect as a cause of mental retardation. In their study, 24 out of the 65 (or 5.5% of the total population of 436) *had strongly suggestive evidence that abuse and/or neglect was the cause of their mental retardation*. Five cases suffered skull injuries with subdural haematoma and subsequent permanent brain injury. Seventeen cases had undernutrition and failure-to-thrive as infants prior to reported evidence of psychomotor retardation[40].

We considered all the 140 children under 16 admitted to, or already resident within the two subnormality hospitals in Wiltshire over the 1972/73 two year period[30]. This study was largely prospective, paralleling routine clinical work. A double system of investigation of files was also used. Firstly, names and alternative names of the children, sibs, parents and other relatives were used to track files in a laborious family record linkage search. Secondly, the records of at least 25 different types of medical and social agency concerned with child welfare were scanned throughout the areas of the child's (or sibs') residence. The following definitions were used:

(1) VIH (Violence-induced handicap): Mental handicap following brain damage caused by assault(s). Assaults included fierce or repetitive shaking and/or throwing of a baby or young toddler – more dangerous practices than simple fist blows. VIH is not so difficult to confirm where a child has previously been entirely normal and healthy. Nevertheless, abnormal children may be most at risk. This definition, therefore, includes doubtfully healthy or abnormal children, whose intellect was *unequivocally further impaired* following assaults affecting the brain. In this latter instance, the VIH must usually have been severe.

(2) Abuse: Independent professional evidence that, before admission to hospital, the child had been a victim of physical assault(s) inappropriate to its age or development, and to an extent which warranted concern and/or intervention on the child's behalf (see Table 6.23).

(3) Neglect: Independent professional evidence that the child was suffering as a result of inadequate parental care, which warranted concern and/or intervention on the child's behalf (see Table 6.24 for instances).

The results can be summarized as follows:
In a survey of 140 children under 16 in two subnormality hospitals:

Table 6.23 Abused children—type of, and age at, abuse among 140 children admitted to subnormality hospital

Type of abuse	Under 2 years	2–5	6+	Total
Abused children with head injuries	6	5	1	12
Fractures associated with physical abuse:				
(A) Numbers of children with skull fractures	2	1	—	3
(Number of skull fractures)	(4)	(1)	—	(5)
(B) Numbers of children with rib fractures	3	1	—	4
(Number of rib fractures)*	(4–7)	(1)	—	(5–8)
(C) Numbers of children with other fractures	3	2	—	5
(Number of other fractures)	(4)	(2)	—	
(D) Total number of children with fractures associated with physical abuse	6	3	—	9
(Total number of fractures)*	(12–15)	(4)	—	(16–19)
Children receiving beatings, or bruisings and other surface injuries associated with abuse	14	11	2	27
Child victims of killing attempts	2	—	—	2
Total numbers of children with evidence of abuse	15	14	2	31

* Sometimes old fractures were uncertain on X-ray. Where there are two figures in brackets, these represent the maximum and minimum numbers of fractures.

Table 6.24 Neglected Children – Type of neglect among
140 children admitted to subnormality hospital

Type of neglect	Total children
1. General low standards of care or neglect specified	33
2. General low standards of care of neglect specified with consequential multi-agency involvement	28
3. Inadequate feeding specified	16
4. Experiential (psycho-social) deprivation	33
5. Failure to seek essential medical care, or co-operate in treatment of child	13
6. Child exposed to unnecessary hazards	5
7. Child exposed to cold with inadequate clothing	5
8. Sexual abuse	2
9. Professional intervention necessary as child was unattended for long periods	6
10. Other forms of neglect or unspecified	12
Habitual pattern of rearing	57
Isolated incident	10
Total children suffering as a result of inadequate parental care	67

1. A confirmed minimum of 4 (2.8% of the total) were previously mentally normal children who had been rendered severely mentally handicapped as a direct result of parental violence. This figure for parental violence induced handicap (PVIH or VIH) compares with a crude independent estimate of 2.5% calculated from the average estimates of 7 Wessex consultants in mental handicap on the probable numbers of children in their hospitals rendered brain damaged as a result of abuse.
2. A possible maximum VIH figure of 11% of the total were apparently normal children at birth and up to at least 3 months, who came from violent homes, and *could* have suffered impairment of intellect as a result of abuse.
3. 22% of the children in the survey had been victims of physical assaults inappropriate to their age or development, warranting concern and/or intervention on the child's behalf. In a further 10% there was evidence of professional concern, but not firm evidence of child abuse. Thus in a total of 32%, there was recorded professional concern that the child was at risk or had been the victim, of physical maltreatment.
4. There was recorded professional concern that the care of the child had been inadequate at home, and this was an habitual pattern of rearing for 41% of the children.

5. In 24% of the children, neglect and deprivation was considered to be a factor contributing to the degree of mental handicap.
6. 21% of the children in the survey had suffered both physical ill-treatment and deprivation. In over three-quarters of this particular group of children, there was no clear cut 'biological' cause for their handicap.

Tables 6.23 and 6.24 give some idea of the types of maltreatment. The rate for children admitted to the subnormality hospitals, who suffered abuse and/or neglect in our survey is approximately 12 times greater than that found in a comparable survey of children in the general population in N.E. Wilts.[41]. That survey used identical definitions and covered a similar area.

The two main conclusions of the study were as follows. Firstly, mentally handicapped children would appear to be more vulnerable to abuse or maltreatment than normal children. Secondly, violence induced (mental) handicap (VIH) should be recognized as a major cause of mental handicap. Children previously normal, but rendered mentally retarded as a result of abuse, account for many more cases than phenylketonuria. The consequences are frequently more severe than those of Down's Syndrome.

References

1. Kempe, C. H., Silverman, F. N., Steele, B. F., Droegemuller, W., and Silver, H. K. (1962). The battered child syndrome. *J. Am. Med. Assoc.*, **181,** 17
2. Oliver, J. E., Cox, J., Taylor, A. and Baldwin, J. A. (1974). Severely Ill-treated Young Children in North-East Wiltshire. Unit of Clinical Epidemiology. Oxford Record Linkage Study. Oxford Regional Health Authority. Research Report No. 4. August 1974
3. Cooper, C. (1975). The Doctors Dilemma. In: *Concerning Child Abuse*, A. W. Franklin; (ed.), (Edinburgh: Churchill-Livingstone)
4. Birrell, R. G. and Birrell, J. H. W. (1968). The Maltreatment Syndrome in Children: A hospital survey. *Med. J. Aust*, **2,** 1023
5. James, H. E. and Schut, L. (1974). The Neurosurgeon and the Battered Child. *Surg. Neurol.*, **2,** 415
6. Guthkelch, A. N. (1971). Infantile Subdural Haematoma and its Relationship to Whiplash Injuries. *Br. Med. J.*, **2,** 430
7. Caffey, J. (1974). The Whiplash Shaken Infant Syndrome. *Pediatrics*, **54,** 396
8. Oliver, J. E. (1975). Microcephaly following Baby Battering and Shaking. *Brit. Med. J.*, **2,** 262
9. Nixon, J. and Pearn, J. (1977). Non-accidental immersion in bath-water: another aspect of child abuse. *Brit. Med. J.*, **1,** 271
10. Winick, M. and Rosso, P. (1969). The Effect of Severe Early Malnutrition on Cellular Growth of Human Brain. *Pediat. Res.*, **3,** 181
11. Watts, G. (1976). Malnutrition in context. *World Med.*, **11,** 57
12. Waterlow, J. C. (1974). Some Aspects of Childhood Malnutrition as a Public Health Problem. *Br. Med. J.*, **4,** 88
13. Lewin, J. (1974). Malnutrition and the human brain. *World Med.*, **10,** 19
14. Hertzig, M. E., Birch, H. G., Richardson, S. H. and Tizard, J. (1972). Intellectual levels of school-children severely malnourished during the first two years of life. *Paediatrics*, **49,** 814
15. Dobbing, J. (1974). The Later Development of the Brain and its Vulnerability. In: *Scientific Foundations of Paediatrics,;* J. A. Davis and J. Dobbing; (eds) (London: Heinemann)

16. Chase, H. P., Canosa, C. A., Dabiere, C. S., Welch, N. N. and O'Brien, D. (1974). Postnatal undernutrition and human brain development. *J. Ment. Defic. Res.*, **18**, 355

17. Editorial (1976). The ultimate cost of malnutrition. *Br. Med. J.*, **2**, 1158

18. Silver, H. K. and Finkelstein, M. (1967). Deprivation Dwarfism. *J. Pediatrics*, **70**, 317

19. Bullard, D. M., Glaser, H. H., Heagarty, M. C. and Pivchik, E. C. (1968). Failure to thrive in the 'neglected' child. *Annual Progress in Child Psychiatry and Child Development*. (New York: Brunner-Mazel)

20. Krieger, I. (1974). Food Restriction as a Form of Child Abuse in Ten Cases of Psychosocial Deprivation Dwarfism. *Clin. Pediat.*, **13**, 127

21. Pringle, M. K. (1977). Parental Deprivation in Under 5s. The Effects of Emotional and Intellectual Deprivation. *Proc. R. Soc. Med.*, **70**, 24

22. Birch, H. G., and Gussow, J. D. (1970). *Disadvantaged Children* (New York: Grune and Stratton)

23. Blackie, J., Forrest, A. and Witcher, G. (1975). Subcultural mental handicap. *Br. J. Psychiat.*, **127** 535

24. Rutter, M. (1972). *Maternal Deprivation Reassessed*. (London: Penguin Books)

25. General Register Office: Studies on Medical and Population Subjects (1968, amended 1973). *A Glossary of Mental Disorders*, No. 22. (London: HMSO)

26. Grossman, H. J. (1973). Manual on Terminology and Classification in Mental Retardation. American Association on Mental Deficiency, Special Publication No. 2. Washington

27. Jones, C. (1978). The Fate of Abused Children. In: *Challenge of Child Abuse*. A. W. Franklin (ed.) (London: Academic Press)

28. Young L. (1964). *Wednesday's Children*. (New York: McGraw-Hill)

29. Dobbing, J. (1974). Intelligence after Malnutrition. *Lancet*, **i**, 802

30. Buchanan, A. and Oliver, J. E. (1978). Abuse and Neglect as a Cause of Mental Retardation: A Study of 140 Children Admitted to Subnormality Hospitals in Wiltshire. *Br. J. Psychiat.* **131**, 458

31. Martin, H. P. (1972). The child and his development. In: *Helping the Battered Child and his Family*. C. H. Kempe and R. E. Helfer (eds.) (Philadelphia: J. B. Lippincot)

32. Martin, H. P. *et al.* (1974). The development of abused children. In: *Advances in Pediatrics*, **21**, (Chicago: Year Book Medical Publishers)

33. Sarsfield, J. K. (1974). The neurological sequelae of non-accidental injury. *Devel. Med. Child Neurol.*, **16**, 826

34. Smith, S. M. and Hanson R. (1974). 134 Battered children: a medical and psychological study. *Br. Med. J.*, **3**, 660

35. Mackeith, R. (1974). Speculations on Non-Accidental Injury as a cause of Chronic Brain Disorder. *Devel. Med. Child Neurol.*, **16**, 216

36. Mackeith, R. (1975). Speculation on some possible long-term effects of child abuse. In: *Concerning Child Abuse*, A. W. Franklin (ed.) (Edinburgh: Churchill-Livingstone)

37. British Paediatric Association (1976). Evidence presented to the Select Committee on Violence in the Family, 8 June 1976

38. Royal College of Psychiatrists (1976). Evidence presented to the Select Committee on Violence in the Family, 8 June 1976

39. Baldwin, J. A. (1976). (Personal communication)

40. Eppler, M. and Brown, G. (1977). 'Child Abuse and Neglect': Preventable Causes of Mental Regardation. From the First International Congress on Child Abuse and Neglect, Geneva

41. Oliver, J. E. (1975). Child abuse. In: *Social Crises in Service Communities*. Proceedings of Triservice Multi-disciplinary Conference, p. 73 (taken from Symposium held at Amport House, Hants, 30 September 1975)

7 The psychiatrist's viewpoint

P. D. SCOTT*

SOME HISTORICAL POINTS

As long ago as 1888 Samuel West, the founder of Great Ormond Street Children's Hospital, had accurately observed and recorded the principal features of what we now call the battered baby syndrome[1]. He noted the very tender age of the child (five weeks), the main symptoms (unexplained painful swelling of an arm), that it was recurrent (there had been previous similar, asymmetrical lesions in the other arm, and one leg), there had been delay in bringing him to hospital, the child was not neglected, three other children of the family irrespective of sex had been similarly affected when they were babies, and two of their cousins had also had swellings of the arms or legs at similar ages, all the lesions cleared up quickly in hospital. He even recognized the traumatic element ('greenstick fractures') but he did not state the origin of the violence. He was in fact demonstrating another, extremely important, feature of the syndrome – the reluctance of observers to enquire into how the trauma happened.

This is perfectly clearly demonstrated by the now well-known history of the condition. It is very interesting to note how large a part radiologists played in facing the awful truth that adults and parents can inflict such damage. The radiologist usually sees little of his patients and views his pictures in a darkened and silent room, far from crying babies and weeping or sullen parents. Possibly it was this isolation which enabled Snedecor (1935), Caffey (1946) and especially Silverman (1953) to reach the point at which the blunt indictment of the parents for deliberately injuring their children and then denying it, could courageously be made[2-5]. It remained for Henry Kempe (1962), well described (*Lancet*, June 1st, 1974) as a latterday Charles Kingsley, to collect the facts, invent a dramatic name for the syndrome, and not only to bring it before the

---

* Dr. Peter Scott died in August 1977.

public, but to go on bringing it before the public[6,7]. Kempe, alarmed by the large number of children coming to his clinic with non-accidental injuries, contacted some eighty district attorneys in an effort to obtain a more accurate picture of the true incidence of the problem[8]. In 1961 the American Academy of Pediatrics held a symposium on this subject at which Kempe launched the term 'battered child syndrome'. This was followed by the British Paediatric Association's report[9] on accidents in childhood in 1966.

DEFINITION

Syndromes, like living organisms, arise, have their day and then disintegrate, leaving a cluster of bright new syndromes behind them. So it is with this one. But the term battered baby has been immensely useful in riveting the attention of a reluctant public to the hard realities of the situation. As such it should live on even though its clinical significance is lost.

The definition of the battered child syndrome has shown interesting changes. Kempe and his colleagues said that it was 'a clinical condition, in young children who have received serious physical abuse, generally from a parent or guardian'. This and the early definitions were concerned to break through the reluctance and inertia shown by the public to face the facts, so that the definitions pulled no punches, and linked parents with words such as severe injuries (note the plural) and with clear motivational implications such as deliberately or wilful and this was justified[10]. But then paediatricians began to realize that the high degree of stigma and opprobrium so engendered, may have a secondary effect of deterring the already reluctant parent from bringing the child to hospital. Definitions then began to soft pedal the motivation involved. Hence Oppé's cautious definition '. . . which cannot be unequivocally explained by natural disease or simple accident'[11]. This process was carried further by the need to encourage reporting of such cases, or at least admission of the child for observation. The casualty officer or paediatric resident or registrar, after a hurried preliminary examination in the outpatient department, is obviously going to hesitate before labelling parents as wilful batterers of their children; hesitation in this field often loses a life. More recent definitions therefore avoid unjustified and potentially dangerous assumptions about causation and motive, and simply state that a battered child is a child under 5 years with unexplained injuries. Clearly abuse does not stop at 5 but, if there must be a cut-off point this is as appropriate as any, especially in view of the child's increasing ability thereafter to give an account of what has happened. Beware, however, the naive idea that children over 5 ought to be able to run away or seek help. Such a belief falls into the category of armchair theories along with such statements as 'Women who are raped must have co-operated to some extent' and 'Battered wives should report their husbands to the police'. Many people have no conception of the degree of violence which is sometimes used, nor of the paralysing effect of very gross or repeated violence. Some have recommended the renaming of the syndrome 'non-accidental injury' in line with this reasoning. One of the most cogent re-christenings, suggested by the Bath Social Services Department (1974), is simply 'CPV' which, of course, offers an immediate challenge to our inquisitiveness; it stands for Concealed Parental Violence[12]. It is the only approach which immediately draws attention to the possibility of parental deceit. Yet clinically it is not as appropriate as it might be, for many battering parents do not conceal it, provided that they are sympathetically approached, and know on what door to knock. We, the observers, are often the concealers.

It is probably best to retain the term 'battered child' for publicity purposes, for it has historical and emotional usefulness but, for teaching medical and social-work students, to use a simple 'non-accidental' definition which, making no assumptions as to causation or severity of lesions, stresses the need for investigation and perhaps offers a reminder about our reluctance to suspect the worst. Such a definition should go some way to revealing the plight of these children, getting them properly examined and investigated, without unduly alarming or antagonizing the parents, and at the same time reminding ourselves of our own inherent blind spots.

A battered child is therefore one who has suffered unexplained physical injury with the following characteristics:

(1) often there are multiple injuries acquired at different times;
(2) often the injuries are concealed by clothing, sometimes the injuries are internal without damage to the skin and may then present as failure to thrive;
(3) coma often with acute abdominal symptoms; such injury should in every case raise the possibility of admission to a children's ward or nursery;
(4) such injury is very likely to recur, as many as 10% are killed and a high proportion suffer permanent damage, all observers tend to be reluctant to recognize the non-accidental nature of the injury;
(5) the immediate stimulus for the battering invariably comes from the victim.

Is there a syndrome? Probably there is a syndrome of physical injury to the child, but amongst injuring agents there are several different varieties. The objective for teaching purposes, therefore, should be to have a check list to cover the immediate examination of the child, designed to help the doctor to decide whether or not to segregate the child, and then a description of the more leisurely team-approach to the family as a whole, designed to help in the making of long term plans. This is a reflection of the fact that the physical signs in this area are more characteristic and definite than the social and psychological findings.

BIOLOGICAL ASPECTS

Whenever studying human behaviour it is always worthwhile first to approach it from a biological point of view, and especially to search for comparable behaviour in lower animals. Animals do not offer us plausible explanations and rationalizations. We have to rely on observation and cannot so readily apply our own introspective experiences to their situation. We can subject them to experimental situations. Their life cycle is sufficiently short for the experimenter or observer to have some knowledge of their whole life experience. We are less likely to become emotionally involved and prejudiced while working with them. There is, of course, no question of transferring conclusions, reached with animals, directly to humans, but it is perfectly reasonable, and often extremely helpful to see if an hypothesis worked out with animals has any application to man. 'Entia,' said Occam, 'non sunt multiplicanda', nor should theories!

Of all the activities of birds and mammals (hunting, gathering, defending territory, eating, sleeping, licking and preening) only the closely related functions of playing, mutual grooming and reproduction require the presence of another member of the species, and of these only reproduction positively demands a very high level of altruism and giving. An animal and even some humans, can exist without much contact with others, but to reproduce successfully there must be a consideration of the other partner, and a great deal of hard work, either filling widely gaping beaks with grubs, or working to buy prams, disposable nappies, baby foods and school fees. Reproduction is without doubt our most difficult and demanding social task. It is not surprising therefore that a number of candidates shy away from it, are late starters or show some degree of failure in the process. One way of failing is to desert the nest, and another is to attack the spouse or offspring. Battering biologically indicates an incapacity, either temporary or permanent, for reproduction.

Biologists learn that if an animal is observed to be behaving in an apparently senseless, non-adaptive way, the first thought should not be to find out what is wrong with that animal, but to ask whether it might be in the wrong environment, or whether something has gone seriously wrong with its environment. A small animal whose natural response to anxiety is to dive down his burrow, may repeatedly precipitate himself from the observer's hand onto the floor, in an apparently suicidal manner. A cat with a litter of kittens, if moved with them to a strange territory, may absolutely reject them, even though apparently suffering great discomfort from swollen mammary glands: restoration to her familiar ground immediately restores a sullen, spitting, starving feline, into the well loved family pussy-cat, once more contented and 'proud' of her kittens. With animals, such as primates, that rely on learning rather than instinct, the picture in complicated in that, although the present environment may be satisfactory, it was not so at some time in the past. Thus Harlow's monkey[13], who battered her baby so severely that it had to be removed in order to save its life, had been brought up in a highly unnatural early environment which had denied her the opportunity of learning normal social responses. Any female monkey subjected to such deprivations would probably show comparable callous behaviour to her offspring. The two deprivations in these monkey experiments were substitution of the real mother by an inanimate effigy and prevention of any contact with other young monkeys. There is no possibility therefore of the now grown up battering mother having been battered herself in infancy. It would be surprising if research in humans revealed (as has been suggested) that all battering parents have themselves been battered.

It is often stated that all puerperal mothers get depressed, and indeed experience in any hospital obstetric ward will reveal a number of weeping mothers, and many others who say that they went through a 'depressive patch'. Yet Dr Martin Richards[14] of Cambridge University, who is completing important research in this area, although confirming depression in the obstetric ward mothers, says that such puerperal tearfulness does not occur in mothers delivered at home. He finds that if inexperienced mothers (whom well-meaning hospital staff may protect) are given responsibility, they rise to it without difficulty. On the other hand he confirms that mothers on new housing estates isolated from the traditional flow of collective experience normally passed on from generation to generation, do show 'a high rate of depression'. Many studies confirm that isolation correlates highly with battering.

Interruption of the chain of interaction between an animal and its newly born offspring is known to be dangerous in many species. Might it not have at least some bearing upon the current practice in obstetric hospitals of keeping mothers and babies apart except at feeding times, and, in the case of premature babies, totally apart? Sheep and goats are likely to kick their offspring to death if they are separated for a while[15] and other forms of rejectant behaviour have been observed in cats, dogs, monkeys and other animals. The moments after birth, during which animals lick or handle, or suckle the baby may be important for the human mother too. 'Not only does this separation of the young from the mother at birth adversely affect the mother's responses and her efficiency as a mother, but it may have an adverse effect on the infant's behaviour for the rest of its life. The rat, sheep, or other animal when it grows up and has its own young is apt to be an inefficient mother, not looking after its young properly, so that there is a high mortality. ... We know[16] that premature babies fare less well at school than full-term babies of the same level of intelligence and suffer more troublesome behaviour problems, but the reason is unknown'[17].

There are sufficient broad hints here, that the causes of battering, or one of the causes, may lie in the immediate or early environment. It is possible also that although clinical research shows that many battering parents were themselves harshly treated in childhood, yet the actual hitting may have been an accompaniment of some deeper factor rather than the direct or essential cause; indeed hitting is so very common that such a conclusion becomes a probability.

To return to lower animals, another view point suggests itself; that if circumstances are sufficiently unfavourable, elimination of offspring is (biologically at least) adaptive. The pregnant rat who smells the presence of a male stranger, may abort. In some species environmental shortages cause resorption of the pregnancy. Disturbance of the nest in some species may (as many of us learnt with childhood pets) result in eating or desertion of the progeny. Particularly in nomadic tribes, control of the economic balance of the group by deliberate elimination is historically not so far off. Aristotle, Plato and Roman law recommended the killing of all imperfect deformed children if the parents wished, though the act was disapproved of. There is much evidence that the attitude to killing of a newly born child is totally different to that of a child accepted as part of the family. Murderers of children who have been allowed to survive their earliest infancy are very rare though not quite unknown among the lower races. Parental destruction of the new born has been common, anthropologically speaking, and was often encouraged, especially if the child was illegitimate, if its mother died, if it was weakly or regarded as unlucky in some way. Even now there is active discussion on the possibility of eliminating mongolism by the destruction of the fetus if tapping of amniotic fluid indicated the possibility of morbidity. Clearly the attitude to survival is still very much evolving in this crowded world. And clearly the finding of modern research that the younger the child the greater its risk from parental attack has ethological and anthropological roots.

We see here the motive of deliberate elimination on expedient grounds, and this, of course, is totally different from battering of children. How many other forms of child injury are there? Can we put battering into its context amongst other deviant behaviours, and is it susceptible to classification?

INTENSITY OR DEGREE OF INJURY

Any piece of behaviour invariably may be reached from a number of different directions and is therefore always susceptible to classification. A great variety of parameters present themselves, each of which has its peculiar shortcomings and advantages.

Castle and Kerr[18] surveying 292 cases of children, under the age of 4 years, suspected of physical abuse, used a classification of their injuries into:

(1) Fatal: resulting in death
(2) Serious: all fractures, head injuries, internal injuries and severe burns
(3) Moderate: soft-tissue injuries of a superficial nature.

They then compared their findings with those of an earlier study by Skinner and Castle[19] of 78 battered children. There were very great differences in the degree of violence which had been applied in those two samples, perhaps partly due to differences in mode of collection and perhaps also to a progressively greater willingness to refer lesser degrees of injury. In the Castle paper 42%, and in the Skinner paper 73%, had been seriously injured. It is very difficult also, even for experienced medical practitioners with the help of psychologists, to assess the severity of brain damage in such young children. Occasionally the post mortem on a battered baby reveals old haemorrhage in the brain tissues, for example within the thalamus, the effects of which had not been recognized and yet which may later on have declared itself as some degree of personality disorder, or other disability. The studies showed that the younger the child, the more serious the injuries are likely to be. The only injury to the great majority of children over the age of 24 months was bruising.

A study by Scott[20] of 29 fatal cases of battering, subsequently extended to 50 cases, shows not only the inevitably greater severity of injuries, but a very marked excess of violence. Thus of the 50 dead children, all under 5 years, 37 (74%) had an intracranial injury (usually subdural haematoma), and 28 (56%) had rupture of some intra-abdominal organ (usually the liver, mesentery or jejuno-duodenal junction); the other causes of death were asphyxia and intra-thoracic complications of violence. There is an overlapping of intra-cranial and intra-abdominal injuries either of which would have been sufficient to cause death. The greater risk for the younger child is confirmed (nearly half of them within their first year), but the degree of violence does not decrease in the older children. Nor is there any difference in the degree of violence (in these fatal cases) between biological parents and substitute parents.

Terms which are descriptive of what has happened, tapping, hitting, thrashing, battering, killing; or not requiring treatment, first aid only, admission to hospital, permanent disability; or fatal, serious, moderate, are useful as a preliminary research approach, but are bound to be subjective and may depend on the existence of good services or observant neighbours influencing the precise point at which the cross-sectional observation is made. Without some longitudinal factor they are unlikely to lead to firm clinical implications, for today's moderate case may very well be tomorrow's fatality, or on the other hand may never recur.

EXTENSITY OF INJURY

A linkage of such grades of intensity with grades of extensity may improve the effectiveness of the classification. The crux of the battering phenomenon does lie in extensity. Anyone who has cared for a difficult baby will understand a single loss of temper, but it is the failure of that one loss of temper to cause such a strong reaction in the parent as never to permit repetition, that is so striking. Clinical practice suggests a division into: threatened or feared attack, a single isolated incident, regular assaults, situational and the crescendo attacks. But here again who can be sure, except after long follow-up, that an isolated incident will remain so?

It would be helpful if it were known what differences there might be between extreme cases in which the child has been killed as compared with lesser degree of damage. Reverting again to Scott's study of 50 fatal cases of child battering and comparing these with Skinner and Castle's 78 cases there are appreciable differences: less of the parents are married to one another, the presence of a substitute parent is more common, more of the mothers go out to work leaving their man in charge, the injuries are excessively severe (even disregarding the lesion which caused death) and there is a higher frequency of, and a higher degree of violence in, the previous convictions of the fathers.

Smith et al.[21] investigated 214 parents of battered babies. They confirmed that the parents are young and predominantly of lower social class. Among the mothers 70% had an abnormal personality and 48% were neurotic. Nearly half were of borderline or subnormal intelligence and 11% had a criminal record. Of the fathers, 64% had an abnormal personality, more than half being psychopaths, 29% had a criminal record. They write 'it is disconcerting to observe that they (the fathers) share similar personality characteristics with a group of fathers who did kill their children'[22,23]. Detailed comparison of the two samples of fathers does show a similar very high incidence of personality disorder.

Bearing in mind the strong correlation between battering and youth of parents and youth of baby it does seem important that research projects should control these two factors. Only one or two studies have done this[24]. The clinical impression, from 50 fatal cases, and rather more non-fatal cases, is that the degree of psychiatric abnormality is less in the very young parents. The group of parents who batter their newly born child seem to contain some of the most severely disturbed personalities as well as some of the most hopeful parents (the very young ones who are unprepared for parenthood and under great environmental stress). Many writers on battered babies do not define what they mean by a battered baby and are inclined to include some psychotic parents who made a single attack upon their child and who ought not really to be in the battering category at all. The occasional mother who is psychiatrically depressed may kill her new born baby, but such a happening is totally unlike the battering of babies[25].

ENVIRONMENTAL PROVOCATION AS A FACTOR IN CLASSIFICATION

It might reasonably be expected that provocation might arise from the material surroundings, from the marital situation or from the child victim. Difficulties in the material surroundings are inevitably present with distressing and monotonous regularity – poor accommodation, hostile neighbours, debts, threats of eviction, unemployment, shortage of money, isolation (perhaps in a high-rise flat) and loneliness. There are of course dangers in inferring too much from such findings. It is less hurtful to pride, to blame a rat-infested home than to admit that your husband is going out with another girl, or that you can't manage to hold down a job for more than a few weeks. The provocation of poor surroundings depends on changes rather than absolute values; it varies with what you expect from life. We know that battering (at least that sector referred to us) occurs in the lower social-class groups, and in the younger sections thereof, and both these factors are known to correlate also with stresses of all kinds. Environmental difficulty falls upon the socially disadvantaged and on them it not only rains but pours. To make any sense of material provocation we would either have to have a control group, or better still study the real meaning of an individual's susceptibility through some form of projection test or Kelly-grid; for even if all the neighbours have similar provocation, yet the final straw of material goading may make the difference between battering and not battering. All that can safely be said about material stress is that it is very widely present amongst non-battering families and that it is unlikely to be the major factor in causing, or even precipitating, battering.

PROVOCATION FROM HUSBAND

The marital situation, and particularly some degree of conflict with the spouse, seems crucial in very many of the cases, especially the mothers. The form of the conflict varies as widely as their personalities. Basically danger arises in the mother when she is angry and cannot effectively or safely express it. An Irish girl repeatedly hit her second daughter (though the first had escaped any such hazard) when her husband began to go out with his business associates and to bring them home, where he would show interest in them rather than her. As long as he was home and attentive to her she felt no impulse to batter. Very frequently the mother is basically ill at ease in her womanly and maternal role, and thus quarrels for supremacy with her husband, but yet gets angry when he leaves the house. A girl who showed unmistakable evidence of 'masculine protest' (having avoided dolls and feminine pastimes, preferred football with the boys, cut her hair short, avoided pretty frocks and make-up) consistently battled with her husband but when he went out to watch a football match (which she longed to see) she pushed needles into her child. Is this not the revenge motive, or displacement of aggression (Medea complex)? Not entirely, for she did not plan the action, and was only precipitated into it by further direct cues from the child – crying and refusal to be fed; but this is a good example of overdetermination, and the overlap of categories. Another and very different variety is the mother who habitually fortified her poor self opinion by ensuring a steady inflow of approval and reassurance (both from others and, narcissistically, from herself), by maintaining a very high degree of material perfection. Such mothers have perfectly tended homes, they themselves are neat, clean and pretty, their children are equally burnished and angelic, any disorder or mess must instantly be cleared up, and any failure of the husband to admire and show approval is met with anxiety and anger. These are not easy houses in which to live, and the strains on the mother are very great; clumsy husbands and messy children are a threat. Retaliation is only possible against the weakest member. The precipitating stimulus here, as in the environmental difficulties, is only really effective if the subject is particularly susceptible or sensitive. By analogy, the body deals with small doses of poisons very smoothly, but if the body is allergically oversensitized, then the attempts to cope are exaggerated and self-destructive, and this may account for the observed fact that other individuals, and even this battering individual, former-ly put up with similar degrees of stress without apparent disturbance. Allergy and anaphylaxis occur in response to social stimuli as well as to foreign proteins!

PROVOCATION FROM WIFE

Battering fathers have a different range of marital responses. The man who has a comparable degree of uncertainty about his masculine identity does not typically batter, he goes out and gets drunk, takes to drugs, steals cars or powerful things, perhaps even capitulates and engages in homosexual behaviour. There are exceptions however: a young man who had had a prolonged homosexual relationship with an older male in late adolescence, and who showed some effeminate characteristics, had cohabited with a motherly and mildly controlling young lady who had been left with four children by her previous partner. He enjoyed this intensely matriarchal setting, feeling happier than with any of his previous girlfriends. But one evening when he was recovering from 'flu', and had just had a quarrel with his mother, he felt he was not getting enough attention, and resented having to help feed and care for the babies. He snatched one of them up by the arm, breaking it, and then let the child fall on the floor causing fatal injuries. Much more common is the man who is essentially unloving, bent upon acquiring attention rather than giving it, who is then left to manage a highly dependent and aggressively demanding baby, he finds the situation quite beyond him and brings it decisively to an end. He is not capable of the generosity and unselfishness which is a biological requirement of parents.

COLLABORATION AND CONNIVANCE

The marital situation has another interesting aspect. To what extent does the other parent collaborate or connive? Some authorities make rather dogmatic assertions that every battering involves some at least covert or 'unconscious' collaboration. This may often, or even usually, be so, for several reasons. First, most marriages are to some degree assortative, with a tendency to complement each other's qualities. This does not mean that they are obviously alike, indeed often quite the contrary, for a dominant woman may select a submissive man or vice versa, but at least they both share a basic problem of difficulty in dealing with aggression, and the solution reached by each is sure to have another side to it. The dominant person has a good understanding of submissiveness, and the submissive person of the dominance which he no doubt rehearses in his fantasy. The woman who is deserted and left with several children has biologically failed and knows it; she is desperate for help and cannot afford to be too choosy about her next partner; a man of low self-regard may feel less threatened by such a woman, yet not above being angry with himself and her for his incapacity to win anyone better; such an association is off to a very poor start. The close interdependence of marital partners favours acceptance of one another's behaviour and attempts to adapt. In the extreme form this reaches the heights of 'folie a deux'. If one partner observes the other abusing the child and inhibits a protective response, then the abusing partner may feel supported in that action and the stage is set for further aggression in one, and further inhibition in the other. In this way, by very gradual stages, a situation of battering may be achieved which would have shocked both at the outset. Many an incredible performance (either of virtuosity or villainy) becomes perfectly understandable once the several steps by which it was achieved are revealed. Sometimes very punitive spouses induce the other to batter the child.

A timid, shy, unassertive man, with a poor work record but no previous convictions, had not been mishandled in any way during his childhood (his parents and siblings were interviewed and gave consistent and good accounts of his early life). His wife's father was very strict and used to beat her frequently and she in turn was punitive with her baby. He frequently witnessed his wife's punitiveness and never managed to complain about it though he had wished to do so. Gradually she encouraged him to be equally punitive, and finally the baby died showing post mortem evidence of many injuries of different ages, which he had inflicted.

It did seem clear in this case that a man whose early handling could not be faulted, had slowly been brought to the point of vicariously satisfying his wife's punitiveness. Such cases must be contrasted with the commoner ones in which the aggression has been handed directly down from generation to generation[26].

WHICH PARTNER DID IT?

It does need to be stressed that it is sometimes extremely difficult (and perhaps fortunately not very essential) to know which of the partners actually carried out the final battering[27]. In one case it was wrongly assumed that a clearly mentally defective woman, married to a highly successful businessman, had been responsible for the battering, and she meekly accepted this. It was not till some six months later that a totally different construction seemed probable for the child was battered again when the mother was not present. The drug taking, unemployed husband inevitably attracted suspicion, but he had been driven to that state by his punitive wife; and was not finally thought to be responsible for the battering, though the matter was never settled firmly one way or the other. Often, innocent wives are coerced by threats of violence into elaborating explanations for their psychopathic husband's behaviour or even into accepting guilt. Very frequently, the battering husband leaves the taking of the child to hospital to his wife and attempts to evade all responsibility. A highly aggressive young man who had systematically abused his small step-son, sought unsuccessfully to blame the child's ultimate death on his epileptic wife. Often the truth is never discovered, but from the scientific point of view it is of considerable significance that in a marital battering couple, one partner of which has a psychiatric diagnosis other than disorder of personality and one partner without such a diagnosis, then there cannot be any assumption about the correlation of battering partner and psychiatric diagnosis. The relationship between psychiatric diagnosis and battering is just as tenuous as it is in all behaviour deviance and crime. Various suggestions, and even assertions, have been made about the high incidence of organic brain dysfunction, or the high level of subnormality, amongst battering parents, but these findings are probably due to peculiarities in sample collection.

BATTERING IN ITS CONTEXT OF OTHER DEVIANCIES

Let us first be quite clear that any relatively weak creature is likely to be assaulted by stronger creatures of the same or different species unless there is adequate group protectiveness or unless it has some defensive or escaping mechanism. This is why in the human species, the law has to protect the weak from exploitation and abuse. Not only babies get battered by humans but also old people and pets. I have a series of cases collected over 18 months in one remand prison of stabbings and clubbings of dogs by their owners, some of them very reminiscent of the features of baby battering. The national press has provided recent evidence of physical abuse to many old people and hospital patients (usually subnormal). It is only possible to guess at the motivation as a venting of frustration on creatures whose dependency was unavoidable, yet distasteful or resented or envied. No doubt if we knew the exact circumstances and personal stresses of each assailant, motivations would be more understandable; for example, society unloads its embarrassing members into institutions and gives little support to the staff, and inadequate facilities for their management. It is not difficult to imagine the stresses imposed on the nurses in these situations. Human children attack and sometimes kill their weaker siblings[28].

The human baby, as Iris Andreski[29] in an article aptly entitled 'The baby as dictator' says that babies come into the world 'not only with Stone Age expectations, but with much of the instinctual equipment to enforce their demands' and are able to make their mothers 'the target for an incomprehensible bombardment of anxiety . . .' Although the babies' cry is impossible to ignore for adults, it is (according to Aldrick[30] not infectious to other babies in the ward who are said not to be disturbed thereby! Perhaps yet another example of the general truth that we only pay attention to stimuli which are significant to us. What protection for the baby other than a postulated maternal instinct is there? It would be difficult to deny an immensely strong self-preservative force in all living creatures, and it is a very small step to suppose that the baby is for a while not distinguished from herself by the mother and thus within her self-protectiveness of the extended family group, which is of course totally lost in most human urban complexes. Admittedly the advice normally handed down abundantly to the mother can be gleaned from the pages of the excellent Dr Spock, but books have no shoulder to cry upon. The baby himself may have appealing features; he has a smile from a very early age, and from 5 to 6 weeks is capable of returning mother's smile with its own[31]; he has a vigorous sucking power and the nipple is an erogenous area.

It is sad to note that we deprive our modern babies of nearly all their natural defences. We artificially separate mother and child in our obstetric wards and nurseries, the primary defences of the extended family have gone; the mother, more often than not, does not breast feed. Like the Cheshire Cat, all that is left is the smile. As well as taking away the baby's natural defences it is very probable that we unwittingly make him positively less attractive, for a crying baby is not the most loveable. Babies cry for a great many different reasons[32] but usually because their needs are not being fully met. Important needs of the very young baby, according to Lawrence Casler[33] may be 'tactile, vestibular and other forms of stimulation' – skin contact with mother, warmth, movement and perhaps even comforting smells. Here we should remember that the rhinencephalon (smell brain) is phylogenetically the oldest part of the brain and quickest to mature. Food derived from a totally different animal, delivered in different quantities, and at a different rate, may cause discomfort; artificially fed babies are the ones that get nappy rash!

Perhaps then, we should be enquiring into the factors which prevent battering, rather than those which cause it, or at least to consider the balance of factors antagonistic to the baby together with those that are protective, for both are represented at least to some extent in the setting of any baby.

DISTINGUISHING BATTERING FROM OTHER FORMS OF BABY INJURY BY PARENTS OR GUARDIANS

The writer has for many years examined and assessed parents of both sexes who have damaged or killed their children, thus gaining experience with a large variety of such problems. In addition, a study has been made of all the 764 men and women[34] and who over a period of $5\frac{3}{4}$ years were indicted in England or Wales for murder; amongst these there were 46 fathers and 39 mothers who had killed their child or children, and these provided a basis for determining the proportions of the different types of child killing which are seen clinically. To put the conclusion before the argument, it is suggested that the source of the immediate provocation in child killing is a very useful criterion for classification. The essential feature of the battered child is that the immediate stimulus for the act always comes from the child. Of parents who have killed their children, the following classification covers all the cases, though the lines between the varieties are of course not always very clear.

(1) Elimination of an unwanted child. The characteristic story here used to be of the servant girl who would lose her post and reputation if she were discovered to have an illegitimate child. But in these days there are few servant girls, and the emphasis (shall we say) on reputation has changed, so that this variety is extremely rare. Parents however still unhappily make the deliberate decision to be rid of a child and do so either by assault or neglect. The stimulus comes from the child who for some reason, usually economic, is thought to threaten the comfort of the parents, but it is not a direct or immediate stimulus. The killing is a matter of policy which, of course, persists when the child is not present.

(2) Mercy killings. Here the parent, or more rarely parents, must have perceived a real disability in the child, and must believe that the disability will cause so much suffering *to the child* as to warrant killing him. There must be no obvious secondary advantage for the parent. This latter clause offers difficulty, for the mercy killer is often a parent of a rather rigid or perfectionist character to whom untidiness, inability to be useful, lack of perfection, is anathema; so that the wish to save suffering may be covertly laced with the wish to avoid personal distress, or perhaps to avoid distress for the spouse. But still, as in the callous eliminator, the act is a considered policy independent of the immediate presence of the baby. This mercy killing group has the highest proportion of fathers (he is most likely to assume responsibility), the highest parental age, the most stable personalities, and (shared with the manic depressive family murderer) the highest proportion of suicides. The method of killing is often drugs or gas, and everything is done to make it speedy. The injuries may be multiple and there may be more than one method of attack (perhaps in a desperate attempt to make the child die quickly) but there are no slight injuries and never injuries of different ages. There is no attempt to evade responsibility, though it is just possible (but psychologically improbable) that there may be a number of mercy killings which do not become known.

(3) A group with gross mental pathology, including organic, toxic, epileptic and functional psychosis, paranoid states, manic depressive psychosis and subnormality. Here perception is often disordered and thinking delusional so that motivation is totally different from that in all the other groups. The child is very unlikely to be the immediate stimulus for the attack, the principal motives being the depressive misplaced altruism and the schizophrenic delusional threat.

(4) Killing in which the immediate stimulus behind the decision arises outside the victim. This is the displaced anger group with or without the Medea or revenge motive[35]. Medea killed her two children to revenge herself on Jason her deserting husband. 'Thy sons are dead and gone, that will stab thy heart.' More common, in fact, than revenge is the situation in which the wife is about to leave

and where, after pleading with her to stay, the husband goes to the (perhaps sleeping) children and kills them, being unable to bear the prospect of losing them. There are several variations of this inability to bear stress, and of the primitive need to destroy rather than lose an object, but in none of them is the child the immediate stimulus for the act[24].

(5) The victim provides the immediate stimulus; a group which includes the momentary loss of temper, the higher grades of punishment and so called corrective chastisement, and the battered baby. In this group the parent never goes to the child in order to beat it, but is for some other reason with the child and is then overtaken by the impulse to hurt it. A theoretical variety in this group would be the misuse of the victim for sexual gratification, but this does not seem to occur between parents and their small children. It is perhaps significant in this connection that the sex ratio of children less than 13 years of age who have been killed by their father is one male to one female, but in sexually mature offspring the ratio is one male to two females. Battered babies often have their genitals damaged, but this is usually by being thumped-down upon hard objects whilst in a sitting position. Very occasionally a baby may be injured or burnt in the genital region as a punishment for urinating but not with any sexual motivation.

The battering parent never uses a lethal weapon, and very rarely anything but his or her hands, though bites are not uncommon[36], cigarettes and other hot objects may be used, and such things as the feeding spoon or bottle may virtually become weapons. In a recent case a young father is alleged to have bound his baby's dummy into place with sticky plaster (this baby had an earlier characteristic limb fracture and other injuries which brought the case within the so-called syndrome). The battering parent does not attempt suicide, but often delays seeking help, and usually tries to avoid responsibility in one way or another.

It might reasonably be asked 'Why not rely on the absence of any intention to kill as the essential criterion for distinguishing the battering parent from the other four categories?' Unhappily it is impossible to say in some cases that there was no intention to kill even though it seems likely that there was no premeditation or planning to that end. If a father in whom no intoxication or mental illness can be found, takes his recently born baby and swings him by the heels so that the child's head is repeatedly smashed against the wall, then it is difficult to deny an intent to kill, even though the father says, as they often do, 'I really loved that child'.

In fathers who kill their child the proportions are approximately one third mentally ill, one third battering parents, one sixth the Medea complex (of displaced aggression), and one sixth are accounted for by the mercy killings and eliminations together. In mothers who kill their child the proportions are less easy to state because there is a strong tendency to deal with them as mentally ill, though this tendency may be diminishing as the facts about battering become better known. The baby of a battering mother is very often less than a year old and the pressures to deal with her under the Infanticide Act 1938 as having 'the balance of her mind . . . disturbed by reason of her not having fully recovered from the effect of giving birth to the child or by reason of the effect of lactation' (whatever that might be) are very great, and often successful. Harder's statement[37] that mothers who kill their children tend to be labelled 'depressed' and fathers 'psychopathic' and that this may be due to prejudice has some force, yet it is likely that there are real differences between mothers and fathers who kill their offspring despite a considerable overlap of similarity.

DIFFERENCES WITHIN THE BATTERING GROUP

We do not really know what the shape of a graph would be if we were to plot incidence against severity of injury to the baby (severe punishment, single loss of temper, repeated battering, battering culminating in death). We do not know whether or not lesser grades of damage would merge imperceptibly with battering, or whether there is some qualitative difference which would support the existence of a battering syndrome as being at least a core-entity. Clinical experience suggests that, although all the intermediate grades exist, yet there is usually something qualitatively different between the parent who actually does batter a baby and those who just want to and quickly break down and seek help after the first excursion into really hurting the child. But we are far from knowing what that difference might be, or even if it is due to the pressure of some factor or to the absence of some defence, or both.

Three arguments give some support to there being a hard core (or perhaps more than one) within the battered baby 'syndrome'. First, battering of babies is a piece of deviant behaviour; whenever other deviant behaviours are carefully studied they all seem to come up with the same answer — that there is a relatively small hard core of subjects who are very difficult to treat and a large penumbra who are, as it were, only peripherally involved with the behaviour. This is true of the addictions, of the more dangerous traffic offences, of sexual misbehaviour, of murder, of juvenile crime, and, one suspects, of every sort of offence. It means that a classification for one type of deviant behaviour works very well with all the others, and that a treatment method which is successful with one will have its application in the others. It would be surprising if this were not so in the battered baby field, especially as there is already much positive experience to confirm it. We should beware then of pessimists who hold every battering parent to be an immediate menace to her children, and likely to progress to further heights of damage; many of them if given a helping hand will readily settle down. At the same time we have to be on the lookout for the 'malignant' case which earns the whole syndrome its dismal reputation.

Second, the lamentably inadequate help which is available to battering families unhappily has one useful effect. It provides a natural control group to the treated cases. Sometimes apparently typical battering cases, though left without any help at all, in very difficult circumstances, yet do very well. A girl was referred for psychiatric assessment by an assize court eight years ago. She was 20 and had killed her daughter aged 9 months. The post mortem showed a succession of serious lesions, and social background indicated many of the common factors (husband in prison, family isolated and living in a caravan, too many children in too short a time). Psychiatrically the mother was child-like in appearance and personality but not otherwise abnormal. The court reduced the charge to manslaughter under the Infanticide Act and put her on probation. She returned to her caravan in a remote area in which effective supervision was not available, and took up the care of her 3 remaining children. Successive follow-up has shown that she made steady progress. Her husband returned to her and they have a further child, now 5 years old (and not battered). What would have happened if she had been imprisoned and her children put into care?

Third, cross-sectional studies of the community have shown that punishment even of very small babies is widespread. The well known studies of John and Elizabeth Newson[38], using a representative sample of 700 mothers of 1 year old children, showed that 62% of the mothers accept the idea of physical punishment and practise it with the children. By the time their children are 4 smacking is almost universal. It is clear then that the punitive, but non-battering, 'penumbra' is abundantly present, and that the relatively few who come to light in the social services may represent some form of special problem or hard-core. Even so that hard-core may be dreadfully large; a figure of 4000 serious assaults upon babies each year, in the United Kingdom, has been given[39] or of 6 per 1000 live births[7]; there is no possible room for complacency.

PROVOCATION BY BABY

In the 'battered child' syndrome, the immediate stimulus for the attack, as we have seen, always comes from the baby. What is the nature of this provocative stimulus. First we must be clear that there are very difficult babies. The difficulty arises in two ways. There are some restless, sleepless, dissatisfied babies who cry persistently and have been like this since birth. The Cambridge research[14] shows that these babies are predictable using data about the pregnancy, labour and the baby's behaviour in the first few days. It may therefore be possible to arrange special care for these particular babies. Yet it is doubtful if these hyperactive, dissatisfied babies will correlate very highly with actual battering. Certainly such babies are exhausting and exasperating. They often reduce the parents to states of frank illness and most certainly stimulate murderous thoughts in hitherto very normal people. They are likely to drive their parents in desperation to the doctor where they announce that they fear they will batter the child. Quite often they may thus be referred to a psychiatrist, social worker of the children's department, or to the NSPCC or other special unit, *as* battering parents, although they have never and probably would never, attain actual battering. The distress that hyperactive, sleepless babies cause is very real, and the parents certainly need help, but it is doubtful if such cases often lead to the characteristic repeated assaults, and the occasional killings which are characteristic of the syndrome. In a series of 50 fatal battered baby cases, killed by their fathers, five were confirmed as particularly difficult, sleepless, crying babies with both parents, but some of these were probably already ill from previous assaults. It is much more common in the hospital out-patient clinic to find that the mother who complains that she fears harming her baby has the hyperactive child. Typically the battered child, though rather more likely to have been premature, and likely to be described perhaps by one parent as difficult, clumsy, bruises easily etc., in fact is found to settle perfectly well in the hospital ward or nursery. The disturbance is often not present when in charge of the other parent. The majority of difficult babies in battering families are frightened and distrustful rather than constitutionally difficult[50]. This is illustrated by one of the fatally injured babies, previously in the care of foster parents who had been prosecuted for battering him. Not infrequently small children are so terrified of their fathers that they vomit when he comes home, or become incapable of eating, or urinate with fear, and these very reactions are the cue for further assaults. It must be remembered that some newly born babies are battered before they have had a chance to indicate what their characteristics might be, whether hyperactive or placid. Indeed the fatal battering of babies provides a control group in the study of murder, in that, in the case of adults, there is always the possibility that the victim knowingly or otherwise invited the attack, and that the assailants might have been involved in some progressive conflict – the unfaithful husband, the masochistic wife, dark hints of blackmail, hidden motivations to eliminate. But with the very small baby almost every incident of its experience may be known, and the opportunity to develop a complex psychopathology or dynamic family interaction has scarcely existed, yet still the innocent may be killed. In the great majority of battering cases the stimulus offered by the child is trivial and its effect on the battering parent idiosyncratic. Why? The Newsons[38] inform us that mothers usually punish for expression of rage and aggression in the child (screaming, kicking, stiffening, breath-holding, head banging, and personal attack on mother); then for destruction or disruption; then for dangerous behaviour (fireplace, domestic appliances, electrical equipment); then at meal times, genital play etc.

Battering is not so rational as punishment; the intellectual reason may often have given way to an altogether primitive reaction. In fatal cases the immediate stimulus was: refusal of food, vomiting, 'sucking the tongue', crying, screaming (especially at night or when the television is on), 'swearing', looking scared or blank, staring, refusal to smile, disobedient, refusal to learn, 'knocked over the pot', spilling things, getting in the way, wet, dirty; many of these factors being inseparable from infancy. The fathers' or mothers' interpretation of these simple stimuli seems all important. Mothers say 'she was playing up', 'I had to shut her up', 'he defied me', 'I don't know what came over me'. Fathers say 'the child was becoming wilful', 'campaigning against me', 'a battle of wills', 'getting the wife down'. Both parents often use the expression (so common in all impulsive aggressive offences) 'I couldn't bear it any longer'. The parents often cannot understand the child not wanting to respond, play, smile, understand 'me' – the familiar role-reversal described by Morris and Gould[41] and in which parents expect the baby to effect the care, not vice versa.

It is tempting to suppose that the parent reacts to such minor incidents as a spilt pot as simply the last straw which breaks her resistance and control; perhaps a mother exhausted by too frequent child-birth, worried about material things, sleepless, perhaps physically ill or hungry. Such extreme factors are uncommon. Just as the battered baby is typically well nourished, its mother and father are also usually physiologically in good shape – the principal reasons are psychological rather than somatic. At least typical battering to death more frequently than otherwise is committed by a parent who is physically well, of adequate intelligence, not psychiatrically ill, under no more stress than others in their social milieu. The most plausible hypothesis to explain these surprising and rather unwelcome facts is by analogy with the allergic response. Although the trigger-pulling stimulus is usually harmless enough in itself, a person may gradually become sensitized to it, with mobilization of more and more emotion, until a trivial event seems a major threat, and the resulting encounter can endanger the parent, child and family.

HOW SPECIFIC IS THE STIMULUS TO BATTER?

Is it just babies that evoke this response or are battered parents impulsive or aggressive in other areas? Skinner and Castle's[19] 78 cases showed that 45% of battering parents have one or more previous criminal convictions. Of fathers who had battered fatally 65.5% had a criminal record as adults, and 27% as juveniles. Twenty seven per cent fatal and 11.5% non-fatal cases have previous records of violent offences, so that as a whole they are distinctly criminal in other ways. Smith and his colleagues[21], from their larger sample of battering parents, determined that 25% of child-battering fathers also batter their wives.

The present author has studied 50 men charged with killing their child. Of these 33 were living with their wife, and 17 with a common-law wife at the time of the killing. Twelve of these men had assaulted their spouse, 29 had not, and in 9 there was insufficient information. There seems no doubt that at least 25% of fatal baby-battering fathers also batter their women – the same figure as determined by Selwyn Smith.

Looking at this problem the other way round, the present author took the last 40 consecutive cases of wife or cohabitee murder seen in HM Prison Brixton and determined whether or not these men had battered their children.

  5 definitely battered a child or children (12.5%)

12 no battering

10 had no children

  7 children grown up or permanently away

  6 insufficient information

---

total: 40

It would be unwise to draw firm conclusions from retrospective study of such a small sample, in such a sensitive area, but at least it is clear that the two sorts of violence (to wife and to children) certainly overlap to some extent.

It is relevant to mention here a very striking and informative clinical fact. If grossly aggressive psychopaths, possessing wives and families, are collected from the practice of a psychiatric teaching hospital then, even though highly aggressive to almost everyone else, they do not attack their small children (nor, happily, do they ever attack their doctor!). This observation is based on a detailed study of 12 cases but is backed by 25 years experience with aggressive patients. I think the explanation rests on two facts. First, the really dangerously aggressive psychopaths, in general, don't have families. They cannot tolerate them and leave, perhaps, in order to avoid killing them. Sometimes they drift into ready-made families and cohabit for a while and this is when some of the tragic batterings occur. Second, the so-called aggressive psychopaths who do have, and maintain, families, seem always to be of the over compensated but basically inferior feeling, self-proving type, who sensitively leap to protect their tender self-regard, and who cannot resist a challenge; they often have a very carefully concealed mothering, protective attitude to underdogs and defenceless creatures. Presumably their small children (and their doctor) offer no threat to such people and are thus perfectly safe. Be this as it may, those who construct theories about parents who batter babies must go further than blaming inferiority feelings (even when combined with long criminal records including offences for violence) for it is quite certain that there are many chronic offenders with gross feelings of inferiority who never batter any one of their often numerous children.

TREATMENT OF BABY BATTERING

Once a syndrome is established it is only a matter of time before it proves inadequate and before a paper appears entitled 'The Myth of the X Syndrome'. This has already occurred with the battered child syndrome[42]. Broadly we find the following sorts of cases described within the syndrome:

(1) Deliberate elimination: a 19 year old mother dumped her 10 month old baby on a lonely track and mutilated her to make it seem that she had been sexually assaulted. A 36 year old mother killed her 4 year old son with a brick and went off

with her lover.

(2) Mental illness in the parent: 3% of mothers and 1% of fathers in one series of battered babies[21] displayed psychotic reactions. The authors remark 'The bizarre nature of the injuries inflicted by the psychotic parents suggest that they form a separate sub-group among baby batterers whose management must differ accordingly'.

(3) Displacement of passion from the other parent to the child: a father whose wife had just left him attempted to assault her but, when she escaped, he rushed to the children's bedroom and killed them.

(4) The commoner situation in which the child offers the immediate stimulus to one or other parent who repeatedly and impulsively assaults it.

Instances of each of these quite different situations are to be found in the battered baby literature.

The experience of each observer is different. Some studies find a high incidence of families in lower social classes, parents of poor intelligence, EEG abnormality[43] and of abnormal babies, but others do not. Workers in general medical practice, in hospitals, in private practice or in remand prisons are likely to see quite different samples of battering parents. Whether we are aware of it or not, each of us has a selection process determining what sort of patients we attract. In general, it is likely that doctors see the more serious problems of battering, though increasing awareness of the problem and favourable publicity may alter this.

There is little certainty about the specific qualities of battering parents or their backgrounds. Most studies indicate that they are likely to be young, a little duller, of lower social class, with a high incidence of abnormal personalities; commonly cited qualities are immaturity, poor ego control, poor self-image, low self-esteem, inability to accept adversity or criticism. Very frequently (but by no means always) battering parents have themselves emerged from punitive households. All these, of course, are precisely those qualities which over and over again have been found in delinquents and criminals generally. Indeed the Birmingham studies of Selwyn Smith and his colleagues have shown that baby battering occurs within a constellation of other social inadequacies and failures of adaptation just as Lee Robins has so conclusively shown to be the case in delinquency[44].

The resemblances which battering adults have with other behavioural deviants is very striking, whether in the sorts of classification which can be used, the correlates, the causes (or their evasiveness) and the range of treatment[24]. If this is accepted then we might save a great deal of disappointment and wasted effort in how we set about investigating and treating the phenomenon. We may confidently expect that the incidence of battering (whether real, apparent or a little of both) will continue in parallel with other crime statistics, that all dogmatic generalizations are likely to be wrong and dangerous, and that within the category there will be a small nucleus of individuals who will be difficult or impossible to help, together with a large penumbra, shading out into the community as a whole, in which even simple methods of treatment, or in some cases none at all, will appear to be eminently satisfactory. A further resemblance will be the negligible relationship of the phenomenon to physical or psychiatric disorder and, as a corrolary, that medical practitioners are really only essential in diagnostic screening, but may be very useful as members of research and treatment teams.

The final resemblance is one which could have been confidently predicted from this close relationship to other deviancies. It is that treatment will often be resisted. The deviant or criminal gladly accepts, even clamours for help in extricating himself from the consequences of his behaviour, but at a deeper level he really believes that he was justified and, when the circumstances again arise, the pattern will be repeated. This is particularly so in those cases which reach the clinic; in fact, it is probably this apparently senseless clinging to an apparently disastrous and self-damaging behaviour which selects the patient for clinical attention. At this point, we have to note that there is a large section of battering parents showing these characteristic resistances.

In summary, we cannot be sure that there is a single battered baby syndrome. Different practitioners may be justified in holding quite different opinions about the phenomenon. There is no universal type of battering adult, and no one common cause or factor to be eradicated so that the medical model has little application. This is not a happy start to a section on the treatment of this phenomenon but, by acknowledging these facts, we are encouraged to think out tactics anew rather than slavishly following old models.

Battering of babies occurs in all sorts of communities irrespective of colour, creed or political structure. It is known to occur also under certain experimental conditions in other primates. It is quite clear also that repeated battering can occur independently of such plausible explanations as low intelligence and mental illness. The wish to batter is reported by very many mothers who are asked in confidence; and the circumstance in which the impulse arises is usually the continuing failure of the baby, despite mother's concerted efforts, to respond in the way in which she wants it to respond (usually to stop crying or to take its feed). The prevailing emotion is invariably and unequivocally reported as anger (unless, of course, the whole thing is denied). It is reasonable to conclude therefore that battering is usually a quantitative, not a qualitative, abnormality which expresses itself through the relationship between parent and child.

Relationships do not occur *in vacuo*, so that the circumstances of both parties will be relevant and, of course, the impact of other family members will be a major element of these circumstances.

With most other forms of deviant behaviour treatment is directed towards understanding, insight and an extended period in which effort is directed to changing the offender in some way, whether through relationship therapy, reality therapy, some form of group or personal analysis or the more recent behaviour therapies. The initial stages of treatment in these other criminals is relatively uncomplicated because the object of the crime is usually inanimate and needs no consideration, or has no dependent relationship and can thus be dismissed, as are the paedophile's children. Only in the strictly family deviancies of pathological jealousy and wife beating is there a situation comparable to our baby battering, and here we deal with adults capable of independent existence. In baby battering, therefore, crisis looms large and demands instant attention which cannot be provided by law enforcement agencies alone. There are always two patients, one of them dependent, and the usual conflict between the offender and society is overshadowed by an infinitely more emotional and dramatic conflict between parents and child. Sides will be taken and the conflict will spread to those concerned with the child and those concerned with the parent. Very important decisions have to be taken in the midst of these tensions. The crisis can last a long time and, once the baby is restored, can break out anew. The treatment of this battering syndrome is then essentially the treatment of the crisis situation. Once that is over, if there is anything left to treat (and often there is not), treatment will resemble that which is appropriate to the other deviant behaviours.

Assuming that stage one (the tactful temporary removal of the injured baby 'for observation') and stage two (the diagnostic elimination of the psychiatric cases: the deluded depressive, the hallucinated schizophrenic and the occasional intoxicated addict) have been satisfactorily completed, then what are the essentials of treatment?

It is generally accepted that the social worker or doctor must approach the parents in a helpful, concerned, non-retributive but not yet reassuring way, and that a standard history of the members of the family should be built up.

There will be denials, defences, explanations and justifications, probably with alternating projection of all blame, remorseful self-criticism and calls for help.

One battering mother scrawled the following while waiting in the hospital:

> I hate you. I hate everybody
> I should be dead
> People can be very cruel
> Some of them make me sick
> I shouldn't have been a mother
> I completely neglect (my children)
> Oh Daniel I wish I was well so
> that I could love you all the time
> You must feel very lonely and lost.

Behind it all, in every battering, the essential feature is unrestrained anger. The task is centred upon this anger and, however much the parent may protest, it must have been present, and it must be faced and coped with. Unrestrained anger is the only common psychological feature of all batterers.

The problem then devolves into identifying and modifying the factors which cause and release anger. This can be tackled at various depths.

The most superficial level is the most important because it is the easiest to influence. A child is hit because the action is gratifying to the adult and because the child is defenceless and cannot retaliate. If someone who will defend the child is present the battering does not occur, so here is something simple and effective which can be aimed at. Combat isolation and arrange for grandmother or a grandmother-substitute to call or to be available. The North American 'Parents Anonymous' Organisation has 55 Chapters; members volunteer to answer telephone calls; 'help is immediate and non-threatening and, therefore, more readily sought than professional help'. Places can be found to which the isolated mother and her baby may go together: under-5 playgroups, special day nurseries, not necessarily only for battering problems, but at least where mothers can remain to help, to meet other mothers and to watch how children can confidently be managed. The weekends are often the periods of greatest isolation and danger, so that specific enquiry and arrangements should, if necessary, be made. The spouse cannot always be relied upon in this context. Not uncommonly resentment of the husband raises the anger which is then displaced (Medea-wise) onto the child, and sometimes parents stimulate one another to gradually increasing heights of aggression when neither reacts against the early moves in the other, mistaking the inactivity of indecision for licence to go further.

Abnormalities in the child are a possible cause of parental anger; prematurity and difficult pregnancies and deliveries[45-47] are well known correlates of behaviour difficulties in the child and of battering[45-47]. The Cambridge studies[48,49] have shown that the restless, sleepless, crying baby may be identified at birth or even during pregnancy, and that by this means supportive measures may be organized and concentrated where most needed.

At the next level, an attempt is made to identify and hopefully to relieve the frustrations which invariably lie beneath the anger; they may arise from either a difficult environment or short-comings in the individual, or both. The environment consists of things and people, and since things are more easily mastered than people, it is sensible first to see what needs to be improved on that front. Many observers have commented upon the ignorance of these young battering parents in matters of practical domesticity and parenthood, so that instruction and sorting out their muddled finances sometimes helps a great deal in reducing frustration. But of course no amount of material manipulation, rehousing and restocking the larder will make up for serious personal defects or serious marital difficulties, which throws us back on people.

R. H. Moos[50] writes 'Our central tasks of understanding, predicting, and changing behaviour compel us to learn more about environmental dimensions and to formulate valid concepts about them. The optimal arrangement of environments is probably the most powerful behaviour modification technique we currently have available.' But here again we cannot escape from the personal relationships which form the principal part of the environment. All our batterers are in the full flood of their reproductive lives and reproduction needs two people who must now show the generosity and unselfishness which is the hallmark of the reproductive process (and only of the reproductive process) throughout Nature. Often enough, young battering parents are still seeking dependency and are in no position to take up the heavy burdens of parenthood. They are disappointed in each other and in themselves and deeply frustrated. If then the baby, who was to have provided the longed-for loving relationship, turns out to be a demanding and insatiable creature who does not understand and gives nothing in return, then disappointment and anger will be inevitable. It is not sufficient to write 'Effective lasting intervention is less a function of therapeutic relationships than of resolving specific problems of parents' lives' because so very often these specific problems turn out to be faulty relationships.

But to erupt into battering, the anger has to be unrestrained, and it is not so easy to understand and empathize with this lack of restraint as it was with the anger. There are two principal sources of lack of restraint, which we cannot distinguish one from the other and which we suspect often exist together. They are first that inherited quality which is sometimes called immaturity, and which is recognized by a lack of firmness and persistence in facing problems, and by a type of emotional incontinence leading to impulsive, apparently rash, behaviour when under stress. Second, there are numerous faults in early social learning which may produce a rather similar picture, though often not so broadly distributed throughout the personality. Some individuals have been taught to use aggression and may have discovered for themselves that resort to aggression reduces anxiety or secures the desired result (conditioned avoidance, and operant conditioning respectively; the former much more difficult to eradicate than the latter).

More characteristic of the battering parent is the situation in which the parent emerged from childhood with low self-esteem, unsure of his or her capacity to love or to be loved, and who is ultra-sensitive to rejection. For the most stable parent, a persistently crying or 'refusing' baby is a trying experience; for the parent handicapped in either or both of these ways it may be intolerable and disastrous. The distress is easily transmitted to others, particularly those to whom an often poorly informed society lightly passes the responsibility for these situations.

Just as the battering parent cannot tolerate this crying baby who will not be pacified and will not allow the parent to feel competent and gratified, so the situation is closely paralleled for the social worker or doctor who must tolerate this adult with whom the rest of society deals by denial or horrified rejection, and who continues to make demands and to maintain a high degree of anxiety in everyone around her, projecting her failure as a parent as the failure of authority to solve the problem.

The social worker must do what the parent has not been able to do, and that is not to panic, to put up with the stress, to wait, to count up to ten and then to go on counting ten as long as the crisis lasts — probably as difficult a task as exists anywhere in the field of social work. Just as the harassed parent must bring this intolerable tension to an end quickly, the social worker and doctor fall under pressure to terminate their intolerable tension by some quick means. Society can be just as punitive as battering parents and for the same reasons.

The British Paediatric Association[51] states that the doctor's ultimate aim is to rehabilitate the family, but this is challenged. Oliver and Cox[52], in a valuable study, have followed families through three generations and find that extensive medical and social help for battering parents does not diminish the tendency to abuse children. They write: 'Many family members showed prolonged, dependent, antisocial and neurotic behaviour throughout their early adult life. Humane and imaginative support was given them by professional and voluntary services. They were not treated as parasites. However, as parents these family members functioned at the emotional level of young children. Their own children were always in profound danger ... The treatment given, though uncoordinated, helped such parents *in time*. Meanwhile, their parents continue to suffer'.

The conclusion that foster homes for such children offer a better solution has to be considered seriously. But there are difficulties. These parents are usually still young and very fertile. Are they also to be sterilized? Are we quite sure that the shortcomings of these parents are conditioned? Perhaps a follow-up study would show that even the fostered children retained these weaknesses. What effect would the removal, perhaps successive removal, of children have upon the parents, and what new hydra-headed problems would they produce? Would the policy be entertained by the courts who would have to make the requisite orders? Would these courts be able to resist the applications for revocation which the parents, backed by civil rights organizations and probably by social workers, would undoubtedly make?

However, there certainly are some parents who seem quite incapable of handling children safely and who are not averse to being relieved of the responsibility. The problem is to know which.

Here the shortcomings of social services and ignorance about the battering problem (particularly some years ago) pay a small dividend, by setting up experimental situations which it would have been totally unethical deliberately to arrange. I have a small series of cases, some of them first seen as long as ten years ago, in which, owing to the lenience of (then) assize courts and of magistrates refusing fit person orders, what appeared to be desperate risks were taken, yet follow-up revealed very satisfactory results. May I briefly recount one such case. A young mother, herself rejected by her divorced parents, on a charge of murdering her middle child aged 2 years, was allowed bail, ultimately was found guilty of manslaughter on grounds of non-intent and was returned home to her caravan (in which the killing had happened), with her two children. Her husband was in prison; she was quite unsupported, except by a probation officer who saw her weekly. Her husband ultimately was released and deserted her. She has found another man who has made a stable home with her. Not only did her two children survive happily, but she has two more, and reports from school and social services are entirely satisfactory.

It is the task of the psychiatrist to try to predict dangerousness and the criteria and methods of going about this are precisely as they are for other criminals and deviants. Thus, the first principle is that we are very incompetent predictors, so that our bungling efforts should whenever possible be qualified by real life tests. This means the well known process of voluntary hospital admission for the child, followed by a care order with perhaps immediate boarding of the child in its own home with nursery attendance and a volunteer to help, particularly at weekends, or else by a more prolonged fostering while the parents prove themselves capable of reorganizing their home. The snag here is that indecisiveness and dithering can be very destructive, particularly to the relationship with the workers concerned, for the child, and for the foster mother. Once the process of restoration of the baby has started, it must (unless, of course, there is renewed battering) go ahead, and should be allowed to do so as quickly as possible, for there is little to suggest that (once the supportive arrangements are made) excessive caution decreases the risk. But where the battering has been prolonged, and where the precipitating causes remain unalleviated, it is very occasionally necessary to influence the case conference to make a clear decision for long-term separation, with a complementary plan, not to abandon the parents, but to help them intensively to heal the scar and perhaps deal effectively with their remaining or future children.

References

1. West, S. (1888). *Brit. Med. J.*, **1**, 856
2. Caffey, J. and Silverman, F. N. (1945). *Am. J. Roentgenol.*, **54**, No. 2
3. Snedecor, S. T., Knapp, R. E. and Wilson, H. B. (1935). *Surg. Gynaec. Obstet.*, **61**, 385
4. Caffey, J. (1946). *Am. J. Roentgenol.*, **56**, 163
5. Silverman, F. N. (1953). *Am. J. Roentgenol.*, **69**, 413
6. Kempe, C. H., Silverman, F. N., Stede, B. F., Droegmuller, W. and Silver, H. K. (1962). *J. Am. Med. Assoc.*, **181**, 17
7. Kempe, C. H. (1971). *Arch. Dis. Child.*, **46**, 28
8. Helfer, R. E. and Kempe, C. H. (1968). *The Battered Child* (Chicago and London: University of Chicago Press)
9. British Paediatric Association (1966). *Br. Med. J.*, **1**, 601
10. Parker, G. E. (1965). The Battered Child Syndrome. *Med. Sci. Law*, **5**, 3, 160
11. Oppé, T. E. (1968). The Battered Child. Address to Annual Council Meeting, NSPCC, London
12. Bath Social Services Dept. (1974). Lewishouse, Bath
13. Harlow, H. F. (1961). In: *Determinants of Infant Behaviour* (B. M. Foss, ed.), Vol. 1, p. 75 (London: Methuen)
14. Richards, Martin (1974). Talk given to DHSS Conference on Non-accidental Injury to Children at Alexander Family House, 19th June
15. Herscher, L., Richmond, J. B. and Moore, A. U. (1963). *Behaviour*, **20**, 311
16. Williams, C. P. S. and Oliver, T. K. jun. (1969). *Pediatrics*, **44**, 640
17. *Br. Med. J.* (1970). Mothers of Premature Babies, **2**, 556
18. Castle, R. L. and Kerr, A. M. (1972). A Study of suspected child abuse. Battered Child Research Dept., NSPCC, London
19. Skinner, A. E. and Castle, R. L. (1969). 78 Battered Children – a Retrospective Study. Battered Child Research Dept., NSPCC, London
20. Scott, P. D. (1973). Fatal Battered Baby Cases. *Med. Sci. Law*, **13**, 197

21. Smith, Selwyn M., Hanson, R. and Noble S. (1973). Parents of Battered Babies: A controlled Study. *Br. Med. J.*, **2**, 388

22. Oliver, J. S. (1973). (Personal communication)

23. Scott, P. D. (1973). Parents who kill their children. *Med. Sci. Law*, **13**, 120

24. Smith, S. M. (1975). *The Battered Child Syndrome*. (London: Butterworth)

25. Smith, S. M. and Hanson, R. (1974). 134 Battered Children: A Medical and Psychological Study. *Br. Med. J.*, **2**, 666

26. Oliver, J. S. and Taylor, A. (1971). Five generations of ill-treated children in one family pedigree. *Br. J. Psychiat.*, **119**, 473

27. Court, J. (1970). Psycho-social Factors in Child Battering. *J. Med. Wom. Fed.*, **52**, 99

28. Adelson, L. (1972). The Battering Child. *J. Am. Med. Assoc.*, **222**, 159

29. Andreski, I. (1966). The Baby as Dictator. *New Society*, 15.12.66, p. 906

30. Aldrich, C. A., Sung, C. and Knop, C. (1945). *J. Paediatr.*, **26**, 313

31. Stone, F. N. (1971). Psychological Aspects of Early Mother-Infant Relationships. *Br. Med. J.*, **2**, 224

32. Illingworth, R. S. (1955). Crying in Infants and Children. *Br. Med. J.*, **1**, 75

33. Casler, L. (1961). Maternal Deprivation: A Critical review of the Literature. Monograph 80. Vol. 26, No. 2. *Soc. Res. Child Devel.*

34. Morris, T. and Blom-Cooper, L. (1964). *A Calendar of Murder*. (London: Michael Joseph)

35. Stern, E. S. (1948). *J. Ment. Sci.*, **94**, 321

36. Sims, B. G., Grant, J. H. and Cameron, J. M. (1973). Bitemarks in the Battered Baby Syndrome. *Med. Sci. Law*, **13**, 3, 207

37. Harder, T. (1967). *Acta Psychiat. Scand.*, **43**, 196

38. Newson, J. and Newson, E. (1963). *Infant Care in an Urban Community*. (London: George Allen and Unwin)

39. Tunbridge Wells Study Group (1973). Non-accidental Injury to Children

40. Smith, S. M. and Hanson, R. (1975). Interpersonal Relationships and Child-Rearing Practices in 214 Parents of Battered Children. *Br. J. Psychiat.*, **127**, 513

41. Morris, M. G. and Gould, R. W. (1963). Role reversal: a concept in dealing with the neglected/battered child syndrome. In: *The Neglected/Battered Child Syndrome*. Child Welfare League of America (New York) 24

42. *Current Medical Dialog* (1973). 40/4, 327

43. Smith, S. M., Honigsberger, L. and Smith, C. A. (1973). EEG and Personality Factors in Baby Batterers. *Br. Med. J.*, **2**, 20

44. Robins, L. (1966). *Deviant Children Grown Up*. (London: Livingstone)

45. Elmer, E. and Gregg, G. D. (1967). Development Characteristics of Abused Children. *Pediatrics*, **40**, 596

46. Klein, M. and Stern, L. (1971). Low Birth Weight and the Battered Child Syndrome. *Am. J. Dis. Child.*, **122**, 15

47. Lynch, M. (1975). Ill-health and Child Abuse. *Lancet.*, **ii**, 317

48. Richards, M. P. M. and Berual, J. F. (1972). A Study of Mother–Infant Interaction. In: *Ethological Studies of Child Behaviour*. N. Blurton Jones (ed.). (Cambridge University Press)

49. Richards, M. (1975). Non-Accidental Injury to Children in a Ecological Perspective. In: *Non-Accidental Injury to Children*, p. 5. (London: HMSO)

50. Moos, R. H. (1974). *Evaluating Treatment Environments: A Social Ecological Approach*. (New York: John Wiley)

51. British Paediatric Association (1973). Non-Accidental Injury to Children. (Introductory comment from BPA and BAPS). *Br. Med. J.*, **4**, 656

52. Oliver, J. E. and Cox, J. (1973). A Family Kindred with Ill-used Children: The Burden on The Community. *Br. J. Psychiat.*, **123**, 81

Recommended Reading on Treatment

Galdston, Richard (1970). Violence Begins at Home. Paper presented at the American Academy of Child Psychiatry. The Parents' Counter Project for the Study and Prevention of Child Abuse

Kempe, C. H. and Helfer, R. E. (1972). *Helping the Battered Child and His Family.* (Philadelphia and Toronto: Lippincott Co.)

Smith, S. M. *The Battered Child Syndrome.* (London: Butterworth)

Szasz, T. (1959). The Communication of Stress between Child and Parent. *Br. J. Med. Psychol.*, **32**, 161

8   The psychological aspects of child abuse

D. R. HENRY

INTRODUCTION

Kempe *et al.*[1] coined the term 'the battered child syndrome' and subsequently a good many articles began to appear in the literature. Because the term 'battered' refers essentially only to physical beating it is somewhat limited in accounting for maltreatment arising out of simple neglect. Therefore, a more inclusive and factually correct term has come into being and that is child abuse. For the purpose of this chapter on the psychological aspects of child abuse it still seems appropriate to employ the definition used by Kempe and Helfer[2] for the battered child. The definition of child abuse employed herewith is 'any child who received physical injury (or injuries) as a result of acts (or omissions) on the part of his parents or guardians'.

This review of the psychological aspects of child abuse covers the period of the past decade. In all, 119 references were examined. Of these, 55 were found to relate to characteristics of child abuse other than psychological. That is, they were concerned with demographic characteristics, incidence of the syndrome, social features of the parents or treatment programmes. Of the remaining 64 references only a handful dealt strictly with the psychological aspects of child abuse. Some of the articles seemed to be repetitious of existing articles, altered only slightly by each particular author's own insights.

One possible explanation why child abuse has not received more thorough psychological investigation may have to do with statistics. While most people would agree that the thought of a defenceless child being bashed, battered and bruised is abhorrent, it appears the incidence of child abuse is comparatively rare. That is, those studies which have reported the incidence of abuse suggest that less than 1% of children are subjected to abuse. Ferguson, Fleming and O'Neill[3] reported that in New Zealand abuse occurs about 3 times in 10 000 children aged 10–16. They reported also that for those children under 1 year of age the risk was slightly greater at $4\frac{1}{2}$ times in 10 000 children. Light[4] estimated that 3 children in 100 in the USA are physically abused, sexually molested or severely neglected. Light's estimate for just physical abuse was less than 1 in 100 children. Baldwin and Oliver[5], for a British population, found the incidence of child abuse to be 1 in 1000 children under 4 years of age. (The death rate was 1 in 10 000 children.)

It may be argued, validly, that if even one child is abused it is cause for concern. But the facts are that sometimes psychological phenomena of one behaviour syndrome do not receive scientific investigation because other syndromes and behaviour anomalies are more pronounced, or more easily identified, or more readily investigated.

The aim of this chapter will be to concentrate on those articles which attempted to elucidate some of the psychological parameters associated with child abuse. Somewhat more attention will be focused on articles which attempted objective study. Wherever psychological tests have been used reference has been made to them in abbreviated form for ease of presentation. A list of these tests, in their full form, is given in Table 8.3 at the end of the chapter.

PROBLEMS ASSOCIATED WITH SOME CHILD ABUSE STUDIES

One manner of studying the psychological aspects of child abuse has been through the case history method. But, if one were to accept the results of case histories, such as those reported by Calef[6], it would be difficult to understand any kind of behaviour, much less child battering behaviour. For example, Calef presents four case histories where parental hostility was shown toward their children. The hostility of these parents was supposedly due to four different types of frustration. They were: (1) being unable to become pregnant, (2) being unable to conduct household duties, (3) suffering severe headaches and neck pains, and (4) being evaluated for abortion purposes. The common element to each of these four independent cases was that the adult had been thrown into a state of disequilibrium either by having goal-directed behaviour thwarted, as in the first two cases, experiencing physiological discomfort as in the third case, or as in the fourth case, fear or anger over evaluation. If one is to predict behaviour, one must be able to identify salient features of behaviour. The fact that each of the four case histories presented refer to behaviour which is not uncommon in our society and does not in other cases lead to child battering indicates these factors are not the salient features of behaviour. Hence, one cannot assume frustration, pain and fear or anger are the psychological predisposing factors that lead to child abuse.

Zadik[7], in studying the social and medical aspects of battered children with vision impairment, discovered that some children are more apt to be battered than others. Even when the batterers are parents, relatives, siblings or babysitters, certain characteristics of the battered children rendered them more susceptible to abuse. These characteristics Zadik has listed as fussiness, being illegitimate, being a stepchild, or being of the opposite sex to that preferred by parents. This study helps slightly in that it emphasizes that the sex of a child and his or her general activity level are important psychological characteristics in child abuse. However, most fussy children do not receive battering. Therefore, it is the personality characteristics of batterers which supersede in importance the characteristics of the child in understanding child abuse. Illegitimacy and being a stepchild may be important factors in predicting child abuse but they cannot be considered psychological components of abuse. Rather, it seems best that they be considered sociological factors.

Goldstein[8] commented that research into identifying the determinants of child abuse has been inconsistent in its conclusions. He stated that there are four major reasons for this. First, it is only after battering or abuse has occurred that abusive parents can be studied. Hence, most of the data gathered on these caretakers consists of interviews and some psychodiagnostic material on a small, select and not necessarily representative sample of any particular population. Conclusions drawn on studies conducted *ex post facto* must always be circumspect. One can never be certain that the observed conditions such as depression, denial, aggressiveness or affect generally were precipitating factors leading to child abuse or are the result of having been detected as an abuser. A second reason for inconsistent findings is the lack of a theory about child abuse and the resulting lack of meaningful and testable hypotheses emanating from the theory. One possible solution to this difficulty may come through the emergence of typologies of abusive parents. As will be seen later on in this chapter, these typologies offer a theoretical means to viewing abusive parents and from these, respective subgroups of abusers may be studied psychodiagnostically. A third reason for inconsistent findings is because of the necessary emphasis placed upon case studies and the correlational data that tend to follow them. The result is that no cause and effect hypotheses are formulated or tested. A final reason for varying conclusions is that without the use of control groups against which to compare the findings on the abusive parents, one is uncertain as to how to interpret the relevance of the results. Fortunately, some advancements have been made in this last instance and a few studies which employed control groups will be reviewed in this chapter.

A good many articles in the literature attempt to describe the psychological characteristics of child abusers. As one example of such articles one might consider that by Lukianowicz[9]. First of all, only 18 cases were studied and it would be erroneous to make sweeping generalizations from so small a sample. Be that as it may, the author goes on to describe abusers with adjectives like aggressive, cold, callous, spiteful, reckless, persistently cruel, hysterical, psychopathic, dull, egocentric, narcissistic, anxious, neurotic, mildly depressive, oversensitive, irritable, immature, dependent, tense, and frustrated. Only two of the 18 abusers were considered to have 'normal' personalities. Children who have been abused are described as listless, withdrawn, apathetic, do not speak, look tired, sad and older than their actual age, wistful and have a blank, emotionless facial expression. It seems apparent that a mere listing of adjectives which describe a clinician's impressions of a patient is lacking in scientific precision. It may be of help in treating the individual case but it is too vague and general if one is attempting to define and indeed, eventually predict, child abusers. Many of the psychological characteristics which Lukianowicz observed in his abusive group apply to persons who (a) do not abuse their children and (b) never require psychological or psychiatric care.

PSYCHOLOGICAL PARAMETERS ASSOCIATED WITH CHILD ABUSE

The most thorough review of the psychological aspects of child abuse is that by Spinetta and Rigler[10]. In it they attempted to summarize all that had appeared in the literature in the preceding decade. They listed 88 references in their bibliography covering what had been learned about child abuse in the 1960s. Their conclusions may be summarized as follows.

1. Economic and social stress may enhance the likelihood of abuse in some families but these are not sufficient nor necessary causes for abuse. The study by Steele and Pollock[11] has shown that child abuse occurs not only at lower socio-economic levels but in middle- and upper middle-class family levels as well.

2. 'The capacity to love is not inherent, it must be taught to the child.' Hence, children raised without adequate love, tolerance and good example may find themselves in positions of parenthood for which they have been either not prepared or, at best, ill-prepared. The result is that they may resort to aggressive and violent means of child rearing, feeling somewhat righteous because this method does not conflict with their own personal experience.

3. Closely related to point 2 above is the observation that abusive parents tend to expect too much of their children and do so prematurely. Based mainly upon the findings of Steele and Pollock[11] and Melnick and Hurley[12], it appeared that parents who abused tended to feel insecure and unsure of being loved. They were often frustrated in attaining support for their own dependency needs. The result was that, unconsciously, they turned to their children for support, understanding, reassurance and gratification, placing their infants in a role which was obviously impossible for them to fulfill. Morris and Gould[13] have coined the term 'role reversal' to describe this aspect of child abuse.

4. Finally, Spinetta and Rigler deduced that '... there is present in the parent (who abuses) a general defect in character structure allowing aggressive impulses to be expressed too freely'. It is as if some parents possess inadequate inhibitions to control the urges that many, if not all, parents feel at some time or another.

The conclusions by Spinetta and Rigler appear to have been reached after a careful analysis of the literature of the sixties and indeed are appealing because they seem so logical. It is tempting to accept them at face value. But alas, at least one group of researchers challenged some of these notions about child abuse. Smith and his co-workers, notably Ruth Hanson and Sheila Noble, have reported in a number of journal articles various aspects of their study of 134 battered infants[14,15]. Smith and Hanson contended right from the start with some of the common criticisms of earlier studies on child abuse[15].

First of all, they included in their data a sufficient number of cases to make generalizations from the results meaningful. These authors utilized a sample from the Birmingham region of England which included 134 battered infants, 53 control children who had been hospitalized but not abused and the multiple parents of all cases making for a total number of 214 parents whose child-rearing practices were evaluated. Some other studies employed an adequate number of cases but paid almost no attention to the psychological aspects of abuse. Included in this category would be studies by Corey, Miller and Widlak[16] (98 cases) and Steele and Pollock[11] (60 cases). The study by Sandgrund, Gaines and Green[17] (60 cases), is an exception. Numerous other studies employed a small number of cases. These are listed in Table 8.1.

Table 8.1 Studies of child abuse employing small numbers of cases

Author	Number of cases
Bender (1976)[18]	2
Clark (1976)[19]	21
Flynn (1970)[20]	2
Forrest (1974)[21]	4
Katz (1976)[22]	22
Kirkpatrick (1976)[23]	20
Lukianowicz (1971)[9]	18
Manciaux and Deschamps (1975)[24]	27
Medvecky and Kafka (1972)[25]	10
Melnick and Hurley (1969)[12]	20
NSPCC (1976)[26]	25
Taipale, Moren, Piha and Valanne (1972)[27]	1
Terr (1970)[28]	10

Additionally, Smith and Hanson employed a control group which allowed them to comment on those essential features of abusive parents that were not common to those in the control group[15].

These authors employed a variety of methods in obtaining their data. The use of interviews is the most common method for gathering information and, while it is the only method employed by some investigators, it was one of many methods used by Smith and Hanson. 'Embedded within the structured interviews were questions requiring self-reports on sensitive or threatening matters. . . .' In addition, a measure of hostility and the direction of that hostility, inward or outward, was obtained by administration of the Foulds Hostility Questionnaire. A measure of extraversion–introversion and neuroticism was obtained using the Eysenck Personality Inventory. The Gibson Spiral Maze was employed to obtain a measure of psychomotor performance. The Vineland Social Maturity Scale was used to assess the child's level of social maturation. And the Griffiths Mental Development Scale was used to measure all children who did not appear brain damaged. Finally, extensive use was made of a seven-point semantic differential scale for comparison of abusive mothers with non-abusive and abusive mothers with abusive fathers.

Smith and Hanson were able to address themselves to many of the proposals which had been put forth regarding child abuse. Morris and Gould[13] had suggested some parents abuse their children because their own dependency needs were not being met. Melnick and Hurley[12] found support for this thesis. Smith and Hanson found partial support in that dependency needs upset some parents who abuse but the same behaviour was present in control mothers who did not abuse their children.

Steele and Pollock[11] had proposed that baby batterers were themselves abused as children and hence had been raised deficient in the sense of basic mothering and being cared for themselves. Here again Smith and Hanson found some support for this thesis but control parents who did not abuse their children also reported experiencing a lack of affection in their own upbringing.

Kempe et al.[1] stated flatly that 'psychiatric factors are probably of prime importance in the pathogenesis of the disorder . . .'. When one hears the phrase psychiatric factors one usually associates it with psychosis and neurosis. Spinetta and Rigler[10] found that several studies in the 1950s and early 1960s seemed to indicate the presence of a frank psychosis in the abusing parent. However, they found too, that by the end of the 1960s several articles, most notably that of Steele and Pollock[11], appeared which '. . . seemed to support the view that only a few of the abusing parents showed severe psychotic tendencies . . .'. Kempe[29] reported that only 5% of a sample of 400 battering parents were psychotic, a finding which would appear to alter his views of a decade earlier. Smith and Hanson again partly supported these earlier findings in that gross psychotic symptoms were apparent in only a small segment of their sample. However, there was an abnormally high incidence of neuroticism as measured by the EPI amongst the parents who abused their children. One of the difficulties here is that having attained a significant neuroticism score on the EPI does not elucidate exactly what are the neurotic character traits present. The EPI is a short, quick-to-administer, reliable test instrument for measuring neuroticism (as well as extraversion-introversion) but it does not provide an index of the neurosis specific enough for one to identify characteristics of child abusers. Further on in this chapter reference will be made to some recent attempts by Paulson and his co-workers to overcome this deficiency.

Smith and Hanson deduced from their psychiatric interview data and from the slowness and clumsiness of parents on the Spiral Maze test that the neuroticism score was likely a reflection of general depression in the abusive parents. These authors found 48% of mothers of battered children and 40% of fathers were neurotic as deduced by psychiatric interviews.

Smith and Hanson obtained a measure of hostility and the direction of that hostility, intropunitively or extrapunitively, in their large sample. They found that abusive mothers were significantly more hostile than control mothers but the authors were unable to specify if this hostility was expressed inwardly or outwardly. Conversely the authors found no statistical difference between abusive fathers and control fathers on the dimension of hostility. Battering parents were found to resort to physical punishment more readily than control parents. This seemed to suggest that abusive parents were undercontrolled rather than overcontrolled. It is as if inhibitions have not been adequately internalized for abusive parents so as to serve as a check on their behaviour at those crucial moments when a child is found to be annoying or when the child provides a ready target for the displacement of aggression. This finding is at odds with that of Melnick and Hurley[12] who were able to support Megargee's[30] contention that overtly aggressive persons are overcontrolled.

Finally, some consideration has been given to the hypothesis that some children are more prone to abuse because of illness or because some characteristic of their personality conflicts with that of their parents. Smith and Hanson approached this aspect of child abuse by attempting to ascertain the social maturity of the child and found that battered children were no more socially mature than were the controls. This finding was interpreted as revealing that if some children are more prone to abuse because they seem mature for their age and more apt to be considered as somewhat akin to adults, they are, in fact, no more socially mature than children who do not suffer abuse. This finding, albeit relevant, does not negate the possibility that other characteristics of the child such as a tendency for colic or obstreperousness could render some children, potentially, the butt of abuse.

THE INTELLECTUAL FACTOR

One persistent characteristic investigated in most psychological studies is the intellectual factor. There may be several reasons for this. First of all, a host of well-validated psychometric tests have been developed for measuring intelligence. In addition these tests are usually quite easy to administer and score and interpretation has been facilitated by the transformation of the raw score results into an intelligence quotient (IQ). Comparatively speaking, dimensions of personality appear to be much more elusive and personality tests do not appear to be as easy to interpret as intelligence tests. A third reason for the general interest shown in the intellectual factor is that purposive behaviour is believed to be largely controlled by cognitive functioning and one of the best ways to infer levels of cognitive functioning is through the use of IQ scores.

An examination of the intellectual factor in child abuse is, like so many other facets of the phenomenon, lacking in unanimous agreement. Steele and Pollock[11] found the IQs of their abusive group of parents ranged from 73 to 130 with most parents falling in the average (90–110) range. Conversely the NSPCC incorrectly quotes Smith, Hanson and Noble[14] as having found over 50% of battering parents to be of borderline mental ability[26]. The rank of borderline indicates the IQs were in the 70s. Actually, Smith et al. found very little difference in IQ between battering parents and non-battering, with most scoring in the low average range. The NSPCC[26], using WAIS scores, found their group of 25 abusive parents to range in IQ from 93–111, generally within the average range. They found no difference in IQ between abusers and non-abusers. Curiously enough, Melnick and Hurley's[12] well-controlled study did not investigate the intellectual component of their abusive and non-abusive sample.

As regards the intelligence of the abused children, Smith and Hanson[15] found a number to be mentally retarded. The NSPCC treated 25 of these children in an appropriate environment for several years and actually found they were able to improve this previously diagnosed condition[26]. It is recognized that mental defectiveness is usually irreversible. Therefore, probably what Smith and Hanson had discovered was that environmental deprivation was being manifested in the intellectual development of some children. Hence, the NSPCC were likely able to obtain improved IQ scores for these children by having altered the environmental conditions that were previously having a psychologically deleterious effect upon them.

PSYCHODYNAMIC EXPLANATIONS

Psychological aspects of behaviour may incorporate psychodynamic formulations of child abuse as well. Flynn[20], in reporting on two young mothers who had severely beaten one of their children, concluded that the defect in motherliness which Steele and Pollock[11] had reported was essentially a defect in ego attitude. Flynn found the women he studied seemed to have an extraordinary reliance on the defence mechanisms of repression, denial and projection which caused them to have '... an incapacity to learn from experience and to appreciate realistically the possible or inevitable consequences of their actions'. Green, Gaines and Sandgrund[31] explain the psychodynamic factors of child abuse as the demands of a particular child intensifying the mother's own unsatisfied dependency needs. The mother turns to the child for satisfaction of these needs and is naturally frustrated because her wishes are incompatible with the child's own urgent demands. The mother then, unconsciously, equates the child with her own rejecting mother. All the stored-up anger, anxiety, guilt and loss of self-esteem rekindle the mother's self-image as a 'bad' person. She then displaces these unacceptable feelings onto the child with the ego defence mechanisms of denial, projection and externalization.

As appealing as the psychodynamic interpretation of behaviour often is, it really only offers the child abuse investigator another hypothetical position which should be amenable to systematic investigation. However, most often, psychodynamic explanations for events are accepted in their original formulation and they rarely become subject to verification through a vigorous, in-depth, experimental investigation.

PSYCHOLOGICAL TESTING

The use of psychometric tests as an adjunct to a psychological investigation of child abuse merits special mention. A number of investigators have used quite a wide variety of tests. A sampling of some of the studies and the tests they used are shown in Table 8.2.

Table 8.2   Psychometric tests used in the study of child abuse

Authors	Tests used*
Steele and Pollock[11]	WAIS, Rorschach, TAT, Incomplete Sentences, HFD, TAT,
Melnick and Hurley[12]	CTP
Taipale, Moren, Piha and Valanne[27]	CAT, WISC
Sandgrund, Gaines and Green[17]	CAT, WPPSI, WISC, Rorschach, B-G, HFD
Smith and Hanson[15]	WAIS, EPI, Foulds H.Q, VSMS,
Katz[22]	Gibson SM, Griffiths MDS, MMPI, Rorschach, DAP, B-G, Rotter

* See Table 8.3.

Some researchers believe that it is through a study of psychological variables that knowledge of child abuse will be advanced. Corey, Miller and Widlak[16], in their study of 48 battered children compared with 50 non-battered, questioned much of the demographic characteristics and medical history items thought to be relevant to child abuse. They proposed '. . . that the causal factors of child abuse will most likely be found through research into the psychological variables underlying the perpetrator's abusive behaviour'. This would appear to be an optimistic statement in light of the number of studies which have employed psychological tests and have come to virtually no consensus as to the essential psychological characteristics of abusive parents. Some studies utilized clinical interview data and made generalizations based upon responses to select questions. This method too appears to have failed to tease out the psychological characteristics of child abusers. These findings, however, cannot and should not be interpreted as indicating that psychometric tests and clinical interview methodology are inappropriate and ineffective means for establishing psychological characteristics. Rather, it should be construed as meaning the antecedents of abuse are sufficiently complex to mean that at this stage of our knowledge investigators have not yet discovered the most efficacious methodology.

NEW DEVELOPMENTS

Two interesting approaches have recently been developing which may eventually prove to be the conceptualizations necessary for clinicians to better understand, diagnose and predict child abuse. The first of these is typologies and the second is prediction scales.

Typologies

A typology is nothing more than a list of types. To classify child abusers according to some characteristic such as the type of abuse is a simple method of counteracting the previously unsuccessful attempts to identify the elusive abusive-parent profile. Four such typologies are presented here.

Merrill[32] made the first major attempt at typology. He distinguished the first three types as applicable to both abusing mothers and fathers. The fourth type he found relevant to abusing fathers only. The four types are as follows:

1. Continually hostile and aggressive parents.
2. Personalities characterized by rigidity, compulsivity and lacking in warmth, reasonableness and flexibility.
3. Passive and dependent personalities.
4. Fathers who had been frustrated due to physical disability or inability to support their families.

Another typology is that by Gil[33]. As part of his nationwide survey on child abuse, a substudy was made which consisted of classifying all cases of child abuse into one of 14 types of abuse. He next subjected the 14 types to a factor analysis and 7 factors emerged. These are:

1. Psychological rejection.
2. Angry and uncontrolled disciplinary response.
3. Male babysitter abuse.
4. Personality deviance and reality stress.
5. Child-originated abuse.
6. Female babysitter abuse.
7. Caretaker quarrel.

The author stated that 'these seven factors reflect the existence of strong associations between certain sets of empirically observed circumstances of physical child abuse and constitute, therefore, a more refined typology of child abuses inflicted upon the children of the sample cohort'. He suggested further that this typology may provide '... a basis for predicting the nature and proportional distribution of future cohorts of physically abused children reported under currently existing, legally established reporting mechanisms of the states'.

Boisvert[34] has suggested another typology, one for uncontrolled battering and one for controlled battering. The following are his classifications:

Uncontrolled battering
1. The psychotic personality.
2. The inadequate personality.
3. The passive aggressive personality.
4. The sadistic personality.

Controlled battering
1. Displacement of aggression.
2. Cold-compulsive disciplinarian.

The fourth and final typology to be presented is that by Walters[35]. He has suggested the following 10 types:

1. Socially and parentally incompetent abuser.
2. Frustrated and displaced abuser.
3. Situational abuser.
4. Neglectful abuser.
5. Accidental or unknowing abuser.
6. Victim-precipitated abuse.
7. Subcultural abuser.
8. Mentally ill abuser.
9. Institutionally prescribed abuse.
10. Self-identified abuse.

Obviously, these typologies include many vague and ambiguous generalizations just as have many of the formulations put forth by other investigators in explaining child abuse. Obvious too, is the fact some abusers will not fall into any one category and where two parents in the home have abused the child two different types may be necessary to categorize adequately. But the advantage in the use of typologies is that it enables professionals to view a situation involving abuse in a more objective manner. It may assist the professional in avoiding the pitfalls of making judgements about environmental factors when he or she has little reliable information to go on.

Prediction Scales

A second innovation which has recently emerged to assist the clinician in the study of child abuse is the development of prediction scales. Particularly, Paulson *et al.*[36,37] have been able to identify existing questionnaire items within the MMPI which show characteristic profiles that differentiate between abusive and non-abusive parents. Furthermore, these items were able to differentiate characteristics within samples of abusing mothers and fathers. In its present form, scales have been developed to identify both male and female abusers. A combined abuser scale is available also. All raw scores are transformed into T scores so that they may be plotted on the MMPI profile sheet. The authors report fewer than 15% of false positives or false negatives identified. A false positive identification refers to the incorrect prediction of someone as an abuser. A false negative identification reflects a test's inability to correctly identify an actual abuser. At the present state of diagnostic sophistication a 15% error rate appears to be within acceptable limits. The fact that different test items are required to identify the male and female abuser highlights the now familiar theme that there are sex differences in the characteristics of abusive parents. Furthermore, it was found that female abusers are often remarkably free of neurotic anxiety, somatizing, self-doubts, depression and expressed insecurity. Their conflicts usually centre around violence, aggression and authority figures. The abusive fathers, on the other hand, are characterized as possessing somewhat paranoid ideation, obsessive–compulsive tendencies and interpersonal difficulties.

It is recognized that, here too, there is a tendency to slip into the use of generalizations in explaining the psychological characteristics of child abusers. But if one were to resist this tendency, one might find that it is through the use of more predictive scales, formulated within the conceptual framework of some typological system, that advancements are going to be made in predicting, and hence preventing, child abuse.

SUMMARY AND CONCLUSIONS

In summary then, it seems safe to make the following cautious conclusions regarding the psychological aspects of child abuse.

1. Socio-economic status may contribute to psychological characteristics. Lower socio-economic status is often prevalent in child abuse and it appears to occur less frequently among the upper-middle class. Low socio-economic status is neither a necessary nor sufficient cause of child abuse since abuse does not occur amongst the majority of low socio-economic persons.

2. When abuse occurs, role reversal may be occurring with the result that the perpetrator of abuse may appear relatively lacking in remorse and may even appear somewhat righteous.

3. Parents who abuse their children are often relatively young, i.e. under 25 years of age, but the majority of young parents do not abuse their children.

4. Recidivism amongst child abusers is common.

5. There appear to be sex differences in the characteristics of abusive parents.

6. The intellectual functioning of the abusive person may be in the borderline mental defective category (IQ in the 70s), but most abusers are in the normal range and child abuse has even been found to occur amongst the superiorly endowed.

7. Abusive parents often were themselves the victims of abuse in their childhood but this is also neither a necessary nor sufficient cause for abuse. Not all who abuse were abused and not all who were abused, abuse.

8. Mental illness may be a contributing factor to child abuse. Rarely is psychotic behaviour a precipitating factor. However, neuroticism, especially depressive neurosis, has been found as a factor in approximately 40–50% of abusive parents. Compulsive tendencies are sometimes also present.

9. Characteristics of the child, such as mental defectiveness, illness or being the result of an unwanted pregnancy, may correlate with abuse but are neither necessary nor sufficient causes for abuse because similar children in different families are not abused.

10. Because child abuse is studied *ex post facto* any investigation of abusive behaviour is in jeopardy. That is, one cannot be certain if the perceived behaviour after the act was a precondition for the abuse or the result of abuse having occurred and been detected.

11. No consistent and homogeneous personality profile of an abusive person has been identified.

12. The conceptualization of typologies acknowledges the inability of investigators to discover any one consistent and homogeneous personality profile of an abusive adult. Typologies allow for categorization of abusers and potentially offer a more fruitful manner of studying their psychological characteristics.

13. Finally, the emergence of scales within existing objective psychometric tests promises some hope for a more efficient detection of potential abusers so that early treatment may avert tragedy.

The future of research into the psychological aspects of child abuse remains unclear. On the one hand, there appears to be some evidence from the available literature to indicate that child abuse is a comparatively rare phenomenon. If these statistics are accepted as reliable, then it is likely that very little interest will be generated in attempting to determine the psychological variables involved. If the statistics are true, there will likely be little effort expended in refining existing scales and developing new ones to predict potential abusers. On the other hand, texts such as the present one may attract increased attention to the child abuse phenomenon. Recommendations put forth by the White House Conference on Children and Youth, to the President of the United States of America[38], even though highly idealistic and possibly impractical, may have a stimulating effect upon investigations. It may be the term 'child abuse' will eventually be expanded to encompass any type of child-rearing behaviour which is potentially detrimental to a child's development into an emotionally healthy, fully functioning adult. Whatever the course of future investigation into this highly interesting and complex phenomenon, one thing is certain. In a socially conscious society, adults are entrusted with the care of persons who are unable to care for themselves. Hence, a responsibility falls to every adult, whether parent or not, to ensure that defenceless children are never the objects of any kind of abuse. It would appear that this obligation can only be met by vigilance. An awareness of the psychological aspects of child abuse would serve as an adjunct to this endeavour.

Table 8.3 Titles of psychological tests used in child abuse studies

Abbreviation	Name
B-G	Bender Motor Gestalt Test
CAT	Children's Apperception Test
CTP	California Test of Personality
DAP	Draw-A-Person (Same as HFD)
EPI	Eysenck Personality Inventory
Foulds	Foulds Hostility Questionnaire
Gibson SM	Gibson Spiral Maze
Griffiths MDS	Griffiths Mental Development Scale
HFD	Human Figure Drawing (Same as DAP)
MMPI	Minnesota Multiphasic Personality Inventory
Rorschach	Rorschach Inkblot Test
Rotter	Rotter Incomplete Sentences Blank
16PF	Sixteen Personality Factor Test
TAT	Thematic Apperception Test
VSMS	Vineland Social Maturity Scale
WAIS	Wechsler Adult Intelligence Scale
WISC	Wechsler Intelligence Scale for Children
WPPSI	Wechsler Pre-school and Primary Scale of Intelligence

References

1. Kempe, C. H., Silverman, F. N., Steele, B. F., Droegemueller, W. and Silver, H. K. (1962). The battered child syndrome. *J. Am. Med. Assoc.,* **181,** 17

2. Kempe, C. H. and Helfer, R. E. (eds.) (1972). *Helping the Battered Child and His Family.* (Philadelphia: Lippincott)

3. Fergusson, D. M., Fleming, J. and O'Neill, D. P. (1972). *Child Abuse in New Zealand: A Report on a Nationwide Survey of the Physical Ill-treatment of Children in New Zealand.* (Wellington, N.Z.: A. R. Shearel)

4. Light, R. (1973). Abused and neglected children in America: A study of alternative policies. *Harvard Ed. Rev.,* **43**(4), 556

5. Baldwin, J. A. and Oliver, J. E. (1975). Epidemiology and family characteristics of severely abused children. *Br. J. Prev. Soc. Med.,* **29,** 205

6. Calef, V. (1972). The hostility of parents to children: some notes on infertility, child abuse and abortion. *Int. J. Psychoanalyt. Psychother.,* **1,** 76

7. Zadik, D. (1973). Social and medical aspects of the battered child with vision impairment. *New Outlook for the Blind,* **67,** 241

8. Goldstein, J. H. (1975). Social and psychological aspects of child abuse: A bibliography. *Catalog Select. Doc. Psychol.,* **5,** 289

9. Lukianowicz, N. (1971). Battered children. *Psychiat. Clin.,* **4,** 257

10. Spinetta, J. and Rigler, D. (1972). The child-abusing parent: A psychological review. *Psychol. Bull.,* **77,** 296

11. Steele, B. F. and Pollock, C. B. (1968). A psychiatric study of parents who abuse infants and small children. In: *The Battered Child.* R. E. Helfer and C. H. Kempe (eds.) (Chicago, Ill.:

University of Chicago Press)

12. Melnick, R. and Hurley, J. R. (1969). Distinctive personality attributes of child abusing mothers. *J. Consult. Clin. Psychol.*, **33**, 746

13. Morris, G. and Gould, R. W. (1963). Role reversal: A concept in dealing with the neglected–battered child syndrome. In: *The Neglected–Battered Child Syndrome* (New York: Child Welfare League of America)

14. Smith, S. M., Hanson, R. and Noble, S. (1973). Parents of battered babies: a controlled study. *Br. Med. J.*, **4**, 388

15. Smith, S. M. and Hanson, R. (1975). Interpersonal relationships and child rearing practices in 214 parents of battered children. *Br. J. Psychiat.*, **127**, 513

16. Corey, E. J., Miller, C. L. and Widlak, F. W. (1975). Factors contributing to child abuse. *Nursing Res.*, **24**, 293

17. Sandgrund, A., Gaines, R. W. and Green, A. H. (1974). Child abuse and mental retardation: A problem of cause and effect. *Am. J. Ment. Deficiency*, **79**, 327

18. Bender, B. (1976). Self-chosen victims: Scapegoating behaviour sequential to battering. *Child Welfare*, **55**, 417

19. Clark, K. N. (1976). Knowledge of child development and behaviour interaction patterns of mothers who abuse their children. *Diss. Abstr. Int.*, **36**, 5784B

20. Flynn, W. R. (1970). Frontier justice: A contribution to the theory of child battery. *Am. J. Psychiat.* **127**, 375

21. Forrest, T. (1974). The family dynamics of maternal violence. *J. Am. Acad. Psychoanal.*, **2**, 215

22. Katz, M. L. (1976). A comparison of ego functioning in filicidal and physically child-abusing mothers. *Diss. Abstr. Int.*, **36**, 5798

23. Kirkpatrick, F. K. (1976). Patterns of role dominance–submission and conflict in parents of abused children. *Diss. Abstr. Int.*, **36**, 5800

24. Manciaux, M. and Deschamps, J. P. (1975). The battered child. *Vie Med. Can. F.*, **4**, 244

25. Medvecky, J. and Kafka, J. (1972). Psychiatric aspects of neonaticide by mothers. *Ceskoslovenska Psychiat.*, **68**, 16

26. NSPCC (1976). *At Risk: An Account of the Work of the Battered Child Research Department, NSPCC.* (London: Routledge and Kegan Paul)

27. Taipale, V., Moren, R., Piha, T. and Valanne, E. (1972). Experiences of an abused child. *Acta Paedopsychiat.*, **39**, 53

28. Terr, L. C. (1970). A family study of child abuse. *Am. J. Psychiat.*, **127**, 665

29. Kempe, C. H. (1971). Paediatric implications of the battered baby syndrome. *Arch. Dis. Child.*, **46**, 28

30. Megargee, E. I. (1966). Undercontrolled and overcontrolled personality types in extreme antisocial aggression. *Psychol. Monog.: Gen. Appl.*, **80**, 611

31. Green, A. H., Gaines, R. W. and Sandgrund, A. (1974). Child abuse: Pathological syndrome of family interaction. *Am. J. Psychiat.*, **131**, 882

32. Merrill, E. (1962). Physical abuse of children: An agency study. In: *Protecting the Battered Child*, V. De Francis (ed.) (Denver, Colo.: American Humane Association)

33. Gil, D. G. (1970). *Violence Against Children: Physical Child Abuse in the United States.* (Cambridge, Mass.: Harvard University Press)

34. Boisvert, M. J. (1972). The battered child syndrome. *Soc. Casework*, **53**, 475

35. Walters, D. R. (1975). *Phyical and Sexual Abuse of Children: Causes and Treatment.* (Bloomington Ind.: Indiana University Press)

36. Paulson, M. J., Afifi, A. A., Thomason, M. L. and Chaleff, A. (1974). The MMPI: A descriptive measure of psychopathology in abusive parents. *J. Clin. Psychol.*, **30**, 387

37. Paulson, M. J., Afifi, A. A., Chaleff, A., Thomason, M. L. and Liu, V. Y. (1975). An MMPI scale for identifying 'at risk' abusive parents. *J. Clin. Child Psychol.*, **4**, 22

38. *Report to the President:* White House Conference on Children (1970). (Washington, DC: US Government Printing Office)

9   The needs of children*

MIA KELLMER PRINGLE

PSYCHOLOGICAL CONSEQUENCES – AN IGNORED ISSUE

It is remarkable that so little attention has been paid to the needs of children who are abused compared with the considerable and still expanding literature on the needs and problems of their parents. There is the same discrepancy between the emphasis on supporting and treating the battering parent on the one hand and, on the other hand, the relative neglect of providing support and treatment services for the child victim (except for physical injuries). Similarly, the parents' socio-economic background, health, personality, personal and marital history have received a good deal of attention[1]. In contrast, very little research has been undertaken into the emotional, social and intellectual effects on children of being subjected to parental violence; or of growing up rejected and ill-treated, even though not to the point of maiming or death which are, after all, only the publicized tip of the iceberg of child abuse. Hence, knowledge about such children's long-term development is woefully inadequate, all the more so since few follow-up studies have been carried out.

This lack of apparent interest in, or concern for, the psycho-social needs of the battered child is quite strikingly demonstrated in the official reports of Committees of Inquiry into fatal cases in the UK. None of them even refer to likely psychological damage arising from physical abuse. Yet surely this must in most cases have been evident before the final tragedy? Though these aspects are more difficult to explore when very young infants are involved, experienced paediatricians and psychologists are nevertheless well able to undertake developmental assessments. Moreover, the first such case which led to a full enquiry concerned a child who was almost eight years old by the time she

---

* This chapter reflects the author's personal views and does not necessarily represent those of the National Children's Bureau.

died[2]; some of the others were also well beyond infancy.

In no case so far has the question even been raised whether and to what extent the killed child's psychological needs had also not previously been met by his family; and whether on these grounds alone earlier intervention should have taken place which might have prevented the subsequent tragedy. However, a recent report recommended that in future the child's psycho-social development must also be considered in suspected cases[3]. For example, 6 year old Maria Colwell[2] changed within a 15 month period from being a happy, responsive, well-behaved child to being withdrawn, sullen, solitary, depressed, unable to communicate, sitting for hours staring into space, and not responding to children or adults. Indeed the descriptions of her behaviour shortly before she died indicated that she was in a state of severe shock, depression and deep mourning for the parents she had lost; and that the treatment being meted out to her was destroying her not only physically but also emotionally.

Yet those professionally concerned (teachers, social workers, health visitors and doctors) did not apparently consider her to be in need of psychological support or treatment. Had she survived, the emotional damage done to her would very probably have had long-term effects on her ability to make relationships. The enquiry report hardly touches on this vital issue, nor does it call for much closer attention to be given in future to early danger signs that a child is being emotionally damaged. Neither does it emphasize the need to provide treatment for the inevitable emotional conquences engendered by physical ill-treatment, nor does any other official report published since.

Another neglected issue is the emotional stress caused to siblings. The likely psychological effects upon brothers and sisters do not appear to have been explored so far, although one would suspect these to be quite profound. Witnessing or being aware of ill-treatment – and in some cases of its fatal outcome – must surely be deeply disturbing to any child and hence at least as deserving of therapeutic support and treatment as offering such facilities to the battering adults.

The 'name game'

It looks as if the full realization of the cruelty meted out by adults to children and its effect on their development is so painful that the mechanisms of avoidance and denial almost invariably come into play. Thus the 'battered child syndrome' – the graphic, strictly accurate but somewhat emotive description coined by Kempe[4] – has come to be replaced by the term 'the abused child' in the United States. In the United Kingdom an even more euphemistic phrase has been invented, namely 'non-accidental injury'; and now this circumlocutory description has been further neutralized by being abbreviated to its mere initials, 'NAI'. Thus the original term has been made totally 'aseptic', devoid of any trace of emotional connotation and compassion. Will this not inevitably diminish professional and administrative sensibility as well as reduce public concern and, indeed, awareness of the problem? Significantly, no-one has suggested substituting these initials in relation to battered wives. Their plight has justifiably been given massive attention even though they are far less helpless than children, expecially the under-fives who are most at risk. Do adults find it easier to identify emotionally with their own age group? And do some adults perhaps have difficulty in reading the silent signs and in understanding the inarticulate cries for help of the assaulted child?

The 'number game'

How many children are injured or killed in various countries by their parents (or permanent substitutes) is not at present known with any degree of certainty[5]. Some argue that it will not be known unless and until there is compulsory notification of all non-accidental injuries. Others, including myself, believe that even then it is unlikely that the true number will come to light for two different sets of reasons.

First, some diseases given as the cause of death in the Registrar General's statistics for England and Wales may not be as innocent as the designation implies[5]. Yet data which were not put into them, can never be revealed by a subsequent search. Parents and others do not always kill their children in easily ascertainable or dramatic ways which can be identified by pathologists and classified into accidental and non-accidental categories. Examples are suffocation by pressing a hand or pillow against the baby's face; deaths following intracerebral and subdural haemorrhages after shaking; deaths from pneumonia or bronchitis in infants who have 'failed to thrive' because of physical or emotional neglect; poisonings[6]; and deaths of severely subnormal children from a multiplicity of causes when the handicap itself originated from a battering episode months or years previously[7].

The second set of reasons relates to attitudes. These include ignorance by the doctor of the syndrome; sheer disbelief or repugnance which may prevent acceptance of the possibility that a parent could kill a child; avoidance of confrontation by ascribing death to an associated existing clinical entity; and the gulf between suspicion and proof[8]. In fact, I believe that the true incidence of child neglect, rejection and abuse will only become apparent if regular health checks for infants and young children were to become compulsory – a suggestion discussed later. Meanwhile, it seems to me that what might be called the 'number game' is another example of the avoidance and denial mechanism in action.

PATTERNS OF PARENTAL VIOLENCE

'Battering parents' are unlikely to be a homogeneous group, either in regard to their personality or social background; nor is there likely to be one set of common causal factors to account for their behaviour. (Dr Peter Scott alludes to this theme in his chapter.) Failure to differentiate between them may well be responsible for the rather confused body of research findings[8]. Before considering the needs of abused children it may be helpful to distinguish, as far as present knowledge allows, between the different motives of parents who violently assault them. Caffey[9] made a beginning by saying 'The prime cause or mechanism are excessive stresses, both social and economic and, in particular, mothers unprepared for motherhood, who succumb to combat fatigue in their struggle with a poverty-stricken environment against material, psychological and social inadequacies which they cannot cope with successfully alone.' However, this view over-emphasizes economic circumstances and social deprivation.

As I see it, there are at least four different sets of circumstances which may lead to a child being seriously neglected, rejected or abused: first, there is the isolated incident which is unlikely to be repeated; second, where one child in the family becomes a 'scapegoat'; third, where parents are markedly inadequate; and fourth, where violence is part and parcel of the parental lifestyle. Each of these circumstances requires, in my view, different treatment, both of the parent and of the child.

The isolated and atypical incident

If it is true that everyone has a breaking point, then it is in this sense – and in this sense only – that every parent could potentially seriously ill-treat a child. In this group is the mother who has no previous history of violence; who has coped adequately with the stresses and strains of everyday life; and who may have brought up other children reasonably well. Then some overwhelming disaster strikes, e.g. postnatal depression, the death of a much loved parent, a husband's unexpected desertion or there is a concentrated accumulation of stressful events, which leads to a sudden outburst of anger in which a hitherto well-cared for and loved child is injured.

Invariably, the assault is followed by horror, shame and remorse; the unjustified ferocity of the act is recognized; and there is unlikely to be a recurrence of this behaviour which is quite out of character. The mother may well need support, not only to help her through the abnormally stressful circumstances which provoked the behaviour in the first place, but also to restore her shaken confidence in her own caring capacity. Provided such support is given, the attacked child can safely be left with her or be returned after hospital treatment.

The 'scapegoat' child

The second pattern, where one child is singled out for ill-treatment, usually represents a persisting parental attitude. Reasons for the 'scapegoating' include the child being an extra-marital 'mistake' who reminds the mother of a despised husband or a hated relative; or it may be regarded as being in some way 'different' from the other children. This 'difference' may be due to a difficult delivery or to prematurity or to early 'bonding failure' because of the baby having to be in an intensive care unit; or he may have some physical or mental handicap which the mother cannot accept.

Thus the rejection and ill-treatment are child-specific, and none of the siblings are at risk. Treatment must depend on the mother's own attitude. If she feels, and indeed wishes, that she could come to love the child, then she should be offered the opportunity to work through her hostility. If she prefers to relinquish it, then she should be supported through this course of action. Future adoptive parents would need to be specially chosen and prepared, since the child – unless still a very young infant – will need to be given additional care and patience while he learns to trust adults and respond to their loving care.

'Inadequate' parents

The third group who are liable to neglect and ill-treat their children are inadequate parents. They include teenage mothers who additionally may be immature for their age; those of limited abilities and insight who themselves have often been neglected, if not ill-treated, in childhood; those who have grown up in institutional care and seek in their babies the loving response and feelings of belonging which were denied to them by their own family.

Mostly such parents also often lack knowledge of normal child development. For example, they do not appreciate the baby's physical inability to stop soiling or wetting; or that nocturnal enuresis is not uncommon among under-fives; or that a terrified infant may fail to acquire sphincter and bowel control just because he is terrified. Frequently too this lack of understanding is compounded by irritability and lack of patience; in turn, these may be due to, or made worse by, environmental pressures including inadequate housing, overcrowding, poverty and too closely spaced and unwanted pregnancies. In many cases, the child has been neither planned nor wanted and, even more crucial, has remained unwanted.

The fathers may be similarly inadequate, in poor physical or mental health, unreliable breadwinners and unreasonable in the marital relationship. Often too they are jealous of the baby, resent its demands for attention and are intolerant of its messiness, crying and helplessness. A violent temper and excessive drinking are further contributory factors. It looks, moreover, as if those unable to achieve and exercise control over their environment are more likely to exercise power in ways closer at hand[10]. Since these features of inadequate parents are chronic, neither quick nor profound change can realistically be expected. Hence the children remain at risk unless really continuous and long-term support can be given, together with intensive training in home making and child rearing skills. Even then, the outlook is not always hopeful.

Violence as a way of life

In the fourth group, violence, both verbal and physical, characterizes the parents' habitual behaviour. Frequently, this is directed not only towards their children but also towards each other, their neighbours, relatives and workmates. Usually only one parent is the actively abusing partner but the other, though submissive, nevertheless fails to protect the child or even colludes in its ill-treatment. People whose life-style is violent include the psychopath who lashes out indiscriminately; the mentally ill, including the delusional schizophrenic; the pathologically authoritarian parent, more often male, who continually punishes a child for failing to come up to his unrealistically high demands; and the sadistic pervert who gains satisfaction from the suffering of the weak and helpless.

Probably most, if not all, such parents were themselves damaged in childhood through an uncaring or violent upbringing. So parental hostility perpetuates itself from one generation to another in what is quite literally a very vicious circle. Thus, to allow a child to remain or return to such a home perpetuates the pattern of violence in the long term. In the short term, it puts even the child's physical welfare at risk. There is no reliable way to ensure his safety since there is no known effective and quick enough treatment which will modify the behaviour of adults for whom violence is a way of life.

Distinguishing features

Parents in the 'inadequate' and 'violent' categories, in contrast to the 'isolated incident' and the 'scapegoat' groups, tend to show little remorse or shame. Instead, they justify their treatment of the child by its naughtiness, dirty habits and other shortcomings. This lack of insight is probably compounded by the fact that, in our society, physical violence against children is widely condoned within the context of disciplining them. Even in relation to very young infants, physical means are surprisingly common. For example, among a normal small town population, 62% of parents were found to smack their one year olds; at four years of age, only 3% were not smacked; and, most significant of all, 7% of this age group were smacked at least once a day, an implement being used in a number of cases[11]. Such general acceptance of physical chastisement is bound to reduce the threshold at which people are prepared to use physical force against even very young children.

The third and fourth patterns of child abuse (the 'inadequate' and the 'violent') are quite different from, and more intractable than, the other two in that they spring from the parents' total personality and way of life. Hence the prognosis for improvement, let alone lasting change, is very unfavourable. At best, it would require long-term, intensive and costly case work support and even then the child's continued safety could not be ensured. Indeed, a very experienced worker has warned against feelings of professional omnipotence and the danger of 'uncritical therapeutic optimism which may result in far too much being expected in the way of improvement of very deprived parents'[12]. Not only is there no proven treatment method, but there is also evidence that children growing up in grossly inadequate or violent homes are themselves likely to perpetuate these same patterns of behaviour with their own children[13-15].

Given that this vicious circle must be broken; given that at present we do not have the means – either in knowledge or manpower – to rehabilitate grossly inadequate or deeply damaged adults within the time scale necessary for the child's future well-being; given that the outlook is much more favourable for the young child 'at risk' if satisfactory substitute parental care is provided; then surely priority must be accorded to the child's needs, even though it deprives adults (who were more often than not themselves 'sinned against' as children and hence deserve compassion rather than punishment) of their parental rights, thus making them victims for the second time.

THE PSYCHOLOGICAL NEEDS OF CHILDREN

In the absence of adequate research evidence, I shall consider the likely consequences of child abuse on long-term development in the light of what is known about the needs of children, how these are normally met and the effects of failure to do so. It used to be believed that developmental needs come into play in a hierarchical sequence, the most basic being those necessary for sheer survival, such as the need for food and water; and that only when these have been satisfied do the higher needs emerge, such as the need for a loving relationship. Now it is held that all human needs are inter-related and interdependent in a subtle, complex and continuous way. For example, an unhappy baby may reject food, and even if he takes it, may fail to thrive; or a child may fight sleep for fear that his mother or father might hurt or desert him.

In scientific terms, love is neither readily defined nor easily measured. However, the elements which go to make up good parental care can be systematically described and many aspects of the parent–child interaction can be assessed and evaluated. Much is now known about the ways in which the quality of family relationships affects children's development; and even more is known about the probable consequences when these relationships are unsatisfactory or actually damaging.

Since physical needs are not only more clearly understood but also more easily and now more generally met, my emphasis will be on psychological needs. As few as two and as many as 60 have been enumerated by different authors. For practical purposes, a four-fold classification seems sufficient: the need for love and security; for new experiences; for praise and recognition; and for responsibility. These needs have to be met from the beginning of life and continue to require fulfilment to enable a child to grow from helpless infancy to mature adulthood. Of course, their relative importance changes during the different stages of growth as do the ways in which they are met[16].

The need for love and security

This need is met by the child experiencing from birth onwards a stable, continuous, dependable relationship with his parents (or permanent substitutes), who themselves enjoy a rewarding relationship with one another. Through this relationship – first with his mother, then father, and gradually an ever-widening circle of adults and contemporaries – the child acquires a sense of personal identity and worthwhileness. Probably it is the most important need because it forms the basis for all later relationships, not only within the family, but with friends, colleagues and eventually his own family. On it depend the healthy development of the personality, the ability to care and respond to affection and, in time, to become a loving, caring parent. Whether a child acquires a constructive or destructive attitude, first to himself, and then to others, depends in the first place on his parents' attitude to him. Their loving acceptance and approval are essential for the development of his self-acceptance; and by imitation or 'modelling' he acquires their standards of personal and moral values.

The basic and all-pervasive feature of parental love is that the child is valued unconditionally and for his own sake, irrespective of his sex, appearance, abilities or personality; that this love is given without expectation of or demand for gratitude; and that the constraints imposed upon parental freedom of movement, upon time and upon finance are accepted without resentment or reproach. (Occasionally begrudging these constraints is, of course, different from a permanent sense of resentment.) Parents communicate this unconditional affection through all their relations with him: from physical care and handling to responding to his first smile and sounds; from protecting him from, and then gradually initiating him into, the social world; and from restraining to eventually punishing him for going beyond the limits they have set for acceptable behaviour.

The need for security is met by providing an environment where attitudes and behaviour are consistent and dependable; and where a familiar place and a known routine make for continuity and predictability. In a world in which the child has to come to terms with so much that is new and changing, a stable family life provides him with a sense of personal and enduring identity. It is the quality of family relationships which is of basic importance to the child's psychological development. This applies not only to the mother's and father's relations with him, but also to those between the parents themselves, as well as to the child's with his siblings and other close relatives. Parental expectation and discipline which are consistent, whether tending to be strict or lenient, enhance his sense of security by providing a dependable and predictable framework. So does a familiar place, as is clearly shown by the contrast between a young child's usual behaviour in his own home and in a strange place.

Thus, the need for security is closely related to clear standards of behaviour being set by the parents. Knowing what is expected of him and, as soon as he can understand, the reasons why, makes growing up a less difficult business. Inevitably the child will transgress, and will be disobedient – partly because he needs to test the consequences of doing so, partly because he is liable to forget rules – but knowing the limits of what is permitted provides the reassurance of both reasonableness and predictability. In contrast, when the same behaviour gives rise to widely different reactions, with the same parent at different times or in either parent, then the child's concept of acceptable conduct becomes linked to individual whim rather than to general principles.

The need for new experiences

Only if this need is adequately met throughout childhood and adolescence will a child's intelligence develop satisfactorily. Just as the body requires food for physical development and just as an appropriately balanced diet is essential for normal growth, so new experiences are needed for the mind. In early childhood, the most vital ingredients of this diet are play and language. Through them, the child explores the world and learns to cope with it. This is as true for the objective outside world of reality as it is for the subjective internal world of thoughts and feelings.

New experiences facilitate the learning of one of the most important lessons of early life: learning how to learn; and learning that mastery brings joy and a sense of achievement. Educability depends not only on inborn capacity, but as much – if not more – on environmental opportunity and encouragement. The emotional and cultural climate of the home, as well as parental involvement and aspirations, can foster, limit or impair mental growth. Play meets the need for new experiences in two major ways: it enables the child to learn about the world; and it provides a means of coping with and resolving conflicting emotions by allowing fantasy to override reality and logic. Probably the single, and in the long run, most crucial factor which promotes intellectual growth is the quality of the child's language environment: not merely how much he is talked to, but how relevant, distinctive and rich the conversation is. Language helps in learning to reason and to think as well as in making relationships.

Going to school is itself a major new experience which opens up a larger and more impersonal world. The child's progress will come to be powerfully affected by his teacher's attitudes, values and beliefs. Wide interests, enthusiasm for things of the mind and receptiveness to new ideas – all these are infectious. Teachers are in a powerful position to preserve, to awaken or to rekindle the curiosity and joy in learning about new things, shown by almost all young children.

The need for praise and recognition

To grow from a helpless infant into a self-reliant, self-accepting adult requires an immense amount of emotional, social and intellectual learning. It is accomplished by the child's modelling himself on the adults who are caring for him. The most effective incentives to sustain this learning, which requires a continuous effort throughout the years of growing up, are praise and recognition. Eventually, a job well done becomes its own reward but that is a very mature stage: and even the most mature adult responds, and indeed blossoms, when given occasionally some praise or other form of recognition.

Because growing up is inevitably beset by difficulties, conflicts and setbacks, a strong incentive is needed. This is provided by the pleasure shown at success and the praise given to achievement by the adults who love the child and whom he in turn loves and wants to please. Encouragement and reasonable demands act as a spur to perseverance. The level of expectation is optimal when success is possible but not without effort. It cannot be the same for all children nor for all time. Rather, it must be geared to the individual child's capabilities at a given point in time and to the particular stage of his growth.

The need for responsibility

This need is met by allowing the child to gain personal independence, at first through learning to look after himself in matters of his everyday care, such as feeding, dressing and washing himself. It is met too by his having possessions, however small and inexpensive, over which he is allowed to exercise absolute ownership. As he gets older, responsibility has to be extended to more important areas, ultimately allowing him freedom over his own actions. Eventually, in full maturity, he should be able to accept responsibility for others.

Granting increasing independence does not mean withholding one's views, tastes and choices, or the reasons for them; nor does it mean opting out from participating and guiding the lives of children; nor, indeed, condoning everything they do. On the contrary, children need a framework of guidance and limits. They are helped by knowing what is expected or permitted, what the rules are, together with the reasons for them, and whether these are in their interests or in the interests of others.

How can responsibility be given to the immature and to the irresponsible? There is no way out of the dilemma that unless it is granted, the child cannot learn how to exercise it. Like every other skill, it needs to be practised under adult guidance which should gradually diminish.

CONSEQUENCES OF FAILURE TO MEET CHILDREN'S NEEDS

If one of the four basic needs remains unmet, or inadequately met, then development may become stunted or distorted. In practice if one need fails to be met, others are likely to be affected too. Of course, all children pass through phases of temporary maladjustment. Transient problem behaviour is so common as to be normal and it has even been argued that a child who has never shown any difficulties should be considered abnormal.

The label 'maladjustment' is applied to a vast variety of troubled and troublesome children. However, the use of the term is only justified when the difficulties are both so pronounced and so prolonged as to handicap the child and distress his family, school or community. The child's age, ability and home background must also be taken into account when assessing the significance of deviant behaviour.

Just like pain, symptoms of maladjustment are a danger signal, a call for help: they indicate that there is intolerable tension between the personality and the environment. Withdrawal is as urgent a danger signal as aggression although the latter is more likely to be heeded because it constitutes a threat to adult authority. The range of possible symptoms is wide but basically they fall into two broad categories: aggression or withdrawal, fight or flight. Some children habitually choose one mode of reaction, others oscillate between retreat and attack.

To some extent, habitual behaviour is determined by personality type. The emotionally robust and outgoing child is likely to adopt aggressive methods whereas the more gentle and retiring will probably choose retreat. To begin with, a child will try-out various means of meeting a difficult situation. Experience then teaches him which is the most effective or least painful way. Thus, the relative success of aggressive or withdrawn behaviour influences which facet of the child's personality subsequently finds predominant expression. If he gains his ends more readily by one mode, he will persevere with this behaviour pattern. Hence, the way in which parents respond to his earliest attempts at non-conformity and independence has a vital influence on shaping later reactions to adult authority.

In practice, nuisance value or social unacceptability are still used as the main criteria of problem behaviour. This has two undesirable consequences: the aggressive child who hits back tends to arouse aggression in the adults concerned; this leads to a vicious circle of increasingly severe punishment calling out increasing aggression in the child who grows hardened to punishment, so that it loses its effectiveness. Secondly, the withdrawn, conforming child, though probably receiving gentler handling, is often overlooked. His needs are likely to remain unmet since the understanding that a child can be 'too good' is still slow in coming.

No generally acceptable definition exists of a mentally healthy child; however, there would probably be general agreement that a confident, enquiring attitude of mind and the ability to make mutually rewarding relationships, both with adults and peers, are essential characteristics. Viewed in this context, the anxious, timid, always obedient child must cause concern. In fact, fight or flight, aggression or withdrawal, should be regarded as equally significant danger signs, indicating that a child's emotional, social or intellectual needs are not being met adequately. Symptoms of maladjustment are perhaps most appropriately likened to a fever: a sign of malaise, requiring careful examination and diagnosis but by itself providing little clue to what is wrong or to effective treatment. Knowing the symptoms does not provide the key to the underlying causes; nor does knowing the underlying causes make it possible to predict likely symptoms. But they do indicate some failure in meeting one of the basic psychological needs and in what follows the probable consequences will be discussed separately for each one.

The need for love and security

When this need is not met adequately then the consequences can be disastrous later on, both for the individual and for society. Prisons, mental hospitals, borstals and schools for the maladjusted, contain a high proportion of individuals who in childhood lacked consistent, continuous and concerned care, or, worse still, were unloved and rejected. Their number is high too among the chronically unemployable and among what I have termed 'able misfits'[17].

Such young people are one example of the fact that parental rejection is neither the prerogative of any social class nor necessarily linked with socio-economic disadvantage. The existence of an unwanted child may more readily come to light in families whose other problems have already led to the involvement of one helping agency or another. In middle- or upper-class homes, emotional deprivation is rarely suspected or detected. To the discerning teacher the signs are quite evident, yet all too often it is the child himself who is blamed for his difficult behaviour and lack of progress, being labelled 'unco-operative', 'disruptive', 'lazy' or 'backward'. Anger, hate and lack of concern for others are probable reactions to being unloved and rejected. Vandalism, violence and delinquency are not infrequently the outward expression of such feelings. In embryo these reactions can be seen when a young child, who has been scolded or smacked, kicks his teddy bear or the table. Through a loving relationship, children learn to control their anger and later to use it constructively during adolescence and adulthood; without affection, it remains primitive and grows more vicious and vengeful with increasing strength.

Not so long ago, it was believed that children became attached to their mothers chiefly because they provided nourishment. This theory of 'cupboard love' has been disproved by the work of the Harlows with monkeys and by Bowlby's studies[21] of attachment behaviour. Now the pendulum may have swung so far in the other direction that there is a risk of the importance of nutrition being overlooked within this context. Recent evidence indicates that impaired food intake is probably an important contributory cause of dwarfism in children from neglectful or rejecting homes[18,19].

It has been suggested that the concept of 'maternal deprivation' should now be abandoned[20]. I doubt whether it is wise to do so until a more discriminating term becomes available. It is more urgent, I believe, to dispel two misconceptions which have had very unfortunate consequences. Both are based on misinterpretations of Bowlby's views[21]. His stress on the need for a warm, intimate and continuous relationship has been taken to imply that the same person must provide care uninterruptedly for 24 hours a day. In fact, he has always held that it is advisable to accustom even quite young babies to being looked after by someone else occasionally; yet some mothers continue to feel guilty about seeking a temporary and brief 'escape'. The second misconception is reflected in the dictum 'better a bad family than a good institution'. While there is no evidence to support this assertion and in any case, institutions are neither the only nor the best alternative, yet this view has bred a reluctance to remove children even from appallingly bad homes. Moreover it ignores the most crucial factors in mothering, namely its quality, stability and intensity. Instead it postulates a powerful bond, commonly referred to as the 'blood tie'. Again there is no evidence for this myth. Rather, present knowledge indicates that good mothering (or fathering for that matter) is neither dependent on, nor necessarily consequent upon, biological parenthood.

That this is so is shown by the generally very satisfactory outcome when children are placed in adoptive homes. Moreover, there is much evidence that this is the case even when a child has, prior to placement, been subjected to potentially damaging experiences, such as pre-natal stress, early institutional care, parental neglect, ill-treatment, or even a combination of these[22-27].

The effects of maternal rejection and deprivation

The evidence for the relationship of maternal care to children's mental health comes primarily from two sources: from the clinical observations of those concerned with emotionally disturbed children; and from retrospective psychological studies which compare the development of family-reared children with those growing up deprived of a loving and secure home. Methodologically, it would be more conclusive if objective studies of intra-family behaviour in the 'natural' environment of the home were possible. Clearly they are not. Controlled experiments to explore the effects of various types of maternal deprivation on human babies are, of course, quite unacceptable.

Just such experiments, however, have been carried out on baby monkeys. The results are clear cut, startling and convincing. Several generations of monkeys were raised under a wide range of depriving conditions: partial or complete deprivation of maternal care; rearing in complete isolation; group care with other motherless infants; and varying the onset of these abnormal situations. This work was continued long enough to see whether infant experiences have effects lasting into adulthood[28-30]. The results show that 'monkeys which have known no affection can never develop either normal sexual behaviour or normal maternal behaviour and are bound to live out their lives as social failures'. This applied equally to male and female monkeys. Those females who did become pregnant – thanks to the persistence of normally reared males – turned out to be 'hopeless, helpless and heartless mothers': they either ignored their babies or else abused them brutally.

Studies with other animals such as rats and goats have produced similar results. These findings are striking enough to lend strong support to the hypothesis that being deprived of love and security in early life may well have similar long-term consequences in man; however, their exact nature must await the findings of further research.

The abused child

It has become fashionable to argue that many children invite parental abuse. This too seems a reflection of current professional attitudes which tend to be more compassionate towards the battering adult than the child victim. Even if abused babies were more often different or deviant from the normal, because of being small at birth, prematurely born or having congenital physical or mental defects, it is nevertheless extraordinary to argue in terms of 'inviting abuse' which implies a deliberate intention. Surely this is quite incompatible with the reality of a completely dependent infant, all the more so if he is particularly vulnerable physically?

Furthermore, now that the development of abused children is at last being given some attention, contrary evidence is emerging[31]. It indicates that it is the adults themselves, whose parenting capacity is inadequate from the outset, who put infants at risk; that few if any of the latter have significant congenital defects; that a relatively small proportion were of very low birthweight; and that neurological dysfunction and mental retardation are more likely to be the results (rather than the cause) of a history of undetected neglect (including malnutrition) and of abuse. The same may well be true of babies who fail to thrive since many improve and put on weight after being hospitalized; some of the neurological malfunctioning also disappears. This is in significant contrast to hospitalized children from loving and caring homes, who tend to fret and regress in behaviour.

The likely psychological concomitants of parental abuse can only be surmised in the absence of research evidence. General principles of child development as well as clinical, but rather anecdotal, reports leave little doubt that these are inevitably profound. In particular, the child's sense of security and of being valued are bound to be undermined, if indeed they have ever been established.

When rejection and ill-treatment are intermittent, then he lives in a state of uncertainty, not knowing what to expect. It may well be that it is these children whose attitude has been characterized as one of 'frozen watchfulness'. Because parental behaviour is unpredictable and contradictory, they live in a constant state of insecurity and apprehension. Moreover, physical chastisement is at times more an outlet for the parent's own anger and frustration rather than a means of ensuring the child's conformity to desired standards of behaviour. Chastisement of this kind only succeeds in teaching its recipient to fear force and later to use it himself; even a verbal berating, coupled with threats of being 'put away', makes a child feel rejected without necessarily enabling him to understand what is expected of him and why.

When abuse is continuous, then either submission or anger will become the typical reaction. The child who submits develops a 'victim' mentality, attempting to appease, to ingratiate himself, even clinging to the abusing parents; or he may withdraw, trying to become inconspicuous, but chronically apprehensive or even paralysed with fear. In a sadistically violent parent, such submissiveness may arouse an even greater desire to humiliate and hurt. On the other hand, the child who responds with anger and defiance provokes a battle of wills where the adult becomes determined 'to show who is master'. Since the infant cannot forcefully be 'made' to do anything – be it to keep down food, stop crying or go to sleep – and since the immature, violent parent finds his own impotence unacceptable, a headlong clash is as inevitable as its tragic outcome.

The ill-treated baby is in an even more desperate plight than the young child because he is as yet physically incapable of responding to force and pain in one or other of the natural ways, namely either fight or flight: he can no more hit back than run away. Hence ill-treatment may well arouse helpless rage and hate, which will then be carried into adult life to become the smouldering anger of the wife or child batterer; or the equivalent of Harlow's female monkeys, 'hopeless, helpless and heartless mothers' who either ignore or brutally abuse their offspring.

'Clinical observations of abused children suggest that many are considerably damaged emotionally as well as physically by the time they come to professional attention. Some have been described as bland in affect, strikingly passive, apathetic and aimless in their behaviour. Others present as anxious, tense, constantly on the alert to gauge adult responses, and attention seeking'[32]. There seems to be a sex difference in that 'the girls ... tend to be passive and withdrawn in contrast to the boys who are aggressive and destructive. However, it does not mean that the girls are any less damaged'[14].

A preliminary study of wife battering concludes that 'Fear must be expressed for the 315 children of the 100 women reported, as many males are developing the prodromal signs of violence while the older age groups manifest a disturbing picture of uncontrolled violence and conflict with the law. Unless an urgent retraining programme can be undertaken with these children a future generation will be subjected to family violence'[33]. This vicious circle of intergenerational neglect and violence has been confirmed by recent evidence, which also shows that children from violent families not only tend to marry early but to have large families[34–36]. Then, they in turn fail to provide love and security for their offspring having been unloved and rejected in their own childhood.

The need for new experiences

When this need is inadequately met, intellectual potentialities and personal growth to some extent too, remain unrealized. In the infant, insufficient sensory

stimulation can retard or even impair development, including later on the ability to think, reason and communicate. In fact, during recent years, the concept
of infant intelligence has been substantially revised. Marked individual
differences have been observed quite early during the baby's first year of life
and there is evidence that these are likely to be due to the effects of social
stimulation[37]. The exact difference which an enriching or depriving upbringing
and home background can make, needs much further research. 'However, a
conservative estimate of the effect of extreme environments on intelligence is
about 20 IQ points. This could make the difference between a life in an institution for the subnormal or a productive life in society. It could mean the
difference between a professional career and an occupation which is at the
semi-skilled or unskilled level'[38].

The normal healthy infant and toddler is alert and curious. His everyday life
is filled with new experiences and challenges to which he responds with eager
vitality. New sounds, sights and tastes – they all arouse his interest and
stimulate his desire to explore and experiment. The more dull and un-
stimulating life is, the more apathetic and bored, or the more restless and
frustrated he becomes; in particular, language skills suffer. Language has two
main roles. First, it is a communication system – a way of relating to others,
sharing ideas and information with them. Its second, and probably more important, role lies in controlling thought and, through it, behaviour. This is not
to say that there can be no thought without language. Rather, thought remains
markedly impoverished without language, perhaps in a real sense sub-human.
Language is to thought what a catalyst is to a chemical reaction: it gets it off,
speeds it up and facilitates it.

The essential element in promoting intellectual growth is the reciprocity of
speech between child and adult, the latter initiating or responding to conversation. The mere presence of adults or just listening to speech (on TV for
example) is insufficient. That this is so is shown by the comparatively limited
verbal ability of those reared in families which are large or where language
skills are very limited[20,39,40].

The abused child

Since the great majority of neglected and ill-treated children come from socially
and culturally deprived families, they would in any case be adversely affected
by the relative lack of stimulation in such homes. However, their plight is likely
to be worse. To begin with, the neglected and abused baby has to spend much
of his time lying in his cot, lonely, uncomfortable and probably in pain; such
conditions stifle exploration and curiosity and, hence, 'learning'.

Next, while trying to cope with new demands – such as to suck more quickly
and less messily, or to become dry and clean – he is bound to be slow and to
make mistakes just because he is immature and a beginner. Yet he will be
meted out punishment for what is seen by the inadequate or violent parent as

naughtiness, defiance or lack of love. The resulting anxiety and fear will inevitably retard or inhibit adequate learning. And so the infant is caught in an unending spiral of unrealistic demands, failure to improve and consequent punishment. If brain damage results, then, of course, improvement becomes even less possible, depending on the severity of the impairment. Once he becomes a mobile toddler, who naturally wants to explore his surroundings, his 'being into everything' is also likely to arouse parental anger as will his normal attempts to assert his own will. Thus the abused child not only lacks adequate stimulation to foster his development but his own striving towards knowledge and independence will be stifled through fear and punishment. Hence it is not unexpected that the few follow-up studies of abused children which have been undertaken, report their development to be retarded, both in the neuro-motor and intellectual fields, as well as in the acquisition of language skills.

The need for praise and recognition

If this need is inadequately met or remains unsatisfied, then in the long term the effects are destructive of self-respect and of confidence in tackling new situations, tasks and relationships. Unfortunately, praise and recognition are almost invariably given for achievement and not for effort. In consequence, this need is most readily and often satisfied in relation to intelligent, healthy, well-adjusted and attractive children (who are praised even for their pleasing appearance!). In contrast, the intellectually slow, the physically handicapped, the culturally disadvantaged and the emotionally neglected get far less, if any, praise and recognition. Yet their need is very much greater. Whatever small successes they may manage to achieve, these have inevitably required far more effort and perseverance. Yet they receive less reward because they achieve less.

The plight of children rejected by their parents is worse since they are wholly deprived of the satisfaction of this need by those from whom they want it most. Parental interest and encouragement are vital and most potent incentives in helping the young to realize their potential. Even ability and talent well above average may never declare themselves if adequate nurture and emotional support are lacking[17]. There can be little doubt that the neglected and abused child will be among the most serious under-achievers since – almost by definition – he is under-valued and rejected. Rather than calling out compassion, his backwardness and under-functioning themselves compound his plight by apparently justifying parental punishment. Thus their rejection carries the seeds of his continued failure to come up to their expectations and so it becomes inexorably a self-fulfilling prophecy.

The need for responsibility

The child who is denied opportunities to exercise responsibility will fail to develop a sense of responsibility for himself, for others and for material objects.

When this denial has gone hand in hand with a lack of training in self-control and in planning ahead, then such youngsters will tend to be impulsive, unwilling to postpone immediate gratification of impulses, and contemptuous of the rights of others – in short, irresponsible.

Equally, to thrust too much responsibility onto a child or to do so too early, may also have harmful effects. Without the necessary understanding of what is involved and of the probable consequences of a particular decision or choice, responsibility will be perceived as a burden. He may nevertheless be prepared to shoulder it but at a high cost in terms of anxiety; or he may refuse to accept it, spending much time and ingenuity in devising ways of avoiding responsibility, perhaps wishing or dreaming, but rarely doing.

Even at best, our society is ambiguous and ambivalent about granting responsibility and independence, particularly during adolescence. This is reflected in the way in which various adult rights are conceded at different ages. Parents differ even more widely in the amount of independence they are prepared to allow or to tolerate; they differ too in the extent to which they expect responsible behaviour, without at the same time granting the right to make responsible decisions.

The neglected and abused child is likely all too often to suffer simultaneously from being given both too little and too much responsibility. On the one hand, he may be deprived of toys over which he can exercise exclusive rights; he may be denied sufficient practice to learn to feed and dress himself because he is considered to be too slow and clumsy; and he may also lack opportunities of acquiring the responsibility of give-and-take in the company of other children. On the other hand, he may far too early be left to fend for himself; also he, or perhaps more often she, may be made into a household drudge. In any case, the child will probably be punished for what is seen to be unhelpful or irresponsible behaviour. Yet he has little chance to improve upon past performance because of being denied the relaxed and unhurried practice of those very skills which would enable him in time to act responsibly. So once again the child is caught in a double-bind of neglect, rejection, punishment and continued failure to satisfy what are in fact unreasonable demands.

ENSURING ESSENTIAL CARE

Actual battering is only the visible tip of the iceberg of emotional rejection and abuse, suffered daily by many thousands of children in many countries. Surely civilized society should strive to eliminate such suffering? The introduction of three measures would go a long way towards achieving this goal.

The right to loving care

The first and most specific would involve tilting the balance in all cases of abuse much more in favour of the child's rather than the biological parents' interests and rights. This means making his long-term need for love and security of paramount or overriding importance instead of, as at present, considering mainly the probability of future repeated ill-treatment. Hence, it would also entail a full examination of the parents' way of life, behaviour and circumstances before an abused child is restored to his home.

Next, if his psychological safety were to be given equal weight, he would not be allowed to return to an environment where his development would continue to be impeded and distorted. The criterion should be that a marked improvement has taken place, or can be expected with a high degree of confidence, in a previously damaging milieu. Clearly the more immature, disturbed or unstable the parents, and the more punitive or depriving their attitude to the child, the less realistic it is to expect such improvement. In these circumstances, the child's need for continuing, consistent and dependable loving care should take precedence in law over the rights of the biological parents.

Developmental check-ups

The second measure would be to introduce regular developmental check-ups, at least for under-fives. To ensure the fullest coverage, these could be linked to the payment of family allowances. Children under the age of three years are the most vulnerable: if ill-treated they can neither 'tell' nor even run away; and they are the age group most at risk of neglect and abuse. Hence the check-ups should be at least once every six months and for three to five year olds at least annually. Once a child goes to school, he comes under the daily care of a trained professional; also he is more visible to neighbours, shopkeepers and the like. Furthermore, unless completely cowed, he can run away from home. Therefore, from then on, regular check-ups, though still desirable, are less essential. The first screening could be carried out by a health visitor or public health nurse. If there is any cause for doubt or anxiety, then a full developmental and medical examination should follow. Some will argue that to operate sanctions against parents is an infringement of their liberty. Others may fear that children of poor parents will be penalized because they may be unable to take them for regular check-ups. But these could take place in their own homes or in day care facilities in which many of the most disadvantaged children are placed. To make this possible, the number of health visitors would need to be considerably increased. However, it would pay to do so since the hospital services required to treat abused children are much more costly. State intrusion into the privacy of family life should clearly not be advocated lightly. In this case, however, it has to be balanced against another major right which should equally concern society: to ensure, and if need be enforce, a child's right to loving care and protection, both of his physical and mental health. Surely the state gives an allowance to parents precisely because it wishes to support good child care. Has it therefore not also a duty to make sure that this is in fact being provided?

For similar reasons, the state provides free education. The parent who refuses to send a child to school, has to show – usually in a court of law – that he is substituting an acceptable alternative. In the same way, it would be open to a parent who refuses to have a regular check-up to show that he is nevertheless giving his child adequate care. The family allowance would then be restored but only after the court had satisfied itself that the child's interests were indeed being safeguarded. Those parents who have the well-being of their children at heart – the vast majority – would surely welcome such a preventive measure. After all, it would also ensure the earliest detection of handicap[41]. Among those who object to it may be some who have something to hide and it is their children who need the protection of a compulsory examination. Incidentally, its introduction would also make it possible to ascertain the true incidence of child neglect and abuse.

Preparation for parenthood

The third measure is not only the most basic but also essentially long-term. Its aim would be to raise the level of children's emotional, social and intellectual development in a way similar to that in which their physical health has been improved beyond measure during the past 30 years. The starting point would be the recognition that modern parenthood is too demanding and complex a task to be performed well merely because every adult has once been a child. Indeed, it is about the only such skilled task for the performance of which no knowledge or training is expected or required. But to improve the quality of family care, wide-ranging changes in the attitudes to parenthood and child rearing will have to be brought about.

Probably the most effective way for this to happen would be to make available for all young people a programme of preparation for parenthood. What is required is neither a narrow course, seen as a branch of biology or home economics, nor a very wide general one in citizenship; the model of sex education is not appropriate either; nor should such a programme be confined to girls and the less able ones at that. An effective programme of preparation for parenthood would have to adopt a wide and comprehensive base, including family planning, child development and the whole area of human relations and motivation. First-hand, practical experience of babies and young children should be an essential and integral part as well as an understanding of their emotional and intellectual needs. Included too should be an appreciation of both parental rights and responsibilities. At present, the father's role is rarely mentioned while home-making and motherhood are simultaneously grossly undervalued and misleadingly over-romanticized. Deglamourizing parenthood may act as a deterrent and a brake on those with unrealistic expectations. Responsible parenthood should come to mean that the parental life-style has been deliberately chosen in the full realization of its demands, constraints, satisfactions and challenges. Since the technical know-how is now available, it should be possible for the slogan 'every child a wanted child' to become eventually a reality. Then just as poliomyelitis has been virtually eliminated, even though it cannot be cured, so child neglect and abuse may become a 'disease' of the past, even though it may never prove possible to 'cure' the inadequate or violent parent.

REFERENCES

1. Jobling, M. (1976). *The Abused Child. An annotated bibliography.* (London: National Children's Bureau)
2. Department of Health and Social Security (1974). *Report of the committee of inquiry into the care and supervision provided in relation to Maria Colwell.* (London: HMSO)
3. Baher, E. *et al.* (1976). *At Risk: an Account of the Work of the Battered Child Research Department of the NSPCC.* (Routledge and Kegan Paul)
4. Kempe, C. H., Silverman, F. N., Steele, B. F., Droegemueller, W. and Silver, H. K. (1962). The battered child syndrome. *J. Am. Med. Assoc.*, **181**
5. Smith, S. M. (1975). *The Battered Child Syndrome.* (London: Butterworths)
6. Rogers, D. *et al.* (1976). Non-accidental poisoning: an extended syndrome of child abuse. *Br. Med. J.*, p. 793
7. Oliver, J. E. (1975). Statistics of child abuse. *Br. Med. J.*, **5975**
8. Howells, J. G. (1975). Deaths from non-accidental injuries in childhood. *Br. Med. J.*, **5984**
9. Caffey, J. (1972). The parent–infant traumatic stress syndrome. *Am. J. Roentgen.*, **114**
10. Carter, J. (ed.) (1974). *The Maltreated Child.* (London: Priory Press)
11. Newson, J. and Newson, E. (1968). *Four year olds in an Urban Community.* (London: Allen and Unwin)
12. Court, J. (1975). Non-accidental injury, a symptom of family crisis and stress. In DHSS *Non-accidental Injury to Children.* (London: HMSO)
13. Frommer, E. A. and O'Shea, G. (1973). Ante-natal identification of women liable to have problems in managing their infants. *Br. J. Psychiat.*, **123**
14. Pizzey, E. (1974). *Scream Quietly or the Neighbours will Hear.* (London: Penguin)
15. Oliver, J. E. and Cox, J. (1973). A family kindred with ill-used children. *Br. J. Psychiat.*, **123**
16. Pringle, M. Kellmer (1975). *The Needs of Children.* (London: Hutchinson, New York: Schocken)
17. Pringle, M. Kellmer (1970). *Able Misfits.* (London: Longman in association with National Children's Bureau)
18. Silver, H. K. and Finkelstein, M. (1967). Deprivation dwarfism. *J. Pediat.*, **70**
19. Talbot, N. B., Kagan, J. and Eisenberg, L. (eds.) (1971). *Behavioral Science in Pediatric Medicine.* (Philadelphia: W. B. Saunders)
20. Rutter, M. and Mittler, P. (1972). Environmental influences on language development. In: *Young Children with Delayed Speech.* M. Rutter and J. A. Martin (eds.). (London: Heinemann)
21. Bowlby, J. (1973). *Attachment and Loss, Vol II. Separation: Anxiety and Anger.* (London: Hogarth Press)
22. Bohman, M. (1971). A comparative study of adopted children, foster children and children in their biological environment born after undesired pregnancies. *Acta Paediatr. Scand.*, **221** (Suppl.)
23. Kadushin, A. (1970). *Adopting Older Children.* (New York: Columbia University Press)
24. Pringle, M. Kellmer (1967). *Adoption – Facts and Fallacies.* (London: Longman in association with National Children's Bureau)
25. Seglow, J., Pringle, M. Kellmer and Wedge, P. (1972). *Growing Up Adopted.* (Windsor, Berks: NFER Publishing Co. for National Children's Bureau)

26. Skeels, H. M. (1966). Adult status of children with contrasting early life experiences. *Monograph of the Society for Research in Child Development*, **31**

27. Skodak, M. and Skeels, H. M. (1949). A final follow-up study of one hundred adopted children. *J. Genetic Psychol.*, **75**

28. Harlow, H. F. and Griffin, G. (1965). Induced mental and social deficits in rhesus monkeys. In: *The Biosocial Basis of Mental Retardation.* S. F. Osler and R. E. Cooke (eds.), (Baltimore: Johns Hopkins University Press)

29. Harlow, H. F. and Harlow, M. K. (1969). Effects of various mother–infant relationships on rhesus monkey behaviour. In: *Determinants of Infant Behaviour.* B. Foss (ed.) (London: Methuen)

30. Harlow, H. F. and Harlow, M. K. (1970). Developmental aspects of emotional behaviour. In: *Physiological Correlates of Emotion.* P. Black (ed.) (London: Academic Press)

31. Martin, H. P., Beezley, P., Conway, E. F. and Kempe, C. H. (1974). The development of abused children. In: *Advances in Pediatrics*, I. Schulman (ed.). Vol 21. (Standford, Ca: Medical Publications Inc.)

32. Jones, C. (1975). Children in violent families. *National Children's Bureau.*

33. Gayford, J. J. (1975). Wife battering – a preliminary survey of 100 cases. *Br. Med. J.*, **5951**

34. Martin, H. P. (1976). Emotional deprivation of abused children. *Develop. Med. Child.*

35. Frommer, E. A. and O'Shea, G. (1973). The importance of childhood experience in relation to problems of marriage and family building. *Br. J. Psychiat.*, **123**

36. Rutter, M. and Madge, N. (eds.) (1976). *Cycles of Disadvantage.* (London: Heinemann Educational)

37. Kagan, J. (1971). *Change and Continuity in Infancy.* (New York: John Wiley)

38. Bloom, B. S. (1964). *Stability and Change in Human Characteristics.* (New York: John Wiley)

39. Douglas, J. W. B., Ross, J. M. and Simpson, H. R. (1968). *All Our Future.* (London: Peter Davies)

40. Wedge, P. and Prosser, H. (1973). *Born to Fail?* (London: Arrow Books in association with National Children's Bureau)

41. Wynn, A. (1976) Health care systems for pre-school children. *Proc. Roy. Soc. Med.*, **69**

Further reading

Bowlby, J. (1969). *Attachment and Loss, Vol I. Attachment.* (London: Hogarth Press)

Cameron, J. M. and Rae, L. J. (1975). *Atlas of the Battered Child Syndrome.* (London: Churchill Livingstone)

Castle, R. L. (1973). *Battered children – myth and reality.* (NSPCC)

Court, J. (1969). Battering parents. *Social Work*, **26**

Court, J. (1974). Nurture and nature. In: *Concerning Child Abuse.* A. White Franklin (ed.). (London: Churchill Livingstone)

Essex Area Health Authority, *and* Essex County Council (1974). *Report of the joint committee set up to consider co-ordination of services concerned with non-accidental injury to children.* (Chelmsford: Essex County Council)

Gil, D. (1971). *Violence against Children.* (Cambridge, Mass: Harvard University Press)

Goodman, L. (1975). Aspects of law in relation to non-accidental injury to children. In Department of Health and Social Security *Non-accidental injury to children. Proceedings of a conference held in June 1974.* (London: HMSO)

Greenland, C. (1973). Reporting child abuse in Ontario. *Reports of Family Law*, **10**, 1

Helfer, R. E. and Kempe, C. H. (eds.) (1974). *The Battered Child.* 2nd ed. (Chicago: University of Chicago Press)

Hotyat, F. (1974). How children learn new skills. In: *Advances in Educational Psychology, Vol. II*; M. Kellmer Pringle and V. P. Varma (eds.). (London: University of London Press)

Hyman, C. A. and Mitchell, R. (1975). A psychological study of child battering. *Health Visitor*, **48**

Jacka, A. (1973). *Adoption in Brief. An annotated bibliography*. (Windsor, Berks: NFER Publishing Co. for the National Children's Bureau)

MacKeith, R. (1974). Speculations on non-accidental injury as a cause of chronic brain disorder. *Developm. Med. Child Neurol.*, **16**

Martin, H. (1972). The child and his development. In: *Helping the Battered Child and his Family*. C. H. Kempe and R. E. Helfer (eds.). (Philadelphia: Lippincott)

Norfolk County Council, *and* Norfolk Area Health Authority (1976). *Report of the review body appointed to enquire into the case of Steven Meurs 1975*. (Norwich: Norfolk County Council)

Pringle, M. Kellmer (1971). *Deprivation and Education*. 2nd ed. (London: Longman in association with National Children's Bureau)

Robins Lee, N. (1966). *Deviant Children Grown Up*. (Baltimore, Md: Williams and Wilkins)

Sturgess, J. (1975). Non-accidental injury to children under the age of 17. *Research Bulletin, Home Office Research Unit*. No 2, p. 36

West, D. J. (1969). *Present Conduct and Future Delinquency*. (London: Heinemann)

West, D. J. and Farington, D. P. (1974). *Who becomes Delinquent?* (London: Heinemann)

10   Child abuse, neglect and deprivation and the family

A perspective from Canada

J. JACOBS

Hear ye deaf and look, ye blind, that ye may see . . . seeing many things, thou observest not; opening the ears, he hearest not. Isaiah; XLII, 18–20.

THE WORLD, CHILDREN AND VIOLENCE

There are many inequalities into which children are born in this unfairly constituted world – inequalities of rank, of riches, of opportunities, of basic endowment, all of which have been with us for so long a time that they are more or less taken for granted. This means that for some the world is secure, stable and predictable; they are born with acceptance, concern and care; they are planned for, hoped for and welcomed. For others, life is short, sharp and brutish. They have parents who hate them from conception, reject them from birth, batter them as infants, neglect them as toddlers, and institutionalize them or have them fostered at the drop of a hat. A seemingly indulgent family from a superior household may camouflage as many cruelties and crudities as an overcrowded tenement basement[1].

Canada shares with its southern neighbour the United States and indeed with the whole of America as well as the Western World, a proclivity within its members to violent interactions. The vast majority of this is actually within the family. In certain areas, for example homicide, perhaps 80% or more occurs within family members, in aggravated assault the percentage is a little less, whereas in forcible rape, just over 50% occurs outside the family. Within armed and unarmed robbery, people outside the family, or strangers are involved in some 80% or more[2]. These American figures can undoubtedly be extrapolated to the Canadian scene varying, perhaps, in different parts of the vast continent. There is equally no doubt, but that children are the recipients of this violence to a major degree. In Canada (or in North America) we are

245

moving into an era that may be historically the most precarious for our children. The evolution of one society from a rural to an urban-based family system, from an extended to a nuclear family system and from a labour intensive to a machine economy, has made the child no longer an economic asset to the family.

Marked increases in the cost of raising a child cause individual parents, and the economy in general, to view childbearing and childrearing as an economic liability, in competition with other values. Moreover, at the ideological level, there has been a downgrading of the sense of personal worth derived from parenthood, especially for a woman. The ego-satisfactions gained from having children are deteriorating[3].

Perhaps some three generations ago, when maybe one in five North American women were employed, the woman who worked violated the Victorian norm of role definition. Even when compelled by sheer economic necessity, she was made to feel that she was neglecting her primary responsibility to her children. Today, when one out of every two married women work and when a new ethic proclaims work a cardinal virtue for the liberated woman, the one who can and chooses to stay at home, begins to feel herself a traitor to her class. A lifestyle that was once defined as deviant has become modal[4]. A mother is severely criticized if all she does is look after her child's body without playing with him, talking to him and stimulating his interests. She is similarly criticized if she neglects his physical needs, is helpless when faced with his illnesses and only concerned with his mental advances. At the same time, she is faced by the reality that during a child's development, before mental pathways via thought and speech are opened up, all excitation is discharged through the body. This means that fear, frustration, loneliness, anger, rage etc., are expressed by the infant, not only by crying but by means of sleep disturbances, food intake, elimination, or cumulatively by a general failure to thrive physically[5].

It is not surprising that we can say that the family is a cradle of violence. We like to think of the family as the abode of love, a home as a safe retreat, where any member of the family can be sure of support and protection[6]. The reality is rather different. Whenever human beings are held together by ties of love, whether that love is primarily erotic or supportive, aggressive tensions are also inescapable. It is our nearest and dearest who are most notably capable of provoking our intensest rage and many of us find ourselves more easily capable of sympathetically identifying ourselves with murderers than with any other type of criminal. Helplessness can easily be made humiliating and dependency necessarily involves restriction. Humiliation and restriction are potent instigators of violence in adults, but we can see there are precursors in normal human infants.

It can be said that ontogeny recapitulates phylogeny, that is to say, that the life history of the individual recapitulates the life history of the race, such recapitulation occurring not only during intrauterine life, but also in terms of environmental and other input, after the child is born. In Canada (just as in North America and many other parts of the world) many ethnic groups have come into the country. It is not surprising that they have brought with them not only their good qualities, but also the varieties of cruelties as it were, that children have been subjected to over many eras. Maltreatment of children has been justified by the belief that severe physical punishment was necessary either to maintain discipline, to transmit educational ideas, to please certain Gods, or to expel evil spirits. Children have always been the victims of mutilation through such practices as castration, circumcision, foot binding and even deformation of the skull[7]. Older children have been beaten, maimed and often killed to discipline, educate and exploit them by parents, teachers, priests, professional beggars and employers in factories and mines. Children in North America are still the exclusive responsibility of their parents, but they have full legal rights. The legal limits of justification are not clear cut, however, and our law must be supplemented by public opinion. With the beginning of industrialization, pauper children from five years of age were abused by the factory system. In the 19th century, the Society for the Prevention of Cruelty to Animals was able to remove a maltreated child from his parents, on the ground that he was a member of the animal kingdom and entitled to protection under the laws against animal cruelty. This case precipitated the formation of the Society for the Prevention of Cruelty to Children in 1871. It is still true that more money is left annually to protectual societies for animals than to societies for the prevention of cruelties to children[8].

Infanticide (that is the wilful destruction of newborn babies through exposure, starvation, strangulation, smothering, poisoning or through the use of some lethal weapon) has been viewed with abhorrence in the Judaeo-Christian concept almost from the beginning of their era. Yet in these days of world population crisis, there can hardly be a more important historical question, than that of the chronically superfluous population growth and the methods by which humanity has dealt with it. Langer[9], in his historical review of the subject, writes that among non-Christian people (with the exception of the Jews) infanticide has from time immemorial been an accepted procedure for disposing not only of deformed or sickly infants, but of all such newborns as might strain the resources of the individual family or the larger community. At the present day it is still employed by so called underdeveloped people, in an effort to keep the population in reasonable adjustment to the available food supply. In ancient times, at least, infanticide was not a legal consideration. It was a practice freely discussed and generally condoned by those in authority, and ordinarily left to the decision of the father as the responsible head of the family. Plato and Aristotle, amongst other philosophers[10], considered the survival of the fittest was needed to strengthen the race, while the Roman law of the twelve tablets forbade rearing of deformed children. Children have been buried alive beneath the doorsteps of new buildings in 16th century Germany, or immured in the dikes of 17th century Oldenberg[11]. The Victorian era seemed to epitomize the 17th century view (extant even now) that 'love is a boy by poets styl'd – then spare the rod and spoil the child'[12].

Resort to expert 'advice' has been proven to be generally unsatisfactory to most parents who cannot, without guidance, extract the sound from the unsound and the realistic from the unrealistic[13-15]. It is of interest that in an interview with Benjamin Spock[16], he said 'My father never showed me the slightest physical affection. It never occurred to me to show any toward my sons. In the neighbourhood I grew up in, I never saw a father being physically affectionate with his son or his wife.' I wonder how this relates to his books?

'Parentage is a most important profession, but no test of fitness for it is ever imposed in the interest of children'[17]. Homan[18] adds 'parenting is the most difficult, the most challenging, the most significant and the least mastered and most promising frontier'.

Discipline

Present day studies in the United States and England show that between 84 and 97% of all parents use physical punishment at some point in their child's life[19], while in West Germany 60% of parents beat (not slap or smack or spank) their children. Perhaps the 'primitive infanticide' can be rationalized in modern thinking to the passive euthanasia approach to a newborn retardate with Down's syndrome being allowed to die, if by chance there is a duodenal obstruction present, which kills in the absence of operative intervention[20]. One can similarly look at the 'abortion on demand' available virtually throughout the Western World.

The accepted mores of the so-called civilized world, tends to enhance concepts leading to the total syndrome of abuse, neglect and deprivation. Children are born the same all over the world, but the societies in which they grow up differ. Adolescence is a luxury, a syndrome of the over-civilized. It is scarcely known in some places where childhood ends abruptly in instant adulthood. In Mexico, where the legal age of adulthood is 18, boys may be expected to assume a grown up's burden at 12 or 14. In Thailand, rural boys of 5 of 6 go to work tending the water buffalo which represents a farm family's wealth and social standing. In Italy, despite a law forbidding child labour under 14, many hundreds of thousands of children are present in the employment field. A Bedouin girl in the Jordanian desert, at eight is relegated to the cook tent with her female relatives, whereas the boy of eight joins the men drinking tea around the fire. In the culture of poverty, the poverty itself shapes the lives of the children.

There are other forms of discipline. Consider these tactics to bend children to the cultural world. In Germany, they tend to be hostile to children and they not uncommonly strap toddlers into cribs and leave them alone without babysitters. In Japan, mothers do not spank, they scold, they tell a child that he will be laughed at or he will be made a fool of, and by the time he is old enough to question the significance of shame, it is already too late. In Israel, discipline comes in the form of withholding love, as parental disapproval, by instilling a sense of guilt for unacceptable behaviour. In France, discipline is present from the early stage of strictly regular feeding, through a military routine at the nursery school, and certainly until the beginning of secondary education. Corporal punishment and severe curtailment of privileges enforce diligent work habits. The father in Buenos Aires says to his children 'I want you to realize that I am not your friend, I am your father. I am the man who gives you love, protection, backing, security, not his confidences. You will deal with me as a father and don't ever forget it.' In North America, the confused, frustrated, infuriated child commits the adult equivalent of his so often successful childhood act of stomping and screaming and throwing his bottle or building blocks; he fights or stabs or shoots.

There are many who say permissive courts and permissive parents are far less responsible for today's climate of violence, than are hostile or indifferent parents, oppressive social conditions and poor prison rehabilitation programmes. Anthropologist Robert Ardrey[21] said 'the evidence is today overwhelming, that in order to become an adequate, healthy, co-operative, loving human being, it is necessary to be loved. No child is born hostile or aggressive. He becomes so only when his desire to be loved and to love, are frustrated.'

Societal care

Margaret Mead[22] points out that in 'primitive' societies, all the functions served by institutions – care of the orphan, care of the child of a sick mother, care of the handicapped or defective child, care of the illegitimate child – are dealt with, either by care of the child within the greater family or neighbourhood group, on an individual basis, which obviates the major 'trauma-inducing' aspects of institutional care; or drastically, by the elimination of the child, by such means as burying the newborn child with the dead mother, or by exposing immediately or extinguishing by a process of slow, low level care, children who show extreme handicaps. She emphasizes that the child who is chosen to live, is cared for personally not impersonally.

In Russia, socialization of the child is a community responsibility. The school addresses itself actively to the process of socialization of the child and all members of the community feel free to step in and address themselves to the child's behaviour. It seems that in modern China, there is a similar situation and each child tends to help his neighbour in the classroom and outside. The extended family extends even into the community and each one has a responsibility to look after children who are their 'intimations of immortality'. This kind of attitude is certainly not prevalent in the United States and Canada, where people are very loath to intervene with other people's children and schools are reluctant to see their role as other than educators. The child is treated as the exclusive property of the individual parents, a situation which seems to many to be conducive to the kinds of child neglect, abuse and deprivation which are allowed to go unchecked and unreported in our society. 'If the function of the family is to love and to nurture and to support its members, then violence in the family would seem to be incompatible with its function'[23].

The feelings of hurt, hate and destruction which lead to aggressive acts are common human feelings. The 'inhumaneness' enters in the manner of expression. The family is the first battleground where one learns to fend for oneself, to find ways of meeting basic needs, to understand and to tolerate feelings, to learn to put some needs aside for the present when it is for the mutual good.

Mother and child

A mother has to be able to tolerate hating her baby, without doing anything about it. She cannot express it to him. If, for fear of what she may do, she cannot hate appropriately when hurt by her child, she must fall back on masochism[24]. The most remarkable thing about a mother is her ability to be hurt so much by her baby and to hate so much, without paying the child out, and her ability to await her rewards that may or may not come at a later date[25]. A mother has to accept and at the same time control what she does about these hate feelings. She has to be able to release these feelings in a non-hurting way and to let the child know when he is old enough to understand that what he does hurts her. The mother has to realize she can feel hate, without taking away the security of her care and loving.

All communities of all degrees of technical sophistication, urbanization and industrialization, have evolved their own cultural patterns, which can be defined as the common way of life shared by all members of the group. This includes not only their preferred life goals, their valued ends and sanctioned means and their attitudes towards life and death, but also all aspects of everyday life, the relationships between different members of the family, customary ways of preparing food, and improved methods of rearing children.

Culture and motherhood

The culture pattern of the group is based on learned behaviour, sometimes partly acquired by deliberate instruction on the part of the parents (rarely perhaps nowadays), but mostly absorbed subconsciously by incidental observation of the behaviour of relations and other close members of the community. This process of learning begins at birth, if not before; it is mediated by every contact the infant has with the surrounding world including, for example, the way young babies are carried, the roles of the parent in childbearing and as a concept that becomes habitual, the foods that are, or are not, eaten within the particular community.

Traditional preparation for motherhood is often more appropriate in pre-literate villages than in a sophisticated urban context. The little girl in a pre-literate type of home, shares fully in the family life and her behaviour is generally governed by fairly strict rules. Both these elements of her upbringing give her security. Almost as soon as she can walk, she begins to share the responsibility in looking after her juniors and of performing the household chores. As she gets older, she has more hard work to do and greater responsibilities. At, or about the age of, puberty she may have to undergo forms of initiation some of which are educational, whilst others may be hideously painful and dangerous, but she may consider herself incomplete without them. The pre-literate mother normally takes marriage, pregnancy, lactation, hard work, child care (and often child mortality) in her stride and is desperately unhappy if she has failed either in producing children, or in any other of her responsibilities[26].

The girl from an advanced culture may belong to a small family. While young, she is protected from the facts of life, but she is soon exposed to loud advertisements, fantastic romanticism and glamour and violence on television. She tends to 'gang up' on her own age group. At school she learns about history, geography and the advertisement of the great world and the physical and theoretical sciences; she may also learn ballet, swimming, typing and tennis. She may learn relatively little about her own personal life and that of her neighbours. She may not even have held a small baby, let alone seen one breast fed, until she has her own. Apart from her own physiological developmental urges, which may or may not be considerable, she may be subjected to flamboyant and irresponsible bullying on the subject of her behaviour, compared with what is currently the norm in a permissive society. She may have episodes of disturbed behaviour when, it is said, she is seeking for her identity.

Violence and TV

The Canadian Commission on Violence on Television[27] in its interim report has called our attention to another facet of violence. In understanding the impact of violence on TV on its viewers, the question arises which theory is most useful? That of the vicarious safety experience? That which pursues the evocation of violent behaviour, or are we mostly confronted by the issues of poor taste and seduction to past gratification? The interim report points out that in the first ten years of life, a child could have viewed 13 000 violent deaths on television. It gives the following definition of violence and a range of complications. 'Violence is action which intrudes painfully or harmfully into the physical, psychological and social well being of persons or groups. Violence or its effects may range from the trivial to catastrophic. Violence may be obvious or subtle. It may arise naturally or by human design. Violence may take place against persons or against property. It may be justified or unjustified, or justified by some standards and not by others. It may be real or symbolic. Violence may be sudden or gradual.'

Violence in the context of sports, to which nowadays virtually the whole world is exposed, can perhaps be best illustrated on the Canadian scene, by quoting from a newspaper[28], 'X is a gun-slinger for hire, pigskin's Clint Eastwood – good, bad and ugly. For a fistful of dollars, he will gladly hurt, maim and otherwise brutalize the opposition. He relishes making trouble, feeds on violence –. "I play with a definite hate for the guy who has the football. I want to hit him and hurt him".' This then is the example to which our youth in Canada are exposed (as is the rest of the world) from very early childhood and this type of message is given in the context of a number of games from early childhood into adult life. It is of interest, that not one letter appeared decrying this description of a game, and of a player, seemingly there was tacit acceptance thereof.

Canadian House of Commons, Child Abuse and Neglect Report

In common with all countries, Canada has indeed a vested interest in endeavouring to look at the problems of child abuse, neglect and deprivation. Perhaps this may be best illustrated in that a standing committee on health, welfare and social affairs was appointed to report to the House of Commons, on the problems[29]. If we look at this report, with or without cynicism, we may see the problems of any part of the world and realize how people are, or are not, dealing with the total situation.

DEFINITIONS

It seems that many of the problems are bedevilled by the context of definitions. How does this report deal with definitions? The Canadian Minister of National Health and Welfare said that he was pleased that the committee included in its terms of reference neglect as well as abuse, and went on to say that it is neither easy nor desirable to separate physical abuse or battering from other more subtle forms of child abuse and neglect[29]. It was difficult to arrive at a definition of these terms. He was not in a position to define them categorically but said that child neglect in the legal sense, constituted all those conditions listed in provincial law and under which a court may find a child neglected, or 'in need of protection'. Thus the term 'child neglect' covers the abused and battered child as well as the child whose parents are unable or unwilling to care for him adequately. Child abuse and battering is the end of a neglect continuum, which ranges from neglect to ignorance on the part of parents to deliberate maltreatment. It is not always possible to distinguish the point at which neglect becomes abuse. Battering tended to be direct physical injury to the child, resulting from intentional use of excessive force by an adult, and such injuries can be identified on medical examination if there are repeated fractures, etc. He ended by saying 'child battering, to use a well known analogy, represents the tip of the iceberg of child abuse and neglect'.

The Solicitor General of Canada brought in the question of psychosomatic dwarfism or 'failure to thrive', saying that emotional abuse was at least as important as physical abuse, and that a word should also be said about sexual abuse. He would tend to use the United States Child Abuse, Prevention and Treatment Act of 1973[30]. Child abuse and neglect is taken to mean 'the physical or mental injury, sexual abuse, negligent treatment or maltreatment of a child under the age of 18 by a person who is responsible for the child's welfare, under circumstances which indicate that the child's health or welfare is harmed or threatened thereby'.

From the Department of Justice it was described as a continuum of potentially damaging behaviour of caretakers towards children in their care:

(a) *Child neglect* usually involves a failure to provide the child with the necessities of life be that food, clothing, medical supplies, or emotional support, or a failure to provide sundry living conditions or adequate supervision. Child neglect may occur because the caretakers are unaware of what is necessary to sustain the child, or unable or unwilling to properly care for the child.

(b) *Child abuse* in a narrow sense is the intentional, non-accidental use of physical force, or intentional non-accidental acts of omission, on the part of a parent or other caretaker interacting with the child in his care, aimed at hurting, injuring or destroying the child. Child abuse includes cruel treatment which leaves no physical scars but produces emotional damage to the child. 'Child abuse' if broadly defined would include child neglect, child battering, sexual abuse of children, emotional abuse, the so-called 'failure to thrive' syndrome, and perhaps nutritional abuse as well.

(c) *'Child battering'* refers to the extreme cases of physical abuse of children.

Greenland[31] regarded child abuse as 'not an isolated and unique phenomenon. Child abuse, in my view, is an extreme form of neglect by parents of their children, but it also represents a gross failure of our child welfare services and also of the community to cope adequately with the needs of children, in particular very young children.'

The Chief Coroner for Ontario quoted the battered child syndrome[32]. He indicated that the term was used in its broadest sense, to include all cases of serious malnutrition, anaemia, vitamin deficiency, bed sores, exposure to excessive heat or cold. Such cases may end up with permanent damage or death and yet show only minor trauma and no battering *per se*. He felt that psychological trauma must be included in the general term of child abuse, although not causing death itself. Any child being beaten or deprived is bound to suffer mentally and in those who do not die, there is no doubt that they suffer from mental trauma and scars of varying degrees, forever. These trauma affect the victims throughout their lives and may lead to a subsequent mental illness, nervous breakdown, delinquency, family problems and, of course, they may abuse their own children in the future. He enumerated fractures, subdural haematoma, multiple bruises of the skin, unusual soft tissue swelling, malnutrition, dehydration, low weight and failure to thrive as instances of child abuse. Also included were severe anaemias, avitaminoses, and varying types and degrees of injuries, bruises or burns found not consistent with the history given as to how they occurred. From the Mental Health Committee of the Canadian Pediatric Society, the definitions offered were those of Kempe of 1962; the Children's Hospital euphemism 'Trauma X'[33], and the description in the Symposium by Oppé[34]:

1. The battered child is an infant who shows clinical or radiological evidence of lesions which are frequently multiple and involve mainly the head, soft tissues or the long bones and thoracic cage, and which cannot be un-equivocally explained.
2. A neglected child.
3. A persecuted child.

At the annual council meeting of the National Society for the Prevention of Cruelty to Children[34] a psychiatrist, B. F. Steele, considered that these criteria were interchangeable.

A further description was given in 1971, giving a spectrum of non-accidental injury and deprivation of children[35]. Kempe[36,37] spoke of child abuse as being psychodynamically related and having nothing to do with race, colour, creed, sex, income, education or anything else. The Mondale Bill of 1973 pointed out that the definition of child abuse and neglect is not what the doctor thinks it should be, or what the social worker thinks it is, but is actually what the courts say it is[30]. The court is, of course, influenced by the public and its definition will change from time to time and may be different in different localities based on the emotional climate of the cities in the area. The parent–infant traumatic stress syndrome[38] includes intentional, non-accidental or physical injury but would not include abandonment, neglect and exploitation, although these may occasionally be concurrent factors. Caffey[38] has pointed out that no definition is perfect but the expression 'battered child' is offensive to some people who fear it may arouse a more punitive response to the parent, than an innocuous word like 'abuse'. Others feel that the trauma is aptly described by the bad term 'battering' as defined in the Oxford Dictionary and euphemisms are deplored. The sense of outrage felt on behalf of the child tends to blind people to the desperate plight of the battering parent who may be subjected to totally inap-propriate retaliatory procedures. To some the term 'battered child' means only the child who has been the victim of the most severe form of physical punish-ment, i.e. the child who represents the far end of the child abuse spectrum. For others the term implies the total spectrum of abuse beginning with the parents (or future parents), who have the potential to abuse their small children, ending with a severely beaten or killed child. This lack of clarity has led to great confu-sion, both in the literature and in the minds of those wishing to help these children and their families. The confusion and the limited communication

between those working in the field are often the primary sources of misunderstanding among those who wish to define the problem more clearly[39]. It
has been suggested that a less emotive title might be 'child abuse, neglect and
deprivation in the family (Child AND Family Syndrome)'[40], which would include 'any act of omission or commission by individuals, institutions or society
and any conditions resulting from such acts or inactions which deprive children
of equal rights or liberties and/or interfere with their optimal development constitute by definition abusive or neglectful acts or condition which may inhibit a
child's development'.

Such a syndrome concept allows workers in the field, in any discipline, to
look at the presenting problems in the context of the child, the parents and the
family. Given adequate help, probably the best possible chance of a favourable
outcome for the abused and abusing members is within an extended family
system.

What then is to be gained in terms of defining and going through definitions
more precisely? Because of the problems of a definition and labelling, we may
only be treating a very narrow portion of the true population of abusers and our
treatment methods may be totally inadequate to deal with the unrecognized
population of abusers and abused.

The spectrum

The concept of child abuse has had a wide variety of definitions as is seen
above, including an occurrence where a caretaker injures a child not by accident, but in anger or deliberately[41–43]. Child abuse can be limited to broken
bones or physical trauma, or can be a wide range of activities which include im-
proper clothing, feeding, or caring for a child[44], abandonment and emotional
mistreatment.

A major problem is defining the phenomenon to be investigated. A corollary
problem which arises is that it is impossible to compare the abundant data that
have been gathered on abuse because of idiosyncratic and varying definitions
on child abuse. Polsky[45] has pointed out that people who are caught in acts of
deviance are systematically different from people who get away with the same
acts (i.e. just getting caught indicates that they are less 'successful' deviants).

The label of 'abuser' is selectively applied. Policemen, physicians, nurses and
social workers who have either read literature on child abuse or had experience
with child abuse cases, build up a mental inventory of characteristics of people
and situations associated with child abuse. They 'know' that abusers are
typically poor and uneducated. Abused children are typically under 3 years of
age. If a person arrives with an injured child and does not fit the stereotype of
abuse, they may be more likely to avoid the label.

The further complications of names and definitions is given by the name the
'maltreatment syndrome in children'[46]. A term also liked in France, 'les enfants victims de s'evictes'[47], and even more difficult, is the present reference to 'non-

accidental injury to children'[48,49]. This brings up very many problems. What is an accidental injury and what is a non-accidental injury? So often the ability to diagnose whether an injury is accidental or not, lies not so much in what one sees in terms of the injury, but in the surrounding circumstances. If, therefore, we do not take a past history (and this has been shown to occur in many instances) but rather ask what has happened in the here and now, it is going to be very difficult to understand what is an accident and what is not. The concept even of 'accident proneness'[50] is a very dubious entity. If we look at a child of five being run over by a car, this can be looked at as an accident, but is it? What was a child of five doing in a neighbourhood or in an area where he might be run over? What instructions has he had? So often, when one goes into the surrounding history, one finds that this type of child comes from a family where both mother and father are rarely home and very few arrangements have been made for the child while the parents are away. When they are home a great deal of conflict, fighting and anger is shown. In other words, when we look at a child who has bruising to his extremities, a subdural haemorrhage or fractured ribs, and we take the history there, we find great difficulties, family violence, intrafamilial communication problems exactly the same as in many of the apparent 'accident' cases.

It would even seem that perhaps more important than having exact definitions of differences in abuse, neglect and deprivation is that any case which presents should be taken and looked at fully, measuring if necessary the bruises (as is so beloved by the lawyer and the law) and finding what goes on in the skeleton and elsewhere. At the same time it would be useful to make enquiries in terms of what sort of family or origin did the mother/father have; what was the consistency of input or discipline in their homes of origin; how indeed were they disciplined and how was obedience ensured? Was there a question of alcoholism in the home as well as overt violence, battering or beating? Was it a home where parents ignored children or where the discipline was so permissive that children of two and three had to take necessary decisions? Are we seeing a background where these children in early years 'failed to thrive' and where the pathology might be in an individual or mother who is able not to feed her child[51,52]. It is easy to discuss in many of these instances, poverty, societal difficulties, ignorance etc. However, there are large numbers of other people, in similar circumstances in whom these accidents do not occur. It is important to note that by using emotive terms one can ignore the needs of the parents and this is very wrong. On the other hand, now to turn and ignore the needs of the abused children, except from the 'therapeutic' approach (which almost bends over backwards to deny that the parents have in fact committed a series of horrific acts), is equally dangerous. Realistically a definition can only help to convey certain impressions, perhaps to lay people, and it may help doctors to put symptoms and signs in a nice group – the 'medical' syndrome; it may allow the social worker to ask for resources and later on the lawyer and judge to mentally allocate to varying definitions varying sequelae. Is this what we want? One would suggest that almost irrespective of the type of neglect, deprivation or battering presented one has to look at the total situation. Can one measure a bruise and say because it is one or two inches in length, or that there are ten such bruises, this is a worse case than one where there is only one bruise? Can one say, there are no bruises but there is a fractured rib, and that is worse? Can one say, because in a child who has haemorrhages in the fundi after shaking and where there may be a haemorrhage in very vital areas near or in the brain causing profound damage, that in fact the harm that was intended in that child was greater than the harm intended when somebody fractures a long bone?

If we can look dispassionately it almost seems that the site of trauma, say the head, may be accidental in the sense that someone has lost his temper and hits a child. He happens to hit the head. On the other hand we remember that people say 'I'm going to knock his (block) head off' which means that we have learned or observed how many people hit children on the head. In many schools even, this is certainly so.

Brain damage

MacKeith[53] points out that some children die of non-accidental injury, but that it is likely that others will survive with chronic neurological disorders, often presenting with cerebral palsy of unrecognized aetiology, the initiating event being possibly some years in the past. The possibility of child abuse is often not considered. Subdural haematomata are easier to detect by routine neurological examination, yet often it is the cerebral contusion association which will probably determine the sequelae. In the follow up of subdural haematomata[54,55], approximately 8% were dead and 30% were moderately and severely incapacitated – for every death there were at least 4 severely incapacitated. In the UK, there are 1600 new cases of cerebral palsy each year and 600 of severe mental handicap, with no adequate cause of the condition being found in half of the cases. MacKeith speculates that after a non-accidental head injury, 5% are severely subnormal and 5% are severely mentally handicapped. Such speculation may well be correct and how do we now relate this to the initiating abusing action?

Physical trauma

I recently saw a child in a 'good' family, whose parents were very angry because their child stole, did antisocial acts within the community and did not learn in school. The father, when he came home, being told by the mother of the happenings, hit the child so that when seen, he had a large bruise covering half the side of his head and face. The child fortunately did not sustain any intracerebral damage, but how different is that from a child who does have intracerebral damage?

Another instance was of a child who came with a haemoptysis after the father hit him on his chest. On the chest wall one could see the marks of the father's hand and the child coughed up blood. Is that better than, or worse than, somebody who has had his ribs fractured? In questioning the father he said that he too was disciplined as a child by his father hitting him on the body with the open hand, but then said that he went wrong because, unlike his father, he did not take the precaution of putting a blanket over the child prior to hitting him. He then said that his memory of his father was that of a big hand coming down to hit him.

Mental trauma

A girl of 10 was brought in because she was failing in school. One year previously she had been taken to a psychiatric-social work group to be seen because of the same symptomatology. Then the group looked into the family psychodynamics and found that the mother–father interactions were poor, with problems in their sex life, and proceeded to help them by marriage counselling and family therapy. After being seen on five or six occasions the parents felt that there was an improvement and that they were managing things better. The child's problems, however, went on unabated. One year later, the parents slept with one another with greater ease but the child had hardly altered. When the mother was asked how it felt to be a mother, her answer was – 'To be a mother is to cook, to wash, to do for, to clean up all the mess, to handle one's husband or children if he or they are ill, but not to be able to carry out one's own life objectives, to complete one's degree'. This told us a great deal. The father concerned was a highschool teacher, administratively involved. When asked whether he was prepared to spend more time with this child as with the sister, he replied that if this interfered with his school work and life, he was afraid that the children were not all that important. The children concerned, very easily showed in their way of not looking, in their way of turning away, in their anger, in their inability to relate to one another, that they were neglected children. This then was a different form of child abuse but did it mean that these children were less seriously damaged than children who had great bruises cr broken limbs? It does seem that these children will bear the scars throughout their lives.

Deprivation and emotional abuse

The point of departure for most definitions is whether or not to include a reference to emotional abuse and/or parental deprivation. The more liberal or broad definitions tend to include these areas despite difficulty in precise definition, since limiting reporting to physical and sexual abuse excludes a large proportion of very serious cases, which lack obvious physical signs of child maltreatment. Broad definitions of child abuse lead to the reporting of all cases involving children coming to the attention of child welfare authorities, the police, school officials and others serving the needs of children and family. The more narrow definition excludes deprivation and/or emotional abuse perhaps because of the difficulty in proving this type of abuse in court and the often conflicting interpretation of what constitutes proper emotional stimulation and home environment. Not only is it very difficult, but maybe it is undesirable to make precise distinctions between neglect and emotional deprivation or abuse. Yet a useful distinction for case management purposes may be made between a narrow legal, and a broader operational, definition of child abuse.

While child abuse is difficult to define in a legal sense, those professionals involved in child health and welfare will often provide interventive and therapeutic services or facilities, where abuse has not been proven, but where high risk or potential abuse seems evident. Again, one must ask whether in terms of proof we are talking about a television camera seeing the event, or whether we are talking about parents whose upbringing has been such that they have never seen or learned how to mother or father; they have never absorbed these skills, do not know how to parent and have indicated in the various parameters of handling themselves, handling pregnancy, the birth and the upbringing of children, that indeed it is a very difficult area. The present event which may bring them to know this can be seen as part of a total family life system. In terms of therapy, what are the aims? Is it to bring the family to the court so that one or other parent can be sent to jail? Should it be more realistically, in the vast majority of cases, to look at what the deficits are in a family and how these can be corrected? Surely, this could be brought even to a court. It can be seen that there are needs in the family which may or may not include removal of the children. What cannot be gainsaid is that these children have a right to be handled in a different way. Many cases are not reported to a registry or to process of the courts, but perhaps that type of restriction should not prevent the Children's Aid worker or other social professionals from providing the family with appropriate services. Many cases of child abuse are not seen or felt to be the result of premeditated malicious behaviour by a parent or caretaker, but seem to be the result of excessive discipline, inadequate parenting skills, carelessness or complete social and cultural strains on the family. If one has these beliefs, then again it is of paramount importance that the total background be looked at and that the life events within these families be investigated. It then becomes less and less important in the context of the majority of cases, as to what premeditation means. Maybe we are looking at this in the context of murder in the adult world, whereby somebody has decided that he is going to kill X. In the child world, we are talking not about premeditation except perhaps in a very small number of cases, but rather about the end result of an accumulated series of feelings of inadequacy, frustration and inability. These feelings culminate in complete loss of control and hence very malicious behaviour. A problem is that the stress placed on the definition, in terms of the determination by the reporter, particularly by a concerned layman, of guilt or wilful intent, may have an adverse effect on the number of reports received by the authorities.

A big problem then, is that the definitions plague legislators, those who provide service and those who seek better understanding of a phenomenon for educational preventive purposes. Can one definition meet all these needs? Are there areas where problems of definition seriously impede the search for solutions, or even treatment of the problem. Perhaps in a way by seeking the minutiae of definition, we are almost tacitly saying that the problem is too big to handle and if we can stay at the level of definitions, then maybe we do not have to deal with it?

Again, are we saying that this is part of society, part of ourselves and our feelings, hence too difficult to alter, so we should not alter our approach? It is refreshing then to hear from a judge[56] 'I think we will accomplish little, if we spend our time trying to devise new definitions of abuse and neglect. It is not without reason that most criticisms of the present definitions do not include alternative proposals.' Much can be said by accepting that the physical discipline of children is common in our society and that the determination of reasonable force and ill-treatment becomes blurred and hazy. Maybe the event itself can be made less of and the pre-existing life events, social situations, upbringing etc. assume a greater importance. A further indication of how people look narrowly at events and use this to hide their anguish or difficulty, discomfort or embarrassment at broadening the outlook is given by the programme initiated by Greenland and his co-workers[57]. This looked at suspected child abuse and neglect (SCAN) cases in hospital. These descriptive words were taken exception to, by the various doctors, nurses and social workers involved. They were considered to be too emotive and too offensive so the project was changed in name to the Home Accident and Injury Study (HAIS).

Although a humane approach to 'help', to both the victims of child abuse and their families, has developed, a theoretical framework to integrate the diverse origin and expression of violence toward children and to inform a rational clinical practice does not exist[58]. It is the general opinion throughout the country that so inadequate are the 'helping' services in most communities, so low the standard of professional action and so distressing the consequences of incompetent intervention for the family, that it has been speculated that punishment is being inflicted in the guise of help[59]. There is a great deal of medical and legal ambiguity concerning the problem and too fundamental, and in some ways irreconcilable, dilemmas about social policy and the social response to families and children.

Children's rights

How children's rights – as opposed to parent's rights – may be defined and protected is currently the subject of vigorous and occasionally rancorous debate[60]. 'Children and youth are no longer, if they ever were, *tabulas rasas*, upon whom we imprint the patterns of our own personalities from realized dreams. Their rights should not threaten ours, even if they are on occasion competitive.'

The rights of very young children should be unconditional. The rights of the older child cannot be quite so absolute because there is the beginning of an interplay between the child and his environment, in which he must learn that his own rights are relative and the rights of others have to be respected[61]. Fromm[62] described as principles:

1. Firm faith in the goodness of the child.
2. The aims of education (life) to work joyfully and to find happiness.
3. In educating, intellectual development is not enough, education must be both intellectual and emotional.
4. Education must be geared to the psychic needs and capacities of the child; the child is not an altruist; altruism develops after childhood.
5. Discipline, dogmatically imposed, and punishment create fear; fear creates hostility.
6. Freedom does not mean licence.
7. Healthy human development makes it necessary that a child eventually cuts the primary ties which connect him with his father and mother, or with later substitutes in society, and that he becomes truly independent.
8. Guilt feelings primarily have the function of binding the child to authority; guilt feelings are an impediment to independence.

Clinging and letting go, are not two distinct stages of growth and development, they overlap and are concurrent for many years. When young parents cannot tolerate the excessive clinging and dependence of the young child, the more it is rejected the more the child clings and so the vicious cycle occurs leading to child abuse.

The family has a traditional autonomy in rearing its offspring. The schools are not, in effect, constrained constitutionally from any type of punishment however cruel. If, indeed, the quality of protective services in Canada is low, it has been suggested that access to such services should be restricted – the reporting of child neglect should be discretionary rather than mandatory and would narrowly define the basis for court jurisdiction. This could well make matters worse, not better, for children and their families. The conflicts of the relation of children to the state, as well as to the family and the relative rights of children independent of their parents, makes for great difficulty of clear articulation of enforcement of rights. It seems that people are unprepared psychologically to accept the possibility of parental atrocities and they are unwilling to become legally responsible for reporting suspected cases of abuse to the authorities[63]. In writing about this as a 'shocking conspiracy of silence', Oettinger[64] says 'when 25–50% of the children returned to unsafe environments by physicians, who fail to report abuse, are maimed or murdered, the conspiracy of silence becomes a conspiracy in crime'.

REPORTING OF ABUSE

At least eight of the ten provinces in Canada have introduced provisions in their legislation making mandatory the reporting of information, even if confidential or privileged, concerning the abandonment, desertion, physical ill-treatment or need for protection of a child. Mainly in such legislation it is specified that no action can be taken against the informant unless it can be proven that the information was provided of malicious intent, or without reasonable and probable cause. Most provinces have established centralized child abuse registries which record all cases of abuse reported to local child welfare authorities. Consultative and follow-up services may then be provided on a case basis. Why are people not reporting cases of child abuse? There seem to be a number of suggested answers. It may be due to the deficiencies in the reporting system, or that people simply do not know about it, or the professionals do not want to use the information. Is it a matter of securing evidence or proving a case? Do we have cultural inhibitions about interfering in the affairs of the family? All of these possibilities are parts of the answer.

Non-reporting and attitude

With regard to physicians, it is said that non-reporting occurs[65] as a result of:

1. Lack of understanding of the seriousness of the problem.
2. Lack of awareness of one's own responsibility in reporting the child.
3. Disbelief that these could be abusing parents.
4. Reluctance to expose prosperous families to a court hearing.
5. Lack of knowledge about how to make a report itself.
6. A wish not to become involved with court proceedings.
7. A belief that the court will not take appropriate action, anyway.
8. Lack of community facilities which can provide a type of help these parents needs.
9. The discomfort and resistance which the reporting person feels when he is confronted with a 'battered' child and his parents.

In the belief that most adults have warm, loving and protective feelings towards children, there is a great tendency to deny that parents also have hostile and negative feelings, often totally unconscious.

Corbett[66] said that in Massachusetts only 9% of wilfully injured children were referred by physicians. In *Look Again*[67] it is suggested that it is a difficult decision for family physicians to make, in that reporting seems to revolve around the point at which discipline and a parent's rights stop and the welfare of the child begins. Many other professions, social work, education and clergy are reluctant to report and there is almost a total lack of publicity with respect to the consequences of reporting. The Ottawa Children's Aid Society rather want to give the message that they seek to serve the family, to aid them in the resolution of their problem, rather than seek revenge and punishment. Doctors have strong enough erroneous convictions about confidentiality in patient–doctor relationships which may discourage the idea of reporting. In the HAIS report[57], the authors point out that 25% of doctors would not report a suspected case to the authorities, (whilst half the physicians did not know the correct reporting procedure in 1967[68]). In their own preliminary assessment of cases reported, they felt that the number of cases in Canada was much less than the States. This was realized to be incorrect but, despite setting up a clear list of indications for screening of patients (physical ill-treatment, dehydration, malnutrition, neglect, repeated injury, unusually fearful children, home accidents, burns, scalds, poisoning and guide lines in terms of the behaviour of the parents) in two hospitals, objections to the project were such that hospital representatives decided not to continue the project. The reasons given were:

1. They never saw abuse in their hospital.
2. This would violate the doctor–patient confidential relationship.
3. They did not want to scare away families who needed their help.
4. They did not have enough staff to do this.
5. The social agencies do not even know what to do with the cases we find.

In hospitals that did use the screening device, it was found that only between 5 and 9% of cases which should have been screened (using the adequate criteria) were in fact screened.

The House of Commons report[29] suggested that there was a need to inform the general public and professionals about child abuse and then develop better systems in order to make use of any reporting mechanism. One view suggested that penalties were needed in order to deal more effectively with those who fail to report such cases, saying that 'it is impossible to prevent further abuse or death unless there is reporting'. It was emphasized that physicians are really the first line of defence indicating that in most of the provinces, if not all, a physician suspecting child abuse must report the case to the Crown Attorney directly, or to the police or Children's Aid Society who then reports it to the Crown. One of the witnesses suggested that what was needed was not so much a sanction-orientated piece of legislation but one that should encourage people to report, despite the fact that many people feel that abuse is a crime and as such it should merit punishment. Such a view would not necessarily effectively represent the rights of children.

The Canadian Council on Social Development in Ottawa suggested that the voluntary cooperation of members of the public and of professional groups could improve the reporting of child abuse or suspected child abuse to appropriate authorities. It indicated that the child abuse registers maintained by provincial governments are an essential part of the arrangements for the surveillance of abused children and that this process of reporting should be made a privileged communication. If appropriate resources and services were made available to parents, perhaps self-reporting might occur. They also indicated the important role of the public health nurse in this detection and the need for enough nurses to provide the constant services needed in the community. Special attention should be given to creating programmes for the detection of child abuse in terms of good screening programmes, in terms of regular medical examinations of young children and on the alertness of all people coming into contact with young children. With regard to a central registry, many witnesses felt that the legislation should provide for a central registry of child abuse cases, giving the opportunity of providing statistical information on a continuous basis showing the extent of the problem in the provinces.

At the present there is a registry but it is not working very effectively and there is nothing much in the legislation about it. Such a registry could provide information for various authorities when they are confronted with suspected child abuse cases. The question of more effectively following families from jurisdiction to jurisdiction and helping to develop more pertinent research was also pointed out, with a proviso given by many people on the alleged interference with the life of such parents, this being regarded as an intrusion into the privacy of people.

Reporting laws

Hepworth[69] wrote that the reporting laws and child abuse registries raised many questions. It is not really apparent if a reporting law is truly mandatory. The Protection of Children Act in British Columbia was amended in 1968 and again in 1974, to make reporting mandatory. Sometimes it seems that 'mandatory' means, when a specific penalty is given in the legislation for failure to report. It is not always clear who is reporting to whom and what is reported and what therefore is ultimately recorded in the child abuse registry. In Ontario, it is mandatory for any individual to report a case of suspected child abuse to a children's aid agency or to a Crown Attorney. At present there is no legislative requirement for agencies to report cases to the central registry in the province. What is reported to the central register in Manitoba comes from the Children's Aid and regional offices of the provincial department but, at least in published documents, there is no indication of the source of the reports to the agencies and regional offices. Alberta, Ontario and Nova Scotia give some information of the source of the regional reports but there is a wide variety of sources identified and again it is not clear whether these are truly primary reporting sources of intermediaries. Sometimes other agencies or another children's aid organization are identified, or a social worker on the staff of the children's aid organization. There is therefore likely to be much variability in the type and quality of the reports made within a province and in the comparability of data between different parts of a province and between provinces. Similarly the types of injuries identified may vary and indeed whether any injury is involved. Some provinces identify emotional and physical neglect, in others (for example in Quebec), physical abuse is specified in legislation. Thus, a lot depends on the legislation and on the administrative practice. However, it is of interest that all provinces with reporting arrangements and registries in operation, indicate very low rates of malicious reporting by the general public. Some provinces make a distinction between the number of reports and the number of cases of probable child abuse. In Quebec, for the first year of operation, the Youth Protection Society received 2241 reports of 'situation'. Of these, 1123 were substantiated, which involved 2464 children who had been victims of physical ill-treatment. In the 1118 situations not substantiated, there were 562 children who, although they had not been physically maltreated, were in urgent need of help[70].

There is no doubt that some of the bureaucratic procedures connected with the reporting and handling of child abuse could be collected and recorded more systematically and that the different provincial registers could be aligned so that they recorded information in more comparable ways. My own view is that mandatory reporting on general lines will achieve little, since it will be too difficult and costly to effect. Where reporting could be mandatory is in the emergency room of any hospital with an automatic filing of a HAIS type of form, which could then be followed through by social worker, paediatrician etc.

The syndrome spectrum

There is clearly a continuum within the total spectrum that is being looked at. It is not at all clear that the majority of children coming into care and staying in care in each year, properly belong in the area of physical and emotional neglect. Many come into care because of economic or housing conditions, where parents are not able to care for their children properly. Improvement of these conditions might alleviate many of the attendant emotional problems which beset poor families. What becomes quite clear, is that neither mandatory reporting laws, nor child abuse registers are a panacea – at best they are tools which need to be properly and wisely used. They are not a substitute for good social services and good therapy. Some provinces are working on more effective liaison arrangements between different services, e.g. the police and child welfare services[71].

Edward A. Park in a preface to the first edition of *Child Psychiatry*[72] wrote 'Of all classes of physicians, a paediatrician is so pre-eminently concerned with preventive medicine. Because the paediatrician has this intimate family relationship and the special responsibilities, it is to him that the problem of abnormal behaviour (real or apparent) first comes. He alone has the chance to encounter the personal difficulties in their incipiency. In the past, paediatricians have not been accustomed to regard the healthy development of the child's personality as their responsibility. With the continued growth of knowledge concerning the child, the paediatrician can no longer escape this obligation.' Despite this, Eisenberg[73] wrote 'Academic paediatrics has, I believe, lagged in its interest in clinical care of the non-hospitalized child (? abused). Its training has moved toward an ever more precious occupation with the exotic; it prepares its house officers exceedingly well for what they rarely see and says hardly a word about what will confront them daily.' Medical students in a hospital setting, until very recently had very little opportunity of studying the socio-economic and cultural determinants of health and illness[74]. Regretfully, when residents and students are exposed to these issues, the glamour of microbiology and the difficult diagnostic problems overshadow all else.

Public and professional attitudes

An aid in altering attitudes and resistance to reporting would be to appreciate that the general public have roles as neighbours, relatives and parents[75], as possible battering and abusing parents themselves and as voters affecting legislature and encouraging the development of services for abusing families. The public needs to know about the factors that contribute to the problem, how to identify an abused child, where to get help or refer parents and children for help and what community resources or legislation needs to be developed and supported. In terms of suggestions, the following should be considered: (1) giving attention to role models, such as TV programmes (reducing emphasis on violence), (2) abolishing corporal punishment in the schools, (3) teaching concepts of healthy home situations and in child rearing concepts in elementary schools, with the expansion of such training in secondary schools, (4) providing specific child development and family practice training as a supervised experience such as cadet training and education for parenthood programme, (5) making family planning education available throughout the high school and open to the general public, (6) giving group education in the immediate post-partum period with supportive services available on a regular basis to all post-partum patients (perhaps more appropriately, this might be started during the antepartum period as well), (7) recognizing that high-risk families particularly those with young mothers with many children close together, single parents, parents with histories of alcoholism, drug addiction, delinquency and parents of handicapped and premature children need ready and individualized support, (8) teaching parents the basics of child development, what to expect of children; that crying is a way for a child to communicate and that a child is not a little adult, (9) perhaps most important of all to teach that the ability to socially parent a child is not totally instinctive – it is a developed and learned behaviour.

It can be seen that attitudes which were developed over many years and are implicit in the training of all professions concerned will not be changed overnight. The first step must be the recognition that these attitudes exist and that unless some changes are made the present barriers to communications will last. At this stage, if an educator communicated directly to a social worker, the principal of the school may resent this very much; the family judge may distrust a doctor because of a different professional approach and at this stage certainly seems to distrust social workers. In turn the social workers, having taken cases before judges who have rejected their views, are very wary of the situation and may not take them back on future occasions. Social workers may feel that public health nurses stress cleanliness too much and do not know much about the family. On the other hand, the public health nurse may feel that the social worker tends to relate too much to the family and not really accomplish any good at all. However, professional attitudes may be beneficial when generic training gives common ground between social worker, psychologist, psychiatrist and some of the other medical and paramedical workers[75]. It is no exaggeration to say that the life of a child might depend to a considerable extent on the overcoming of professional rivalries and tensions.

Service systems

When one asks what are the problems in service delivery models this has been presented[76] as the internecine warfare which exists between the various professionals in the systems involved. If we have any difficulty in recognizing the characteristics of the battering families, we need only look at the interrelationship pertaining between the following systems: (1) the medical system (doctors, nurses, hospital administrators), (2) the social service system (public and private agencies which provide services to families and individuals), (3) the criminal justice service (the police, the lawyers, the judges and the courts), (4) the school system (teachers and counsellors), (5) the neighbourhood and friendship system and, (6) the family and kin system[77].

All these systems are involved in identifying, labelling, treating and attempting to prevent child abuse within the professional world. We recognize failure to develop a sense of confidence or basic trust, lack of security and a sense of personal identity, unreal expectations and demands one of the other agency, and lack of consideration. It is not surprising that the professional 'bruises, fractures, scalds, poisonings, malnourishment and failure to thrive' highlight our inability to work together and indeed reflect our battering upbringings.

RECOMMENDATIONS OF THE REPORT TO THE HOUSE OF COMMONS[29]

(a) Preventive services – that there be a commitment on the part of government at all levels to the concept of assisting families in the child rearing process and thereby strengthen family life. To comment on this, what really does commitment mean? Governments often make statements of intent but the real need is for specific proposals, programmes and implementation machinery.

(b) That government at all levels encourage and assist the development of community resources for families with children. One can say that they always do this but that in fact, it is not enough; it is not taken proper care of and it is inadequately supervised and evaluated.

(c) That every child be entitled to adequate protective services in his own home and that these services include support services to parents as well as health and other community services to the child in his own right. Many charters of children's rights have been drawn up but to what degree they are legally enforceable, how much they are dependent on the prevailing economics, and how much remains at the level of exhortation, are open questions.

(d) That communities consider a block parents' programme such as those which have been operating in several communities for a number of years, in which block parents offer their homes to children needing assistance in emergencies (i.e. lost, have been molested or followed by strangers). One can make many reservations about block parents' programmes. Not enough care has been taken in selecting block parents – '*quis custodiet ipsos custodes?*' (who guards the guardians?). There is little supervision; the commitment of block parents is vague in that often signs are left in windows when people are out. If indeed this is a valuable programme, it has to be properly assessed; the personnel being taken on have themselves to be evaluated very much as one evaluates any possible abusing parent.

(e) That community health and social service centres be established to provide a range of coordinated services appropriate to community needs. With such centres, there have been problems in terms of citizen participation, legitimacy, democratic mandate and so on in many provinces. Certainly, they could be part of the caring services but again, there is a need for proper organizational linkages and a relationship between the services at every level. At this time the organization even of services such as the Children's Aid group and other social agencies, is so poorly done and the quality of care and of personnel so uniformly poor that it is hard to introduce a further area of difficult communication.

(f) That such centres consider the feasibility of providing home visits to every new parent, with such subsequent visits as are necessary with a view to giving support and assistance to the parents, to making any referral which the parent may request which may seem desirable and to outlining the services available to parents. Surely, this should be a regular service and part of the programmes that governments arrange irrespective of such centres.

(g) That the Federal Government consider the advisability of ensuring cost-sharing with the provinces for the kind of assistance plan, the proposed new Social Services Act or otherwise in:

(1) respite, remedial and other supportive services to families and children, designed to assist parents to care for their children more adequately;

(2) programmes designed to involve parents and prospective parents in discussions, meetings, courses on child rearing and training;

(3) interprofessional and interagency seminars and staff training projects on child abuse. Realistically, what is going to happen in terms of providing the money which such a programme requires?

Certainly it would be very desirable. Certainly it is needed, but in terms of money and services, implementation at the local level is what counts and perhaps the federal government should do much more to support specific programmes or projects adequately and give adequate grants.

(h) That there should be encouragement of the development of preventive health and social services through integrated community health and social services centres. Perhaps the federal government should seek a greater mandate in this area as it has already started.

(i) Recommendations were made in the context of the advisability of research into the interaction of personality of the parents, the characteristics of the child and environmental stresses; in the area of early identification of high-risk children; then the positive effect of ethno-cultural differences and patterns on the aetiology of child abuse and neglect; and in the periodic follow-up evaluation of cost-effectiveness of the programme of preventive services.

(j) That there should be consideration of the advisability of the establishment of a common data base, promoting information exchange by having meetings on the subject of child abuse registries and providing a resource service to the provinces on developments in legislation, programmes and services in child and family welfare (including the prevention of abuse and neglect and for abused and neglected children).

(k) The Canada Evidence Act and the Criminal Code – it was suggested that it would be desirable to amend the Canada Evidence Act to permit a spouse to give evidence in criminal cases, in accordance with recent recommendations and in fact in criminal cases involving child abuse.

(l) That mandatory reporting requirements exist in provincial and territorial legislation and that it should not be included in the Criminal Code.

(m) That central registries be established at provincial levels, then there would be no need for a federal registry.

(n) Public and professional education – that the government consider the advisability of extending public education through media such as the Radio Canada, The National Film Board and television with such programmes as *Challenge for Change*, by including programmes on child rearing, child care, family living and child abuse. Again, the appropriate professional schools broaden their curricula to include material on aetiology of child abuse and neglect.

(o) The training of child care should begin in primary schools with further courses in secondary and post-secondary schools.

Voluntary organizations

Since then, a task force of the national voluntary organizations concerned with child abuse and neglect was called to a meeting in February of 1977 in Toronto by the federal government, with initial discussion amongst representatives of a number of the national voluntary organizations concerned with the welfare of children. It had been suggested that there was a need for ongoing surveillance in the making of provisions and services for abused and neglected children or children at risk of abuse and neglect. The national voluntary organizations can and do promote some of the monitoring required. However, a very much more systematic approach is required to be effective at the local level where the problem of child abuse occurs. It was suggested that a permanent task force consisting of representatives of a national voluntary organization should be created as a vehicle for the more systematic monitoring of services. The task force would seek to reach an agreement on promotional activities which member organizations might wish to endorse as their own formal policy, but which would not automatically require such endorsement before their undertaking.

The task force might seek to act as a umbrella group with which local inter- and multi-disciplinary groups concerned with child abuse and neglect, both in an active service and a promotional context, might be allied or maintain contact. It might have as one of its objectives the formation of further local inter- and multi-disciplinary groups concerned with the problems, where such groups do not at the present exist. At the national level, the task force could act as a watchdog in relation to social policies which have relevance to the welfare or broad well-being of children and families. Again, it could have regard to social policies and programmes in the areas of income, security, housing, health and the personal social services at the national and provincial levels. It could comment from time to time on such policies and programmes and suggest changes or improvements as appropriate. As a relatively unstructured vehicle, it might be in a better position to make representations to government and agencies at all levels, than would some of the separate national voluntary organizations. It should be a vehicle for the expression of concerns of every kind about child abuse, neglect, deprivation and the welfare of children in general. It should not necessarily be formally structured, but be a flexible vehicle which is not bound by the terms of reference of the interested national voluntary organizations. Funding for specific activities or project meetings should be sought either in the name of the task force or in the name of the various organizations. The task force should have an action-orientation in which practical short-term goals take preference over long-term goals which belong more properly to the concerns of some of the national voluntary organizations. The term 'task force' might not be satisfactory but the creation and existence of the task force should be a demonstration and a symbol of ongoing concerns about child abuse, neglect and deprivation. It was enunciated that child abuse was a very personal challenge to everybody. It is a challenge to ordinary members of the public, as much as it is a challenge to professionals, administrators or politicians. It is a challenge that at times each of us might have to face. Each one of us might be an abuser; each one of us might be the witness of abuse. Each one of us might have to ensure, regardless of the embarrassment or social consequences for ourselves, that an abused child or a child at risk is adequately protected. It has to be said that in the matter of child abuse, 'each and every one is our neighbour's keeper'.

Canadian child abuse programmes

Programmes are now existing virtually over all the provinces in Canada[78]. In British Columbia–Victoria, there is a child abuse committee dealing with prevention, community education, self-help programmes, films and video tapes on treatment teams and statistics. In other areas, there are child abuse consultation teams, post-partum counselling, self-help group meetings, crisis homemaker services, community education and services for parents in crisis.

In Vancouver, there is a child abuse team for professional training, assessment of family, clinic involvement with family, resource development, research and material. Another project which is hospital based provides consultation and assessment and education of medical staff. There is a proposed programme for a task and talk group for single mothers, a high school education programme and a parental stress line.

The Parents in Crisis Programme (on the Parents Anonymous and the Alcoholics Anonymous models) has United Way funding and it gives a safe place for parents with a child abuse problem. Post-partum counselling is dealt with by professionals and volunteers who give support and treat parents fearful of hurting their children or who are aggressive towards their children. The Parent Aid Programme is based on the Denver Lay Therapist Model, where volunteers are trained in child abuse and assigned to the mother or father who need training in parenthood. There is a task and talk group for single mothers, dealing with a high-risk group, with volunteers for extra support. There is a centre for a self-help therapeutically oriented group which meets regularly and is led by a social worker and a volunteer. The focus is on child care and the centre is open to mothers to attend and learn specific child caring skills. There is a project parent, in which they work with parents whose mothering ability is in question. In Alberta, there is a child abuse project at the Children's Hospital with a three-year pilot project started in August 1974. There is a multidisciplinary team which consults, assesses, treats and follows-up. The modalities used are family therapy, group therapy, a mothering skills group, a parenting programme and a parent support programme. Calgary has a specialized foster parent programme for abused children, with assessment and selection criteria of prospective foster parents using questionnaires and interviews. There is also a family aid programme. In Saskatchewan, the Department of Health has implemented a child abuse team in some Hospitals. In the Department of Social Services, it plans for a provincial registry with telephone access with a public relations programme. The hospital programme is an interdisciplinary team. There is continuing medical education with provision for physicians under public programmes. In Manitoba, there is an advisory committee on battered children, which has had mandatory reporting since 1970 and had a registry in July 1971. In Winnipeg, there is a child abuse committee with volunteers. In Nova Scotia, there is a suspected child abuse and neglect committee, which is multi-disciplinary with the aims of advocacy, education and clinical conferencing. There is a teaching home-makers programme in Halifax Children's Aid. In New Brunswick, the Department of Social Services administer the Child Welfare Act and Child Protective Services.

Taking Ontario as an example, the Ministry of Community and Social Services has funded a series of demonstration projects in 1976–1977:

1. The use of extended foster families to provide support to the young, abusive parents and their children – this is done by the Children's Aid.
2. Parent aids to work with abusing and potentially abusing parents. Day nurseries to be used for crisis placement. To be used by currently functioning multi-disciplinary treatment teams under the Children's Aid.
3. Weekly group therapy sessions for the parents of 'failure to thrive' infants (from age 6 to 18 months) under the mental health clinic.
4. Utilization of professional and mature (mothering) aids to assist abusing parents through parent education and problem solving training through group discussions at the Children's Aid.
5. Parents Anonymous – a two-stage project to measure the effectiveness of a self-help approach as a means of dealing with child abuse.
6. Children's Aid utilization of play therapists and home-makers as support to case workers and treatment of abusing parents.
7. A University Group uses family volunteers and treatment sessions for potentially abusing parents of premature infants who have received intensive neonatal care. 'The project to demonstrate that, with some compassionate support, the young mother will develop more positive attitudes towards herself and her child.'

Parenthetically, it must be realized that the spreading of very limited funds over a number of projects almost ensures that major changes cannot and will not occur, reflecting the ambivalence pervading the whole field.

A child abuse training programme called 'We Can Help' is a curriculum for multi-disciplinary training of child abuse workers, prepared by the National Centre on Child Abuse and Neglect (NCCAN), Children's Bureau, Office of Child Development and the United States Department of Health, Education and Welfare. In September 1976, it was distributed throughout the United States and at the same time was made available to the Ministry of Community and Social Services, Ontario, for use and testing in this province. The training package was designed:

(a) for multiprofessional use;
(b) to be used as a package, or in part, or as adapted for local use;
(c) so that it can be used by inexperienced trainees, as well as experienced ones;
(d) to be supplemented by guest lectures and audiovisual resources.

The programme includes both didactic and experiential methods of teaching. This programme is well laid out and it has much of the field covered in terms of theory and of the variety of needs of children, parents, the types of children who are produced in the varying categories, the types of parent problems and so on.

There has been a meeting of the Federation of Women's Teachers Association of Toronto which gave a report[79] with emphasis on the recommendation that schools undertake the development of educational response to the problem in the hope that the cycle which has led to abuse may be broken. They quoted that possibly 2000 children are abused each year in Ontario, although, in fact, only 769 were reported in 1975. They use the *Harvard Review*[80] definition as well as pointing out Gil's definition[41]. They suggest that many professionals involved in the treatment of problem children now believe that the only way to ensure better parenting in the coming generations is to offer a course in parenting at all levels in the school system. Here, the greatest number of prospective parents could be influenced. They point out that parenting implies love, nurture, sheltering, protection, help, encouragement, guidance, counselling, discipline and teaching in such a way as to develop a feeling of self worth, respect for self and others, repect for individual differences and an understanding of the value of cooperation.

A seminar on child abuse was held in February 1976, at Queen's Park Toronto[76]. Representation was ensured from the major professional and volunteer groups across the province involved in the detection, treatment and prevention of child abuse. The conditions were that all were familiar with the position; papers were distributed in advance of the meeting; all had specialized personal knowledge of the problems; a belief that solutions could be found only in collaborative interprofessional efforts; and an assumption that the seminar was a single but significant step in a continuing process. The goal was the mobilization of provincial resources to deal more effectively with problems of child abuse. This group echoed many of the recommendations of the Report to the House of Commons[29] and urged among other things, the promotion of support of the establishment of local inter-professional child abuse teams to include resource material and consultation. It urged the various relevant professional associations to recognize publicly the responsibility to understand and deal with the phenomenon of child abuse, to report cases and to collaborate with other professional groups and community approaches to improved management. It suggested exploration of ways of improving its central child abuse registry, for operational research purposes and suggested the amendment of the Child Welfare Act to delete reporting to the Crown Attorney and confine it to the Children's Aid, so that there would only be one referral point. It agreed that the Children's Aid Agencies should usefully provide all their staff members with basic instructions in the detection of actual and potential abuse situations; that child abuse specialists should have expert supervision and protection against the 'burn out' so prevalent amongst such workers; that initiatives should be provided to cooperate with other agencies to establish abuse teams and to assure after-hour emergency services and availability of staff. It suggested that a hospital or community-based child abuse team should work in collaboration with the Children's Aid, police, public health etc.; that the professional associations of doctors (especially paediatricians and family doctors), nurses (especially public health nurses), psychologists, social workers, lawyers, teachers and other relevant helping professionals should ensure that basic instruction in the detection, treatment and the referral of child abuse cases should be part of both professional education and in-service training. The proposal was also made that such associations should publicly recognize their individual and collective responsibility to report cases of child abuse and to cooperate in case management.

Of interest, it was asked that given 'it should be used only in severe cases', and 'as a last resort', what alternatives are there when a legal process is being initiated? What resources can be brought to bear to avoid unnecessary entry into the adversary system? What possibilities lie in the extended use of negotiation and arbitration case conferences? What experts should be involved and how should they be used? How can such strategies avoid over-treatment in some cases at the risk of under-treatment in others, particularly when resources are limited? Questions were raised about the adversary system and the use of professional and lay persons.

In Alberta, Bell[81] looked at some of the cases that were being referred and dealt with and then tried to look at the characteristics of the parents who tend to abuse. McRae[82] looked at the varied aspects of the battered child, as it appeared in his province and was able to add to some of the descriptions, perhaps especially in the context of the type of bone injuries that were received.

The reports of the Royal Commission of Family and Children's Law (especially part five)[83], look through the various aspects of emotional neglect and abuse, the need for empathy, the needs in the hospital setting, the prevention of the tendency to child abuse and the recurrence of child abuse. It also tends to give statements of children's rights.

Emotional neglect

Perhaps one of the most important areas described[83] is on emotional neglect and abuse. Stevenson indicates that an attack on the widespread problem of emotional neglect needs: (1) an increase in the spectrum of service resources available with coordinated delivery pattern, (2) change in attitudes and awareness; children's rights and needs must be well publicized and presented in a way which enables parents to feel comfortable asking for help, (3) a widened court mandate to provide back-up for voluntary services and effect involvement by a summons and court conference, (4) a definition of emotional neglect (and abuse) that allows a judge and panel in an outlying area to come readily to a conclusion and which applies equally well to a native population.

Nova Scotia[84] recommended, (1) the establishment of a central registry, (2) a system of child advocacy (to ensure that all relevant evidence is placed before the court trial and before disposition) and that the interest and rights of the individual are safeguarded, (3) a legislated bill of rights for children including enforcement procedures, (4) elimination of corporal punishment in the schools, (5) strengthening and improving of the family court, (6) provision of legal council for all parties, (7) extensive development of preventive services, (8) provision of more and better qualified social workers for child care work, (9) adoption of the team approach in the treatment of battered and abused children, (10) greater use of community, public health personnel, (11) limited removal of abused children from their homes, (12) increased support for unwed mothers who keep their children, (13) improved case documentation, (14) development of social diagnostic indices, (15) increased public health knowledge of reporting legislation and continuing education programmes on child abuse, (16) need for a higher index of a physician's suspicion, (17) standardization of hospital record systems, (18) development of interdisciplinary approaches of education with concerned professionals, (19) increased surveillance of siblings of abused children, (20) concentration of further research in preventive aspects and, (21) regular review of status and plans for all children in care. As in other countries it will be seen that a great deal of work is going on in Canada.

THE RIGHTS OF CHILDREN

Let us look at the child as such, the diagnosis of the situation in all its aspects, the types of expertise needed etc. The rights of children[85] is a developing concept, diverse in scope and content and ranging from reference to deeply psychological states to basic environmental necessities and legal status. It is a concept for international concern. The immediate requirement for implementation is a social guarantee, different in various parts of the world. The rights to emotional security, to education, to sound custody decisions and to meaningful visitation with the separated or divorced parent reflect a certain level of cultural development of a country. A statement of these rights for the Western child is appropriate because the knowledge and resources make them clearly a present possibility. Emphasis put on some of these rights would seem utopian in underdeveloped countries where the rights to childhood, survival, minimal parental care and elementary public health services are of critical import. The rights of children must become a concept widely accepted as a primary social value, but influencing social policy and social planning at every level. The family is a unit most immediately affected by attitudes, policies and guarantees as to children's rights, and to speak of the concept is to wrestle with the deep psychological feelings aroused by the terms 'parent' and 'family'. While making available to parents the range of resources necessary for effective parenting, we need to be more explicit about the social expectations of parents and parental accountabilities to the community for the form and quality of child rearing.

An acceptance of the child as a person, not a parental property or a cherished creature in the process of becoming an adult, admits fully to his human legal rights. At certain ages and under certain circumstances, the child cannot care for himself, protect himself, speak for himself, or make prudent choices in his own best interest. The problems greatly needing exploration, policy decisions and means for policy implementation, are the rights to protection through prenatal care, to economic support such as National Children's Allowances programme, to appropriate a maximum of educational opportunities, to medical treatment in mental illness, mental retardation and other severe handicaps, and to truly rehabilitative services for the delinquent child. The question of the age of emancipation of the child requires comprehensive study, leading to uniformity in province and state statutes. When we ask 'what is care?' one can say physical care is food, shelter, housing and is easy to measure. Supervisory care is the awareness and control over the child's conduct and teaching him self discipline, which can also be measured, though far too often they are measured in a delinquency proceeding rather than a neglect proceeding. (Parental neglect, excessive weakness, categorical leniency destroy respect for the law and for those charged with its enforcement.)

Emotional care is giving the child love, an identity and a sense of security. These parameters are difficult to measure and yet they are possibly the most important elements for a stable society so as not to hear from a child that 'my parents just did not care very much about me, when I did something good, I was never praised and when I did something wrong, I was punished sometimes too much, sometimes too little'. We know that the family is the first society that any human being can become aware of. Symbolically it represents society in miniature, to the young, it acts as the declared representative of the community as a whole; the concepts of the rights of children as it wants an ethical judgement about the nature and value of the human being and a statement affirming both the legal assurances or under provision of social resources that a democratic society needs to guarantee its citizens. One can say regretfully that, whilst rhetoric reflects the North American mythology about children as our most precious resource, our actions conform to a pathology which allows blindness to deprivation that brand children with stigma and leave them feeling neither wanted nor needed. It is this pathological blindness that alienates and destroys the capacity in children for caring for others or having hope for themselves. Myths of equality, of universal justice, of human brotherhood and even myths about parental love and natural rights, all require examination, cross-examination and validation. Improvements for children would provide the key to the doorway for broader social change. Paradoxically the self-image of 'a child centred' society has failed to open the pathway to protection, to care, to support and to the recognition that children, too, have rights. It is difficult to understand and even accept that North American society has been the least generous towards its children and the judicial as well as the legislative and executive branches of government have been most reluctant and tardy in protecting the constitutional rights of children, indeed the Canadian Criminal Code virtually gives its blessing to the violation of the security of the person of minor children[76]. In general despite rationalizations, state intervention in family life, particularly with respect to child–parent relationships, has historically been orientated towards *ex post facto* action focusing on punishment of parents and placement of the child outside the family group. This pivots action on what is a presenting symptom of family dysfunction and delays remedial steps beyond the optimal point of time.

SYNDROME RECOGNITION

It is vital that everyone concerned with children of all ages should be alert to the early signs of non-accidental injury, neglect or deprivation. Many of the signs may be very slight although if looked for they can be found. Suspicion is aroused:

(1) by the character and distribution of the injury (or the difficulty of equating the clinical findings with the history given);
(2) by the history of the injury;
(3) by inquiry into the personality, background and behaviours portrayed by the parents;
(4) by the total social circumstances and intrafamilial dynamics of the family;
(5) by the history of the child[86].

The above suspicions can be aroused in the doctor's office, in the emergency room of a hospital, in the private office of the paediatrician and perhaps these are the major sources. However if we now look at any injury as an injury and cease making the possible classifications of accidental and non-accidental injury, rather believing that it is very difficult to differentiate between the two, then we can see that it is mandatory when facing a child in almost any situation, with almost any complaint, with almost any symptomatology, that one of the questions that must be asked is 'Can this injury be produced by other than an inflammatory situation, a neoplastic situation or a natural event?' When asking any of these questions one has to look at the surrounding care. If we believe that a child is a member of a family, is a member of society, and if we believe in the rights of children and their needs to be looked after, protected and their problems anticipated and prevented, then a natural part of the history-taking in any medical student, nursing student, social work student and certainly in the postgraduate professional, must be a dispassionate look at the total situation. If this becomes a uniform part of looking at any child at any time of reference, the discomfort in asking many of the questions will become less, and in turn parents will begin to expect that others have feelings for them and for their children, and reflect on how fortunate it is that people ask the type of questions that must be asked. It is essential that we take a proper background history in the context of the total pregnancy, delivery, feelings, handling and so on. In terms of injury, there can be:

(1) Bruises at any age – any bruises on a baby especially on the cheek or head (but also elsewhere) in the first few months or year of life.
(2) Bruises compatible with adult human bites.
(3) Black eyes, especially bilateral (without gross bruising of the forehead).
(4) Petechial haemorrhages (tiny multiple 'asphyxial' haemorrhages in the skin, from rough handling of a young baby, or bruises from a belt or hard object) or bizarre marks.
(5) Evidence of bruises in varying stages of resolution.
(6) Hand marks (finger and thumb) on face, trunk or limbs suggesting gripping followed by violent shaking.
(7) Multiple subungual haemorrhages.
(8) Fractures – any fracture whether associated with road accidents or home accidents must be checked in the context of the situation, how the child happened to be at the site of trauma, the degree of surveillance exercised and the family situation (age, especially the first year but also any age within childhood). Additional unsuspected fractures of the ribs, long bones and skull may be revealed on X-ray and are often easily overlooked; especially noteworthy are multiple-aged healing fractures. Radiological signs arousing suspicion; a single fracture in a young infant, spiral fracture in a young child, multiple fractures, various stages of healing, metaphyseal fracture or fragmentation, double contour lines of the periosteum, massive cortical thickening (a late sign), avulsion of provisional zone of calcification.

Joints. A tender, swollen joint with a normal X-ray may require further radiology in ten to fourteen days to exclude subperiosteal bleeding or a fracture.
Burns and scalds. Any burns or scalds in young children. Sores or scars from cigarette burns. These may be of different ages and multiple.
Mouth. Lacerations or bruises around the mouth in a baby – tear of frenulum or damage to gum as a result of bottle, fist or object forced into the mouth of a crying baby.
Brain. Subdural haemorrhage (irritability, vomiting, increase in coma), tense fontanelle, seizures, increasing pallor in the 'acutely sick' child, failure to thrive, stroke, developing coma (seizures in the chronic case).
Eyes. Retinal haemorrhages from shaking and asphyxial states (and any subsequent odd abnormality of the eyes having an origin associated with trauma of any sort).
Viscera. Intra-abdominal origin or injuries to solid or hollow viscera with signs of bleeding, shock etc.
Chest. Haemoptysis, cough, dyspnoea, lacerations.
Poisoning. Ingestion of tablets, medicines or domestic fluids in any age group.

Unexplained failure to thrive[87], undernutrition, repeated apparent diarrhoea, (hypernatremic) dehydration[88], emotional deprivation (should be carefully considered with the relevant differential diagnosis). Sexual abuse. Any case of drowning (or near drowning)[89,90] and any case of suffocation.

Extended syndrome in childhood and adolescence

A similar situation occurs in children and adolescents in terms of truancy, bullying, lying, stealing, swearing, acting out (sexually or otherwise), school failure, attendance at special classes in perhaps ordinary, even extraordinary situations, and children who are excluded from school. All of these indicate how virtually any child coming with any symptom, to any doctor, is worthy of a total growth and development history in terms of the child, of child rearing habits, a history of both parents and their upbringings with perhaps special reference to methods of discipline, rearing attitudes, alcoholism, violence etc. In the past history, there may be an unexplained or inadequately explained injury, or even a previously known child abuse of this child or other children in the family. Sometimes these injuries have not been mentioned in the history. There may be inconsistencies in the history with little or no mention even made of the present injury. The explanation and mechanism of the injury may be implausible or contradictory. There may be delay in seeking help. The informant may be reluctant to give information. Consent is refused for further diagnostic studies. There is a complaint of irrelevant problems unrelated to the injury. Cause of the injury is described by a sibling or a third party. The parents cannot be found. The adult accompanying the child is drunk or violent. The child is in the care of the step-father, foster parent or child worker. There have been visits to multiple doctors and multiple hospitals.

The parents

The parents come from a battering, non-supportive, punitive or very permissive home with very little parenting demonstrated. They were battered themselves; have a poor self-image, live in stressful social circumstances, poor housing, are out of work, young, emotionally immature, have frequent pregnancies, have no relatives or close friends with whom to share problems, difficulties and a crying, hard to manage child, they have unrealistic expectations of the child, they are inexplicably and inappropriately angry and violent, they show apathy and lack of concern about the child. They are oversolicitous about common events and may frequent clinics or physician's offices very frequently without 'convincing reasons'. The child may have been premature or born with an abnormality and/or separated from the mother for some time after birth. The child may watch with an expression of 'frozen watchfulness'. The child may be mentally retarded. Any of the above may be extant.

Hospital 'accidents'

We can look at trauma and regard it as a leading childhood killer in Canada and elsewhere[91]. In the Sick Children's Hospital, Toronto, the emergency out-patients saw 20 103 patients in that hospital (together with those admitted directly in the hospital of which vehicle accidents were 1403), 381 were struck by a car and others were 7000 falls, 72 suicides. In terms of burns there are 100 new burns per year admitted to the Sick Children's Hospital, of which two-thirds occurred at home in children under ten, 15% due to flammable material and 85% due to scalds. Head injuries under the age of 15 – over a period of eight years there were some 4465 cases of which 68.2% were males, 31.8% were females; 5.2% of these were subdural. There was brain damage in 3.2% and mortality was 5.4%. Falls accounted for 50% and 23% were struck by cars. With their child abuse team at the Sick Children's Hospital, Toronto, 410 abused and neglected children were examined[92]. Among these, bruises accounted for 60%; fractures were 15% (of which 2/5 were skull fractures only); lacerations were 7%, burns were 4%, subdural haemorrhages 5%; failure to thrive were 6% and retinal haemorrhages were found in 2%. One has to comment on these figures in that in a hospital treating as many cases of fractures as it does in one year, to have a total of 60 abused over three years in whom 24 had skull fractures must mean that they cannot be exploring the total abuse situation. Other events determine whether the children are regarded as abused or not. It is relatively easy perhaps if the type of person, the type of story, the type of child makes one think of the possibility of battering. Perhaps the main reason why we have no idea of the composition of battering parents, the battered child or the battered family is that nowhere does one see a total community questionnaire on child rearing etc. It will be noted that there are no cases of poisoning at all but fortunately this is now being pursued actively. Looking at other segments of the report, in a personal retrospective survey of some 32 cases of burns in a routine unit admitting burns and scalds, in 18 sufficient evidence was found in records which were kept by plastic surgeons (who are not usually noted for their good records from a psychosocial point of view), it was very easy to determine that if nothing else the whole situation should have been investigated but was not.

With the number of deaths reported by drowning in 1972, each presumably looked like an 'accident', again it is clear that the relevant questioning has not occurred and the relevant questions have not been asked[90]. One must assume that even in a team labelled a child abuse team, there are areas which people do not want to pursue. It is fairly obvious that the ability to influence other members of the medical and nursing professions is, to say the least, very difficult and that such influencing has to be done consistently and regularly in order to counteract the various internal and external reasons why doctors, perhaps as individuals and members of society, do not want to 'see' the possibility of this family dysfunction whenever they encounter cases.

Fit for the Future

Lest this should be seen as a North American and Canadian problem only, if one looks at *Fit for the Future*[93], while agreeing that the home is more dangerous than the roads, especially with limited space and with limited parental understanding, it says that in the UK in 1971, 25 000 children were admitted with 'accidental poisoning' with 30–40 deaths per year. The comment is made that 'since accidents are, in the main preventable, it is distressing to find that they are the main cause of death between the first birthday and leaving school'. 'They are the result of the encounter of developmentally immature children with a dangerous environment', and the risk becomes greater as social circumstances become less favourable. The real annotation that they should be looked at as an indication of family dysfunction and a part of the child abuse, neglect and deprivation syndrome is not present even in this excellent report. Sibert[94], looked at 100 families of children under five years admitted to Cardiff Hospitals after accidentally ingesting poisons and compared them with 100 controlled families matched for socio-economic class, age and sex of the child. He found significantly more stress in the affected families than in the controls, however, in no place does he then suggest that he was seeing symptomatology referable to the child abuse, neglect and deprivation syndrome. Suitable references are Sobel who indicated the psychiatric implications of accidental poisoning describing the intrafamilial psychopathology, which could well lead to the child demonstrating the problems within the family[95] and Rogers describing 'forced poisoning'[96]. The prevailing desire to describe the need for safe containers but not even mention psychosocial or psychiatric family factors is shown in the report by Calman[97]. This demonstrates very clearly how blind we are when we want to be.

Death. Child abuse. Tragedy

To consider one case of child abuse and death[98], *The Globe and Mail* describes V.E., a child who died at age 1 month. This young baby girl had severe gastroenteritis, diarrhoea and dehydration, hypernatremia with a state of terminal shock. The events, they said, included all the elements of a Greek tragedy and also included all the elements of a system which was meant to ensure the child's preservation but which instead unremittingly continued her destruction, through neglect, confusion and the exercise of incredible self-confidence. The players, the child born to a mother aged 28, who herself was abused and neglected as a child, who hated her own mother and grew to be capable of childbearing, but hopelessly inadequate as a mother. Psychiatrists described her as psychopathic, paranoid, antisocial and passive aggressive. The mother concerned had given birth to five children; two were made wards of the Children's Aid, and three died (one was left unattended in a bathtub and two, including this child, died of neglect leading to disease and were treated too late). The mother was convicted of child neglect in 1971, and in 1973 a coroner's jury recommended that all subsequent children be made wards of the court. The mother refused to receive psychiatric help or to cooperate with the Children's Aid. The mother and father fought a legal battle with the Children's Aid for the custody of this child at birth. A Family Court judge granted custody to the parents when the child was 9 days old. Less than one month before this, the same family judge had apparently refused them custody of their son, citing the family's history of neglecting and maltreating its children. In the present court enquiry, however, he refused to admit evidence relating to the family history for his ruling on the custody of V.E. He appeared to rely almost exclusively upon the recommendations of a social worker, R.P. (who can be regarded as a very skilled social worker, in that she is supported by a psychiatrist of repute and has now become head of a very reputable psychiatric agency). She had developed what she called a 'relationship of trust' with the family and advised the judge that they posed no threat to V.E. provided they were given supervision which she agreed to give. R.P., the social worker, had never read the entire Children's Aid file on the family (even though it was in her office), and was not aware of any psychiatric information. She relied on her feelings, that under her supervision, V.E. would be safe. She was supported by the psychiatrist in charge of the clinic, who did not attempt to get the past history or further knowledge of the family. R.P. visited the family on the morning of death and found 'a healthy normal baby'. Two hours later, the child was rushed to hospital, where a paediatrician found the child convulsing, lethargic, extremely dehydrated from the diarrhoea, having a diaper rash covering 15% of the body and having gross impairment of the central nervous system. That night, the child died. On follow up, the social worker as indicated is now the chief of a big department and the psychiatrist is a chief policy advisor on children's services (and probably quite rightly so, except in the area of his knowledge of the child abuse). The judge continues to sit on the bench of the Family Court.

History and information

In looking at any similar case, we can say that we need the following information:

1. the parent's age, sex, socio-economic status;
2. the values and norms regarding violence in the sub-culture, within the class and community;
3. the role made of violence and abuse, within the family of origin of the parents within the community. The aggression pattern, both leading to the socialization experience;
4. the mental health of the parents. Their personality and character traits, neurological status and controllability, psychopathic status;

5. (a) the stress within the marriage partners, marital disputes, dysfunctioning, affect, communication;
   (b) structural stress – unemployment, social isolation, excess children, stress to parental authority, values, self-esteem;
   (c) stress emanating from the child:
      1. unwanted child;
      2. reality child different from fantasy child;
      3. problem child, crying, colicky, ill discipline problem, physical abnormality, retarded and the varying combinations of 1–5;
6. what the immediate precipitating situations are, the child's misbehaviour, argument, anger etc. resulting in;
7. child abuse, neglect or deprivation:
   1. single or repeated physical acts;
   2. neglect in providing proper care, to prevent poisoning, accidents, burns etc;
   3. deprivation of adequate food, shelter, mental and physical stimulation.

Resources and needed expertise

We have done that, and now? Whoever primarily recognizes the situation then has to report to the necessary authority who then finds the necessary resources and expertise. In the case described, on the final day, the first expert required was the doctor and there we can say that in his role as family doctor, paediatrician, emergency room doctor, psychiatrist or sub-specialist, whether it is orthopaedist, neurologist, ophthalmologist, haematologist or any doctor handling children who may be traumatized in any particular area, his duty is to physically assess the case and make the appropriate diagnosis in the context of the interference with body homeostasis, the organ disturbed, the system disturbed and the body disturbed. Ideally, he ought to be able to take an adequate family history and do a psychosocial assessment but in practice, if he can at least recognize that this is needed and have with him a nurse practitioner, public health nurse or a social worker, who can do this, that is sufficient. In other cases, a follow-up must be arranged. In general terms, having looked for a situation and having enough insight to get others involved from an academic point of view, it is probably the doctor who can act as a source of stimulation to the various members of the team with whom he is associated, be this an in-hospital team, or a community team.

The expertise of *the nurse* in the hospital can really resemble very much that of the doctor, in terms of looking at the happening, but perhaps more importantly, she can look at the surrounding situations more easily, and with a more detached eye, enabling the doctor to look at the existing problems.

The *social worker's* areas of expertise lie in an ability to assess the family, to assess the background and the support system available to the individual and family. Subsequently he must begin to look at what other resources are needed.

There are social worker problems[99]. In talking of relationship therapy, the philosophy of the treatment process includes the following:

1. the determining aspects of the process of relationship;
2. the emphasis on experiencing emotional dynamics rather than on insight or interpretations;
3. the focus is on the dynamics of the here and now relationship rather than on past relationship;
4. resistance in the patient is viewed as a positive statement of a will striving for independence and a force to be encouraged, strengthened and directed;
5. there is a recognition of the individual as a social being who needs another person or persons, for self-realization and development. It is a step by step process of building self-esteem in small increments and involves using the parent relationship to rebuild and remedy previously damaging interpersonal encounters.

Yet 'during the course of our project, we became more and more disenchanted with the frequently superficial and crisis orientated nature of social services to these families. Agencies were reluctant to go to court because of the lack of "hard evidence" '[100].

If we now go back to the V.E. case, it is clear that the social worker developed a relationship situation or an idea of a relationship with the mother. She was not able to see that although family therapy, which she may have been using, might help in getting the parents to relate better to one another, it did nothing to improve the all important area of child rearing. It is probable that since their own upbringing had been so damaging knowledge of child rearing was in fact absent. The social worker could not recognize this (which is not surprising, since this is not within her area of expertise) and yet these defects have not been clearly acknowledged. She has been expected to know all that is happening within a family. Somewhat naively, with apparently a family therapy background, or a similar individualistic psychotherapeutic style, there has been the belief that working on, say, a once a week visiting monitoring basis, one can alter the feelings and ways of reaction of a lifetime (extending from the birth of the mother in which her ingestion, her absorption and her growth has been surrounded by negative influences from her family). The mother may never have understood what being a child means, what it is to have a real mother and has the wrong concepts of what is proper under stress circumstances.

Children's Aid

Of the social worker in the above case, it cannot be said that she is unskilled, but in many other circumstances only 25–40% of the Children's Aid staff are trained social workers and many may have just come out of their social work school to be plunged into the fury of multiple-problem cases. The majority of such cases belong to the child abuse syndrome, even though they are artificially separated and segregated. So frequently there is the choice of the 'least detrimental alternative' or the 'lesser of evils' for the child[101]. Thus, there are difficult situations, difficult backgrounds, in which one has to use each and every skill and technique to help the child and family. The supervision that such a worker obtains (contrary to the supervision which is prescribed and thought a very essential part of growth and development in the social work world) is often of very poor calibre, and usually the supervisor is someone who has grown old in the service, rather than someone who has grown through an academic, theoretical, as well as practical, contact with various problems in the field of dealing with people. This tends to give a very negative input and the young workers are overwhelmed. They find themselves inadequate, feel themselves inadequate and in contact with other agencies, look over their shoulders and do not collaborate. Unfortunately, the Children's Aid services have accepted the total load of looking after 'syndrome families' which is most unrealistic.

Table 10.1   Child abuse statistics, April 1973–June 1977

Total no. of children abused 179   *Died* 6
   Actual 145   *Suspected* 34
Physical 156   *Sexual* 8   *Neglect* 15   (M 95, F 84)

Age range 0–3, 85   4–5, 30   6–12, 32   13+, 32

Active cases 88
No. of months open 1–9; 2–7; 3–4; 4–5; 5–2; 6–3; 7–5; 8–6; 9–6; 10–2; 11–3; 12–1; 13–3;
                14–2; 15–5; 16–4; 17–2; 19+ over months 19

Inactive cases 100
No. of months open 1–21; 2–8; 3–5; 4–7; 5–4; 6–1; 7–6; 8–3; 9–9; 10–1; 11–4; 12–1; 13–5;
                14–1; 15–3; 16–1; 18–3; 19-over months 18

To illustrate

A follow-up study (Table 10.1) reflects statistics obtained from a Children's Aid Society dealing with a population of some 200 000. The criteria for acceptance of the diagnosis are very strict and all cases in all categories must be regarded as very severe. It will be seen that 21 cases were out of follow-up by one month and 64 by nine months. This clearly reflects how a Children's Aid Society (typical of the vast majority of such societies) views the therapeutic needs of abused families. The cost of such inadequate intervention can be at least $1500–2000 (£1000 or so), per month. It would seem that the format or procedure is good – as everywhere – the ability to handle is poor. Regretfully, this is exactly what one has seen in most centres throughout the Western world – namely that greater and greater effort and skill is being applied to the diagnostic procedures and to the format of the management team. However, the actual working with the child and family is of a very poor calibre and it is not surprising that the fallout rate in follow-up is high, reflecting the poverty of the learning and growing. This does not deny the efficacy of the field projects (Denver, Oxford (UK) etc.), but the cost in terms of resources, personnel and numbers involved in such projects virtually excludes their general extrapolation.

Role of a social worker

Many descriptions are available of the *role of a social worker*. There is a need to draw up an efficient system, within which these workers can operate to the best of their capacity, having adequate post-graduate training with the continuing input of good supervision. There needs to be formal chains of communication to secure the passage of information, the emphasis being on personal, formal and informal contacts between the social workers and their colleagues and other disciplines, to increase general awareness of the problems of the child workers who play a part in the full social worker's role.

There is a real need, however, to realize that the parents involved have experienced inadequate or harmful mothering and that they need a period of good mothering themselves, before they are ready to provide good and loving care for their own children. It can take a long time to build up a mother's confidence and enable her to feel that someone does care for her and wants to help her. In the less difficult areas, there is a need for a practical demonstration of concern, such as help in housing, finances, transport to hospital and day care. A day care nursery may provide care, stimulation and a degree of safety for the child and may relieve the mother of the strain which total responsibilities entail[102].

The psychiatrist and deprivation

Should the social worker ask for psychiatric help? Examine a case report[113]. A six year old girl, a severe behaviour and management problem from birth was referred. The overall picture was that of a child who had suffered severe emotional deprivation. (The mother was deprived by a destructive, non-giving paranoid mother and separated parents. The father had severe emotional trauma and deprivation from an ambivalent relationship with a domineering, cold and suspicious mother.) It is said that during the family interview, an attempt was made to achieve an understanding of the dynamics and pathology operative in the family. This would include the following information:

(a) The family structure and organization.
(b) The intrafamilial transactions, past and present.

(c) The way in which the various family members fulfil the role expected of them.

(d) The meaning of the 'illness' of the particular members presented to the family.

(e) A superficial picture of the individual psychodynamics and psychopathology of the family members, including those not present at the interview.

The therapeutic programmes available would be:

(a) The treatment of the family unit as a group by one therapist; occasionally one or other member might also be seen in individual sessions.

(b) A very loosely defined approach where one, two or several members of the family might be seen as a group depending on the exigencies and

(c) child treatment in individual psychotherapy with minimal parental involvement.

(d) Treatment of the significant dyad, mother–child, father–child, mother–father, others being seen periodically.

(e) The child placed in a group or individual and group treatment. The parents seen as a pair individually or in a group.

In effect, the child was seen three times weekly, the mother, once weekly, but a few months later this was found not to work, so the mother was given analytic therapy, three to four times a week, the child, play therapy, once a week, and the father was seen conjointly with the mother on many occasions. This was carried on for three years with seeming gains and some improvement and the family has occasionally been seen since.

It can be pointed out that the psychiatrist concerned is a superb exponent of the art and undoubtedly achieved a great deal, but in what way could such expensive (time and people) therapy be carried on for three years especially as at the end of that time, there was a need for ongoing work and especially as, in order to be sure that what happened was good, one would have to see what this child becomes when she grows up.

One can also notice that the concept of the mother–father abusing (the child) is not raised. One only really looks at the severe emotional deprivation and assumes that this can be overcome even though a situation altering so slowly must still be quite dangerous.

Systems approach

To many psychiatrists it would be proper to speak of the total systems approach as opposed to the interactional, interpersonal or interpsychic approach where one is required to work across many disciplines in the central systems[104]. This approach is an attempt to develop a conceptual system that integrates the pertinent features of the various systems. It focuses precisely on the interfaces and the communication processes taking place there. It begins with an analysis of the structure of the field, using the common structure and operational properties of systems as criteria for identifying the systems and sub-systems within it. By tracing the communications within and between the systems, it insists that the structure, sources, pathways, repository sites and integrated functions and messages become clear, in addition to their content. This, together with the holistic non-exclusive nature of the approach, minimizes the danger of excessive activity in the collection of data and allows for much more clarity in the contextual contributions to its analysis. The prescription and planning of strategies and techniques which follow, gain in clarity and are more likely to be clothed in concrete reality. The family looked at as an open system, its structure, organization and transactional pattern displayed, are regarded as the important variables determining the behaviour of the members. Treatment focuses on the disturbances in the system, from the standpoint of its structure, organization or transactional patterns. The intrapsychic processes of the members of the system are of secondary importance, if indeed attention is paid to them at all.

It will be seen that if the therapist belongs to this school and if he is able to handle the total systems approach, it does arrange for good communication and the use of other personnel. If indeed the intrapsychic process in the context of growth and development, nurturing, mothering, attachment, is not being looked at (and unfortunately in the training and development of most psychiatrists, even child psychiatrists, while the theoretical situation may be known to them, the amount of practice that has been given via 'growth and development' paediatrics is small), the majority of psychiatrists are of little value in the context of child abuse. It is of interest that following the V.E. case, it has been suggested that every family who is suspected of being part of the syndrome should have a psychiatric evaluation. This might, in fact, be less desirable than might at first be apparent.

Abusing family characteristics

Steele and Pollock[105] described the child abuse family as immature, impulse ridden, dependent, sadomasochistic, egocentric, narcissistic and demanding and then went on to say that these were qualities prevalent among people in general, so that they add little to specific understanding. They have their share of widespread emotional disorders seen in any clinic population, namely, hysteria, hysterical psychosis, obsessive–compulsive neurosis, anxiety state, depressive schizoid personality trait, schizophrenia and character neurosis, but stated that overt psychosis or the schizoid type of individual accounted for a very small percentage, probably between 3 and 10%. This would mean that if a particular case has to be presented either to a group – say a child abuse management team consisting of lawyer, social worker, doctor, psychologist and others, it would be seen that in the vast majority of cases, they would not be given a psychiatric diagnosis which would be helpful. On the contrary, if it went to court, the judge would be left with the concept that from a psychiatric point of view, there is a major problem similar to the situation one might find in the general population. In that sense, therefore, the only value of a psychiatrist (apart from psychiatrists who are interested and knowledgeable in the syndrome situation and will be involved) is for a 'psychosis' diagnosis which could clearly be validated by a psychiatrist, but which probably can be made by almost any member of the team in the avowed situation of the person concerned. In the child abuse training programme (*We Can Help*) they tended to speak of abusive families as having:

1. unfulfilled needs for nurturing and dependence;
2. fears of relationships;
3. lack of support system;
4. marital problems;
5. life crises;
6. inability to care for or protect a child;
7. lack of nurturing and child care practices.

Very few of these qualities can be assessed adequately by the usual psychiatrist or indeed the usual social worker. In some instances they can be assessed by a psychologist in that field, but often not; they may well be assessed by a nurse or possibly a paediatrician, but perhaps more adequately by somebody involved in the care of children at an early age.

Oliver and Cox[106] divided parents into four groups:

1. *some 5–10%* either psychotic, out of touch with reality or whose behaviour is liable to be unpredictable (due to post-natal insanity, epileptiform type of conditions, chronic alcoholism, schizophrenia);
2. *5–15%* likely to be of sub-normal intelligence, whose retardation may be the result of psychosocial deprivation when they were children;
3. *1%* act from sadistic motives, the target often being an older child, who might be illegitimate; sometimes drug abuse;
4. *70–80%*, the largest of people with fundamental personality disturbances, usually coming from disturbed environments themselves;
   (a) habitually aggressive personalities including extreme cases of aggressive psychopaths;
   (b) emotionally impoverished, immature, seeking constant love and reassurance from their own children even when the child is a young baby and even failing to respond to that young baby;
   (c) motivated by primitive emotions, finding moral reasons to justify cruelties and restraints within the family.

Robertson[107] describes three groups of parents:

1. Those who actively seek and use help, who are self-motivated, who use help

provided that they are heard and that their need is appropriately responded to.

2. Those who will use help if they are found and referred by family doctors, other doctors, public health nurses, teachers etc.; who are somewhat resistant to help, largely because of their lack of trust and their fear; who need reassurance and time to learn how to trust.

3. Parents who will not accept help of any kind, even though there is evidence and awareness in the community that the children are suffering from some form of abuse. These children should be removed from the home. This group demanded the most time, energy and attention; this group have contributed to the stereotype of the abusing parent and it is this group who are largely responsible for our feelings of anger and helplessness.

The abusing parent

Parents are angry, frightened, defensive, apologetic and/or immature[108]. Perhaps more importantly, we should remember that the abusing parent may be the parent in our house or the parent next door, and when we begin to see that many parents can be part of this syndrome, we may be able to help. A we/they construct occurs, consciously or unconsciously, in most people who see abusing parents as somewhat different, 'not-like me', or in short, as abnormal. I want to clarify, however, that I do not believe that we should then teach that any of us can become abusers. It seems to me that throughout our toning down of definitions, of reporting, of adequate examination, by not searching for the possibility of abuse, yet on the other hand suggesting that anyone can abuse, we deny or minimize the reality of the influence of child rearing practices and family environmental impute. To suggest that a person can hit a child and because of the site of the blow, the effect of the trauma can be overwhelming is true. That this in itself represents the continuum of abuse, neglect and deprivation, need not be quite so true. It is possible to sit with parents and families and find out whether their general plan of life and living is a loving and good one; irrespective of their rigid and forceful concept of discipline (whether one approves of this or not) but that is not necessarily the entity of child abuse, neglect and deprivation, and we should not forget this. Once we say that 'there but for the grace of God, go I', we will in fact either step back and do nothing or step forward and 'maim and kill'.

To return to the V.E. case, what other resources might the social worker have looked for? She should have seen that this mother and father required mothering and fathering skills. If she were not daunted by the past history, then she could have looked for the following possibilities. Firstly, that the whole family could have been taken into 'foster care'. In Oxford[109] they have a unit which contains the whole range of paediatric, psychiatric and legal problems within the scope of one closely integrated team. This gives it the authority to provide comprehensive help to each family and to deal with the closely inter-related emotional, practical and medical problems. Such programmes are being evaluated and attempted elsewhere on a minor scale, and perhaps this could have been found within the area concerned.

Foster parents and foster homes

However, maybe there was a need to separate the mother and the father from the child and put the child in a foster parent home. Arrangements could be made for daily visiting by the mother and father to the home, the mother during the day and the father with the mother in the evening, when he was back from work. In that way perhaps they could have absorbed the therapeutic parenting skills of the foster parents and begun to learn over a period of time what it is to be a parent and what this means. This would have meant the searching for and evaluation of a foster parent home. This home would need to be scrutinized in exactly the same way that one would scrutinize the home of an abuser or potential abuser. It is a sad state of affairs that children are abused more frequently in foster homes than they are in natural homes. This may reflect the type of child that goes into a foster home, but equally reflects the poverty of the examination of the foster home situation. Sometimes, as is perceived by the courts, children in foster homes are put 'out of the frying pan into the fire'. Eisenberg[110] documented his disillusionment with foster care as a means of providing for children who have to be removed from their families. He pointed out that the pathology is sometimes increased rather than ameliorated. Wolins[111] stressed the fact that foster care has been questioned for more than a decade but continues to be the major focus in North America. He cites many studies of the failure of foster homes to meet the needs of all children.

A report[112] in one of the newspapers states 'the ideal situation would be the availability of enough foster homes to allow selection by the Children's Aid of a proper home for each individual teenager. With few families willing now to have teenage foster children, we have no choice. Sometimes when there is no other solution, we must place a teenager with a family where we know there could be difficulties in personality or life-style'. It is still true that a foster home could probably have been found and with special care, could have been an adequate foster home.

In the V.E. case the problem of adoption was considered and in terms of the other children in the family had been initiated.

The courts

The case was, however, brought to the courts. Ours is an adversary system[113] still feeling the after effects of a violent revulsion from the authoritarian in-terrogatory method of the Star Chamber. How can the adversary system best be used so that all parties comprehend the process or are represented by those who do? Should there be an advocate for the child other than, or in addition to, the Children's Aid? Should there be different rules regarding the kind of evidence that is admissible?

The allegations and the evidence on which the court is to decide, must be put in the presence of those accused and be open to test by cross-examination. A problem can exist, because the proceedings are being brought by a body which is also going to be the caring agency if powers are granted. (This may produce a situation in which some of the evidence available is not given, for fear of damage to the social worker/client situation.) I think this has been exaggerated in terms of its ill effects, since it is terribly difficult to believe that one can put to parents that indeed their parenting skills are poor, even if they themselves have suspected this, unless they are willing to receive such information. It is necessary to deal empathetically with such parents, but the concept that one can gently tell them that they are 'terrible' parents, is unreal. It is much more important to give the concept that one wants to give oneself and the services that are available to help them; that one appreciates the difficulties that they are in and the needs they have, bearing in mind that these needs have arisen because of the upbringing that they have received. One can realistically say that to take up any profession or vocation or trade a training is required. If that training is unsuitable there is a need for further training (for example if doctors come to the United Kingdom, United States or Canada from areas where training is dubious then they undergo a period of supervision and training prior to their being allowed to practise medicine). Yet this is not a requisite in terms of parenting skills even though, with superficial examination of the background, the parenting paradigms are seen to have been most inadequate. I think with this type of approach, with the desire to help, the tremendous emphasis which has been placed on the damage to the relationship situation can be superseded. The question of the welfare of the child[114] sounds a simple concept, but is very confused because of the legal, professional and administrative implications, together with the smattering of sentimentality which exists. The following factors operate in determining action relating to the deprived child:

1. The child needs to be protected.
2. It is better to protect the child by the use of voluntary methods rather than the force of the court.
3. The natural parents' right of the child must be taken into account.
4. When using the sanctions, the onus of proof needs to be similar to that which appertains in criminal proceedings.

The above objectives are conflicting and as a result the law is equally confused in its directives. Since juvenile court actions on behalf of the child[115] are not criminal prosecutions against any person, 'proof of guilt beyond a reasonable doubt' is not required, but court decisions must be based upon a preponderance of the evidence and reasonable doubt may be resolved in favour of the child's protection. All of the relevant facts must be presented if a wise decision is to be made. Social workers and physicians must be prepared to present well documented evidence and they may need the assistance of legal council to do so.

The judges

A major difficulty is that many judges do not allow past history to be produced in the court. In other words, just as in any other criminal event the problem is related to the here and now situation and to the actual event. If this is in the sense of depriving, neglecting or battering, then the event which has brought this to attention is looked at and many judges will not allow the history of the parents, of child rearing etc. to be brought to the court. One can understand this in a criminal case, where if someone is to be held responsible for a particular event (excluding child abuse altogether), then it is probably unfair to refer to the fact that he did commit a burglary some time ago, but we are not really dealing with that sort of situation. Realistically judges and lawyers should have some concept of the total situation which is examined, namely the child and family and that early legislation has been clearly for the protection of the parent or the society and not for the benefit of the child. In the V.E. case on the facts as reported it is very difficult to understand how the Family Court judge compartmentalized his mind. He knew what had happened one month before and yet he was able to divorce himself completely from that and apply himself only to the here and now situation of a social worker's judgement. In terms of penalties, assuming that one accepts that there should be penalties for non-reporting individuals in the community or even accepting that perhaps it should be restricted to professionals, should there not be a penalty for someone, say a social worker who blindly has gone along without looking at the full notes? Should there not also be a penalty for a judge who can ignore the knowledge of previous babies who have died or who have been taken into care and yet make a decision as though the abusing background for this child had arisen *de novo* in the community?

Medical and legal conflicts

This can lead to other medical and legal conflicts.

1. The abuser's mental state. To the lawyer, whether the injury is an accident or whether it is intentional is a very important variable, whereas to the doctor, the mental state of the participants may require a difficult or impossible diagnostic formulation. The family dynamics in accidents or inflicted injuries may be the same. The trauma may depend to some degree on the ethnic status and social class of people responsible.

2. The seriousness of the injury. To the lawyer there has to be serious harm.

To the doctor any injury justifies protective response.

3. To the lawyer, it is important that he should know whether the mother did it or the father did it, whereas to the doctor it is the total happening that is important. Moreover one can, if one sits with a family, soon realize that if the father batters, it is the mother who may be giving tacit consent and vice versa.

There may be situations where, through fear of financial consequences and fear of the husband, the wife may not say anything when he is the abuser and even vice versa but this is hard to believe, since primarily if a parent is a 'good parent' he/she may even be willing to lay down his/her life for their child. This accentuates the futility of exact knowledge of the abuser which in any event consumes an inordinate amount of time. It is much more fruitful to regard the injury as such or the depriving or the neglect as part of the total family situation and to express it as such.

4. The role of the law. To the doctor this is an instrument to achieve a particular therapeutic or dispositional objective, i.e. to get services or social welfare involvement, subjective or intuitive. The lawyer demands evidence, not impressions. Equally however, if the judge has seen many cases whereby the removal of the child from the home or the use of foster homes has really achieved nothing, it is not surprising that he turns a deaf ear, as it were, to many of the statements that are given. Many judges have been critical of the ability of social workers to judge when a child requires the protection of the court and they fail to realize that these are not easy decisions to make. In general we are back to the concept of whether punishing the parent helps to change behaviour[116] or whether threats of punishment seem to deter him or her from further acts of abuse or whether we want to partake in a total rehabilitation situation, assuming that this is possible. One might also present the concept that, since so many of these parents have never really been given the love of a parent, as expressed in an authoritarian manner but with love and without violence, it could well be that a day in the court, which is their right, could indeed put this in perspective. This could give the father figure a loving situation but in a firm disciplinarian setting, demanding that in order to expiate crimes committed on the parents by their forebears and abuse of the child by themselves they should undergo all the therapeutic help which is available and can be given. Many will not respond but equally perhaps, those that can be helped should not be deprived of that help, because of the few who will not respond. This then means that in the few parents who under no circumstances are going to change, their children perhaps should be looked at very early on and clear decisions should be made as to whether they should come into care in the sense of being removed, adopted and so on, rather than waiting for later events. If the Bench were reinforced with specialists in relevant disciplines who are not lawyers, one could get a rather better level of management of cases[76]. A system works badly, perhaps because of the way people are using it. An effort is made in the Child and Family Court to marry the legal and the social, but it does not work because the judge cannot be involved in a friendly way for a time and

then, in the end, come down with the club[76]. To illustrate, some of the difficulties of the internecine warfare between the courts and the Children's Aid and others, result in some cases which have not been proceeded with, mainly because of professional problems.

Professional difficulties in cases

1. A child of six was seen in the emergency room having limped in with a fractured femur. X-ray also showed a dislocated hip on the opposite side, with the implication of the use of tremendous force, enough indeed to alert even the orthopaedic people to the syndrome. The hospital Abuse Team looked at the situation, using all of their available resources and referred to the Children's Aid indicating that they felt that the family (consisting of a mother and her common-law husband) were in great difficulties. The mother had a background of abuse and violence. The common-law husband had not really finalized his relationship with his legal wife, having two children with her. He was a man of great violence and an alcoholic. The mother herself had very difficult ways of relating to her two children. It was not very clear from the history as to who had actually manhandled the child. Nevertheless, the Children's Aid took over the case and believing that they could get a relationship with the 'husband and wife' agreed to do family case work with them. The case was brought to the Community Child Abuse Management Committee who indicated their disapproval of the inadequacy of what was happening, feeling that the children should be taken into a foster care situation emphasizing the need for adequate contact between the mother and children. The Children's Aid objected to this partly on the grounds of their fear of alienating the parents. In the meantime, the husband and wife separated and the mother called up saying that in no way could she handle the children, who were then taken into care.

2. Another child, seen at six months, from the history was noted to have fallen on the head at the age of six weeks having a slight fracture and being observed in hospital overnight. At the age of four months, the family was going to sue one of the major stores, because an electric point had somehow been left alive and the child had burnt his hand. The child was seen by an observant nurse from the point of view of a surgical operation and feeling that the situation was difficult, she referred the case for further investigation. One found a past history of violence within the family; the mother and father had married after pregnancy and their parents did not really approve of the marriage. In a verbal battle between the husband and his parents, physical violence ensued with his mother receiving a black eye and even a wall being battered. When the child was examined, marks were found on both forearms indicating how tightly elastic bands had been placed around them. If nothing else, these were enough indicators of the fact that the background was a difficult one and that this young couple needed help. The Children's Aid were notified. The family doctor refused to accept that this could be a battering family and the Children's Aid,

not getting support from him, despite the offered support of other professionals, continued to visit the family, but within three months the visiting ceased.

3. Another case, a boy of eleven, presented with school difficulties. In taking his past history it was seen that at one year he was scalded, at two years he took tablets and was admitted because of poisoning, at four years he fractured his leg, at six years he fractured his clavicle, at seven years he fractured his humerus and at nine years he fractured his wrist. This was in the context of a mother who was not very bright and a father who was abusive and alcoholic. The boy was one of the brightest members of the family and he became virtually the head of the household on the parental separation, again indicating a very difficult situation. This reflected the missed child abuse, neglect etc., situation and presented, in the older age group, with school failure.

4. A child of 8 years was referred because he was difficult to handle and not learning. In taking the history, it was found that a previous child had been killed in a road accident. Because the history included a background of violence in disciplining, in child rearing, as well as alcoholism, the question was asked as to what was happening in the car when the crash occurred whereby this boy was killed. The mother's response was to look up and say; 'yes, it was our fault. We (my husband and I) were quarrelling in the car and had been fighting previously. Things were very difficult, and always had been so. I believe it is our fault that the child died.' She subsequently divorced her husband.

5. A boy of 5 referred because in school he was very active and would not sit still. He did not seem to be working well with other children. Within a very short time, the maternal background of violence and the paternal background of alcoholism presented itself, but in this instance the mother said that both she and her husband had felt that they were wanting in parenting skills, and had decided that they would try and seek help to become better parents. The backgrounds were exactly the same, the mode of discipline in this house was via a belt, which created marks on the children, but the mother did not consider that this was bad, even though she herself had hated the punishment that had been given to her. In this instance, however, the type of entry and the willingness to cooperate made it easier to arrange the various helping resources which could be given.

The follow-up of abused children

For any programme to be considered, we have to know something about the follow-up of abused children[117]. Lynch's paper discusses a five year follow-up, from the family unit in Oxford, Britain, and highlighted the difficulties of carrying out a long-term follow-up, in terms of the inability to locate; adoption and inability to obtain the names of the adoptive parents; the deceased, the institutionalized; distances to be covered; the refusals and uncooperative parents. Despite this, a large number were located but interestingly enough, there is no report on what exactly was found. In Australia, the Birrells[118] were unable to locate 33% of their 42 children after 2 years. Friedman and Morse[119] were unable to trace 25% of 54 injured children. Of 88 children, McRae[82] located 39% only, that is to say 34 cases – 18 were lost, 8 were dead, 4 were institutionalized and 26 refused or lived too far away, or failed to attend. Gregg[120] found of 50 children, 19, that is 28%, were not available for evaluation. Smith wrote[121] that no study has convincingly shown that any treatment of battering parents is effective. In fact, all of the studies are poor in terms of assessment of outcome (including the Denver study)[122]. One has still seen that in individual cases, where adequate input has been given even to very serious cases of neglect and abuse, good end results can be obtained[123-125].

Illustrative case

A child's X-rays showed fractures of both upper arms, the differential diagnosis being scurvy or child abuse. Whilst scurvy does represent a possible differential diagnosis, clinically there is rarely a real problem[126]. The child abuse part was real although not admitted. The father came from a home where he was deprived in terms of communication and affection, beaten in terms of restriction to almost anything that happened and a mother and father who drank and related very badly to one another. He had a very poor self-image of himself, communicated poorly and expressed himself poorly. The mother belonged to a family of 8 children, all of whom had had very poor relationships with one another and with their parents. Drunkenness was present and from the age of 12 years, this girl went out to work, regarding this to be very normal, even on the Canadian scene. Discipline was of a very strict order. Love and feelings normally flowing between members of any family, was minimal. When seen, the mother presented a frozen appearance, appearing to be quite ugly and emitting tremendous anger. An initial contract was achieved by laying down very clearly what the exact problems were and how they had come about. This involved the social worker seeing the parents weekly, arranging for the parents to go daily with the child to a suitable foster home as well as regular medical supervision of all facets. Within a very short time it was seen that this arrangement was not working. After confrontation (with empathy and love, but with firmness), it was arranged that the child would leave the parental home to live in a good foster home. The mother went to the same foster home every morning, the father and mother went each night. At the weekends they also visited and related with the foster parents. A great deal of anger was shown by both parents who initially were very loath to get involved. However, a good relationship developed with the foster mother and father and gradually the relationships and the interpersonal problems were dealt with. Over the weeks to months, improvement occurred. At the end of 9 months the child returned home for weekends and then in a further few months returned home permanently. The mother ceased to be ugly and became what she was basically, a very

beautiful girl. The parents learned to relate to one another, to expect appropriately of the child and to ask for help prior to a crisis. They became much
better social and community individuals. An important but in some ways tragic
event occurred in the foster home. The foster mother's children brought her
some wild flowers as a present on her birthday and the mother gave equal
prominence to this as to other very expensive presents. The 'abusing mother'
said that for the first time she began to realize what it was that a mother should
do and be and that this feeling had never been given or shown to her by her
parents. I think this does indicate that help can be given and that the possibility of so doing is real.

Child and parents needs

What is needed so that we can give in this type of situation? In any syndrome case, the needs of the child have to be paramount and may therefore
have to be looked at in the context of:

(a) Removal from the parental home and placing in a foster home.
(b) Using therapeutic foster parents. Here the foster parents could come to
    the parental home, to help the real parents handle their child or children,
    daily acting as models, not by didactic training, but by examining the
    alternatives available for any situation and showing how they would
    handle the difficulties of a child's life, no matter what the provocation
    might be.
(c) Adoption, which must be considered.
(d) The use of a day care centre or a nursery school for the child.

There is a need to look carefully at such centres and check that personnel are
adequately trained, not only because they have done the requisite courses, but
also because as people they are experts at handling babies and children as a
result of their own good experiences.

One of the prerequisites, then, of gaining mothering and fathering skills,
would be to have available a 'fostering parent or grandparent' within the family. This could well subserve other needs, in that there are many people aged 60
and over, who are vegetating in nursing homes who have given of themselves
very adequately to their own children and are still capable of giving love and
affection. Mothers and fathers could go to day care centres, but not to the
routine day care centres where people have been trained to be child care
workers but where they may not have been screened for their ability to give, in
the sense of being adequate parents[127].

(e) Providing a therapeutic home maker, namely somebody who will go into
    the parental home and help the parents look at the various deficits.
    Pragmatically the mother may need to be taught how to budget, how to
    cook, but more than that how to react and relate to ongoing needs.

Similarly, a community aid might be of value in this context.

GENERAL NEEDS

(a) *Parenting model needs*

Since so many of these families have had very poor paradigms, this would seem to be the biggest single need of fathers and mothers. Eventually this may prove to be the most fruitful area for producing change within the family (although it may still prove as frustrating as the very expert social work and medical input has tended to be). Maybe the most hopeful and helpful role can be played by the 'community professional' – trained in life for the job, being a mature, capable, self-sufficient person able to care for a helpless, needy, dependent, immature individual. He or she must also impart the 'practical' or 'mechanical' basic ingredients of feeding, clothing, holding, cleaning (the infant), protecting from harm and providing motility for the infant. Along with these can be shown the more subtle ingredients of tenderness, awareness and considerations of the needs and desires of the infant and of appropriate emotional interaction with it. This ordinary mother and father should be known and judged by the teacher in the local school who has seen all the children coming through, by the public health nurse, the minister, the family doctor and the neighbours, to have brought up their own children in a praiseworthy manner. In rediscovering the value of people (as foster parents or foster grandparents) to the parents in trouble, as well as the child, a means of showing people how to parent by example can be initiated. A real effort can be made to find peers from the same socioeconomic group, possibly ethnic, possibly age group, who might act in this capacity. Efforts could be made using the public health nurses to find the effective people in any street, in any community who would and could help their neighbours. The financial inducements would not need to be of the order of social workers or other paraprofessionals input ... but the yield might be greater.

(b) *Day care centres*

It has long been suggested that schools should become community centres as some churches are at present. This would be the beginning of initiating an increase in the present numbers of such centres, allowing sufficient numbers for young parents with their first, second or even third children to get some relief at times of stress. By setting a centre in the school, a programme of child growth and development, learning the skills of responsibility to and for others, could be included in an educational programme so that all grades in the school could relate and be involved to this area. This might help replace some of the missing extended family teaching which is ceasing to be a feature of present day life. Thus, using elderly members of society (as well as community professionals), male or female, people who have a great deal of skill can be used and made to feel valuable in society.

(c) *Infant stimulation programmes*

As an adjunct to (b), the development of infant stimulation programmes to include handicapped children from birth to 2–3 years of age, so that parents in difficulties (emotional and other) can receive help and learn from the examples being shown.

(d) *Family therapy*

Family therapy for the parents using an identified member of the Unit when agreed upon by the primary therapist from the Community Team (who may be the Unit therapist).

(e) *Individual therapy*

Individual therapy for one or other, or both parents, sometimes the child or sibling in the family.

(f) *Day nursery centre*

Where the mother can go with the child and partake in the caretaking, and learning how to handle anger, fear, isolation etc.

(g) *Group therapy*

For single parents, mothers, parents.

With removal of the child to a place of safety:
1. Temporarily to hospital for assessment and/or
2. to a foster home, ideally where foster parents have been helped to look at the problems involved, the battering of the parents as well as the battering of the child (children). Ideally, again, the child's parents should be allowed adequate daily visiting so that the loving part of the relationship could be allowed to grow while the negative 'hating' part can be dealt with.
3. *Permanent removal*, if danger on returning home can never be removed.
4. Allowing the child to go back home with arrangements for:
   (i) *Foster parents/grandparents/volunteer community aides* to visit daily to help by showing (not by taking over) what difficulties can be dealt with.
   (ii) *Visiting home makers* to help parents look at alternatives available in budgeting, cooking, cleaning pragmatically in the home, whilst adding to parenting skills. At the same time, parenting skills to be added to in day care centre, nursery school, kindergarten, etc.

(iii) *Social worker* to help to coordinate activities for the parents to aid their communication pattern, discipline concepts, problem solving etc.

It is important that gains should be measured in small amounts so that expectations of success will be looked at in terms of months rather than days or weeks.

Table 10.2 The outcome in missed syndrome cases

Problems	Behavioural difficulties, stealing, aggression, acting out, running away	Routine – retardation, family difficulties, physical handicap, developmental delay
Age range	5–15 yrs.	0–15 yrs
Referral source	Community agencies	physicians, teachers, parents
Number of cases	120	150
Family violence (present)	50%	60%
Alcoholism	45%	40%
Suicide attempts	8.5%	2%
Abuse, neglect, deprivation (in past history)	60%	50%

In studies of Hamilton[135], Table 10.2 refers to cases seen at a centre evaluating and treating problems involving brain, behaviour, special senses and rehabilitation. This tends to suggest that early signs and symptoms of child abuse, neglect and deprivation are not being recognized and past histories of poisoning, fractures, bruises, scalds and injuries are being ignored. The above are usually regarded as reflecting family dysfunction by social worker, psychiatrist and paediatrician and nurturing and child rearing habits not appreciated. These findings reflect those of Steele and Hopkins[136] where with 100 delinquents, 84% had been abused before the age of 6 years and 92% in the previous year or so prior to apprehension. It is not surprising, in view of the above findings, that no study or documentation has been made of problems associated with rehabilitation or the return of the child to its original home after initial diagnosis and therapy for the abusing family.

PREDICTION AND PREVENTION OF CHILD ABUSE, NEGLECT AND DEPRIVATION

Can we predict and prevent child abuse and hence deal with this worldwide hazard? Kempe[128] speaks of the health visitor as being someone who can help to predict child abuse and to prevent this. His health visitor is a little different from the English health visitor, in that she will not be a nurse beforehand but in many ways resembles the community professional parent. In that context she may be very helpful. One wonders, however, whether that type of person, if good, could not be much better used as a paradigm and model rather than in terms of the predictions which could be carried out by people with less overall therapeutic skills.

Questionnaire and approach

More appropriately problems of prediction should be commenced antenatally. In a given population, we could do antenatal questionnaires (on the lines of the Kempe questionnaires[129], in terms of how they relate to the needs of the child in hospital and what they expect from the child) bearing in mind their past family and rearing histories.

The Denver group[130] have now a four year study, following up the use of antenatal and perinatal evaluations producing a high-risk group. This was divided into two groups; to one being given normal paediatric and maternity care, and to the other special attention from paediatricians and specially trained non-medical workers who visited families and helped care for the babies. After about $3\frac{1}{2}$ years they found no abused children in the control group (i.e. a third group outside the high-risk group) but there were cases of child abuse in the other two groups. The more serious cases were found among the risk families who had not received special attention.

This approach can be extrapolated into a total questionnaire approach for all people having their babies in hospital (which in North America means almost everyone) and evaluate them using criteria, during their hospital stay and post-natally[131-134].

Nuclear family

Since the nuclear family is our major focus in the syndrome, hence the need for prophylaxis, the widespread disturbance in parenting and the fragmentation of families in North America suggest the need for re-examination of medical practices that effect the involvement of parents with their children[137]. Maternity hospital teams have denied the need or the capacity of the neonate for social interaction or for initiation of parent–infant involvement. The work of Spitz[138], Bowlby[139] and Ainsworth[140] showed certainly with institutionalization and otherwise, that babies need intimate involvement with other human beings for their immediate survival as well as for their long term emotional health. The interactions promote social stimulation, protection from pain or danger and satisfaction of physical needs. Neonates still recognize and prefer their own mother, recognize smell, will selectively turn to a breast at 6 to 10 days and may be upset by an unusual maternal appearance or behaviour. Thus, through both preference and avoidance behaviour, the infant indicates recognition of the mother's familiar presence, odour, appearance and behaviour.

Mother–infant interactions

The capacities for mothers and newborn infants for social interactions evolved over many centuries, when infant care practices were vastly different from those of contemporary industrialized society. Thus, feeding has been an invariable feature of infant care. Until this century an infant was unlikely to survive without a lactating mother (and it may still be so in many parts of the world). Elaborate anatomical, physiological and behavioural adaptations of breast feeding have developed over the long courses of evolution in both mother and infant. Nowadays the infant is provided with nutrition, temperature regulation, protection, early education and social stimulation, outside the mother–infant relationship. The carrying pattern has been replaced by the resting or caching pattern. Infants spend little time in contact with the caregiver, are fed at 2–4 hourly intervals and are laid horizontally out of sight for many hours. Maternity hospital practices interfere with breast feeding and early maternal affection[141], by routine post-partum separation which may disrupt the mothers, especially when there is a problem (prematurity, malformation, inexperience, emotional disturbance or social isolation). The relationship is even more susceptible to early disruption[132,142,143].

Intrapartum medication, delayed nursing, separating mother and infants, providing supplementary bottles, enforced 4 hour schedules, weighing babies before and after nursing, excluding fathers and giving little support to the breast-feeding mother, all impair breast feeding. This is not to deny that good attachment can occur with artificial feeding, but the modern practice which has imposed a pattern of early separation of mother and neonate certainly can interfere with the attachment situation, especially in mothers at risk. Harlow's studies[144] of young rhesus monkeys indicate that love derives mainly from close bodily contact. In our perinatal care in the maternity hospital we have to be aware of this and be on the lookout for signs of non-bonding but more than that, be sure that the negative input from the hospital experience will not add to an already negative situation. If the parents already have difficulties in terms of their relationship, if they are badly in need of help in their parenting abilities, if they have many problems with life and living, if there are many feelings of inadequacy and even fear of what might happen, then the maternity hospital attitude can be enough to deviate the parents from positive attachment and can negatively detach them. Further difficult situations occur in infants at environmental risk consequent to depriving life experiences, infants manifesting early-appearing aberrant behaviour related to diagnosed medical disorders, and those at biological risk as determined by increased probability for delayed or aberrant development as a consequence of biological insult.

Infants at risk (biological environmental)

The categories of risk are not naturally exclusive and the determining elements of each case can, and often do, occur in interaction to still further increase the degree of, or probability for, delayed or aberrant development for many children. Sources of such interaction are readily evident. They are found in the biologically vulnerable premature and low-birth-weight infants born to adolescent mothers, themselves living in and victims of poverty. They occur in the placement, in infancy, of Down's syndrome infants in the impersonal care of some custodial institutions. They are manifest in the hearing-impaired infant born into a poverty-stricken home deficient in language stimulation, without systematic health care and without knowledge of and motivation to seek corrective resources. They function subtly in affluent homes in which an infant's early problem is met by low parental involvement, non-acceptance and withdrawal of relationship by the parents. In these and other conditions, the synergistic interaction of environmental with biological risk factors serves to further limit the infant's cognitive and non-cognitive development, confounds early diagnosis and poses unique and difficult problems for early corrective intervention. The interactions of environmental and biological risk factors that act to limit the development of established and biological risk infants are pervasive. Precipitated by early developmental flaws, they are often found sequentially in the life of a child to establish interactive patterns that systematically act to diminish his developmental potential and opportunities for normal life experiences. Thus, as can occur, a newborn infant made vulnerable by biological insult from a faulty pregnancy, experiences separation from the mother for intensive newborn care. Returned to the mother with altered and deviant behavioural capabilities, the infant is unresponsive to the mother, who cannot interpret his altered behaviour and therefore does not respond appropriately to his signals of need[145,146]. There may follow then a failure of mother and child to communicate effectively, and the synchrony of their behaviour necessary to optimal development may not be established. Sensing mutual rejection, each withdraws from the relationship, still further diminishing opportunities for their positive interaction to guide the child's development and with the necessary background may lead to the syndrome of child abuse, neglect and deprivation.

'Native' population

In Canada, we have a further problem in the context of child abuse relating to the 'native' population. Many Indians have lost their craft and hunting skills etc., many are on reservations where the amount of work that they can do is minimal and with more frustration and boredom, together with subsidies, many turn to drink. In this sort of atmosphere it is not surprising that a great deal of abuse goes on. The amount of extended family input tends to partially counteract this, nevertheless it is undoubtedly quite a problem and, with an inadequate number of social agencies, social workers, doctors etc., the total syndrome situation is difficult to annotate.

With regard to Eskimos, whilst they maintained their original nomadic style, work problems were less obvious, but with the advent of an urban type of existence, reduced work, reduced stimulation for life and living, again a similar abuse problem is seen (as well as in the Meti population). Accurate figures are not easily obtained, perhaps being less accurate even than in other segments of society (1% in care and 3.4% not living at home in one area)[147]. However, even with slight problems, many children are taken into care, so that relatively greater numbers of Indian children are in care at a particular time, relative to other population groups[148].

Since many youngsters do leave the villages to get adequate education, it is probable that the situation mimics what has been said to occur among the Indian population of Arizona, USA. There, when youngsters left the parental home for education and later returned after being educated, since they were unable to get adequate jobs and careers, they became disillusioned and disgruntled, and started to drink. Apparently at the same time, child abuse was seen. It was said that child abuse had been unknown in this area prior to the initiation of this external educational scheme[149].

Incest

Looking at the area of incest, as part of the child abuse, neglect and deprivation syndrome (which indeed it is), here too we see how so many members of society blind themselves to the events occurring. It has been suggested that 3.9% of the average population of North America has experienced incest and so has some 13.1% of the prison population with a probable incidence generally of 200 per million. Yet, the number of cases that are reported are minimal and even when these are looked at from psychiatric or psychosocial viewpoints methods of therapy are adopted which seem to be superficial. In a report[150], Ingrid Cooper of Montreal suggested that if it were father–daughter incest (as in the majority of situations), separation of the father and child either by taking the child or the father out of the home for a limited period of time, then engaging the family, resulted in 'cure'. The emphasis seemed to be on the amount of recidivism qua sexual abuse without much looking at the family problems initiating the event. Yet precipitating situations, the return after separation after a long time of a husband, the loss of spouse by divorce, separation or death, overcrowding, alcoholism, physical proximity, poverty, rural isolation, intellectual inferiority, personality disorders, marital stress, disharmony and lack of control are known concomitants of the problem, which did not seem to be dealt with. A report by Manchester[151] gave much of the legal views, numbers etc. but again, in terms of how to deal with the total situation little was forthcoming. Another speaker at the same conference, Bluglass[152] gave a historical viewpoint showing the life history of incest within society with some expression of doubt as to whether harm was done to the individual. Once more we see that the denial of the problem, with concepts of child fantasy as a part of the taboo, is common to teachers, social workers, school clinic doctors and psychiatrists[153]. We see how the definition, annotation and precision surrounding an event is looked at but the follow-up and dealing with it is almost cursory[154].

To understand child abuse and to help in dealing with it, one has to reflect with Gil who writes of the serious obstacles to understanding the syndrome and to effective intervention, where people have little belief in social problems as other than isolated fragmented phenomena, rather than as consequences of the societal context in which they evolve and as related to, and interacting with, other social problems generated in the same societal context[155]. He points out that 'explanatory dimensions frequently tend to correspond to the academic discipline or to the professional field of the investigation rather than the multidimensional nature of the phenomena. We are thus caught up in the short term immediate handling of the result and the long term attempt to vent and to give prophylaxis.'

Long term prevention of child abuse really relates to the family as a unit, the family within society and the world itself. Unless there are going to be changes, not only from a country but from a world point of view, to expect that there will be changes within the family is perhaps unreal. Politics, economics, comprehensive education, decent housing, cultural and recreational facilities, comprehensive health care and social services, all of these undoubtedly have roles to be reflected in societal terms and political activism.

However, we can look at a model whereby one may be able to better annotate people at varying stages of their lives and would like to suggest one such model (very similar to the described Kempe model in Denver).

1. *The antenatal area* – perhaps a questionnaire approach[129] to high-risk families. Especially in areas where almost the whole population has a baby in hospital.

Such questionnaires[156] would include personal, family history of life event, life lines, illnesses and attachment concepts, the aim being to anticipate the high-risk family in the context of child abuse, neglect and deprivation[157,158]. Such parents-to-be could then be approached and perhaps provided with life lines of supports which can be described more fully in the post-natal period[159-161].

2. *The perinatal area* – the delivery room and post-delivery observation area should be used to see how people tend to attach and to use the sort of guidelines developed by Klaus[132] and others[162,163] of assessing mother–father interactions and mother–father–child reactions. Always there is a need to assess the three elements in the syndrome, (a) the parental characteristics, (b) the possible initiating factors in the child, (c) the environmental precipitating events.

Babies born prematurely or with congenital abnormalities and other defects can be looked at and in the context of these observations necessary supports can be added. The antenatal high-risk annotation can then be added to the perinatal high-risk observations, to be succeeded by:

3. *Post-natal follow up.* Here, one can use the public health nurse with her skills to relate to the mother on a regular basis. The skills expected from her will be that of assessment of the family ability to parent, the parent–child relationship that has been established, screening for developmental status (the type of surroundings), advice on common well-child problems and nutrition, knowledge of the community and liaison with available health resources and life supports.

The Kempe concept of the health visitor[164] could be extrapolated to the professional mother (as described before) with people who have been annotated to be at risk. This professional mother (to repeat, assessed by the teacher, neighbour, doctor, minister, public health nurse) can be added to the repertoire available to the mother antenatally, perinatally and post-natally.

In addition, social work input should be available so that the intrapsychic, intrapersonal, interpersonal problems and marriage problems can be dealt with and proper case work be done[165]. Making sure that knowledgeable and trained people are making use of their proper skills, rather than as an overall helper, one person might be expected to carry out all functions including being seen as an 'agent of change' in the therapy life of people and trying to understand the compelling, frightening, conscious and unconscious hatred within the parent that is seeking an outlet. In this context, one would then be able to see what are the needs of the various families with whom we are dealing and whether we respond to their parenting and psychosocial needs etc.

To this we would add the possibility of having infant stimulation programmes from birth to 2, where parents in difficulties as well as handicapped children can go, be part of a group and see how 'professional mothers' and child care workers and others handle children (emphasizing, in every instance, that the types of workers used have to really know about parenting and preferably be good parents themselves). Day care centres from 2 years[166] until 4–5 years, even from birth, arranging then for the mother, father too if possible, to go in on a daily basis and partake in the total process, so that they can absorb the types of skills that are needed. In cases diagnosed as very severe cases, in which the child being at home can be more than a difficulty, the possibility of foster parents, grandparents, volunteer and community visiting or living in or vice versa would also be evaluated.

In the context of the neighbourhood, to take up empty classrooms in the schools, within the churches etc. and to develop neighbourhood groups, with the professional mother as the guide, teacher, etc. using other agencies (Family Service agencies, Children's Aid social workers) to act as the coordinators and individual and family therapists. With regard to the day nursery (crisis relief) centre where the mother can take the child and leave him there for a part of the day, this is necessary, but if regarded as a major part of the answer, then it is a further denial of the malignancy of the family problems. This feeds into the concept that parents are alright, it is only when things get overwhelming that they batter their children. To me, this is an inappropriate concept. Whilst there is need for a place for parents who have little in the way of extended family or community support, to leave their children while they go shopping etc., or if indeed a syndrome situation is present, they need much more than that.

A lot of money is being expended by the Ministry at federal and provincial level, to provide programmes designed to involve parents and prospective parents in discussions, meetings, courses on child rearing and training. There is no doubt that these programmes will be of value, but one has to resist the suggestion that one can talk people through their life-long problems of not being able to parent, to relate and handle life. This is of value in the minimal situation where people need some support but to have the concept that this is of maximal value other than as an adjunct to a full programme of individual support, family support etc. on a day to day basis is erroneous. This reflects our long established beliefs that someone can enter a household once a week and monitor the members and then 'everything will be alright'.

Parents Anonymous

Let us look at the Parents Anonymous groups. In many instances they have themselves been battering parents. How then can one believe that their input can be other than at a superficial level? In many ways, if people can pick up a telephone and talk to someone else, they have enough strength, perhaps, not to batter their child. More important than that is the question of whether they are going to batter their child, not just do they feel like it, but are they of that type of material in terms of their upbringing etc. If the latter is real then the anonymous situation is untenable in its present implications. The appeal of Parents Anonymous no doubt results from the many inadequacies in our present ways of offering help to abusing parents. Anonymity suggests the problem being still viewed as a moral issue. Parents also appreciate its openness and honesty, easy accessibility in crisis and finding concrete 'do-it-now' approaches. These parents once more have to be brought into the total therapeutic milieu and guided to appropriate channels[167]. Many of these superficial approaches attempt to bring a 'touch of help' to a situation, which requires very powerful and long-term medicine. One can equate this help with giving an aspirin for a pneumonia which really requires antibiotics. We have to set up within hospitals, child abuse teams, within community child abuse teams, with proper disposal systems and proper lines of communications and very active involvement with the courts so that one can realistically assess what can be done. Time and time again it is being said that all those involved with this problem need to know the various facets of the problem and not to sit bureaucratically with corridor or tunnel vision.

There may be a need to set up a separate admitting procedure whereby the whole family can be taken into care, their needs adequately assessed and a follow-up community health programme available which can deal with problems. Any family 'syndrome' needs to be assessed in terms of its communication patterns, problem solving skills, effective expression, role behaviour and role expectations, autonomy and behavioural controls[168].

The following are some of the difficulties in setting up effective inter-disciplinary action:

1. The lack of understanding by the members of one discipline of the conceptual basis, aims and objectives, standards and ethics of the others.
2. The lack of effective communication from members of one discipline to members of another.
3. The lack of clarity in allocating management responsibility to what group, at which time.
4. Professional chauvinism (doctor to social worker, public health nurse to agency etc.).
5. A sense of despair and hopelessness in the face of overwhelming problems, unsympathetic colleagues and too large case loads.
6. Institutional relationships limiting interprofessional contact (hospitals competing for prestige and patients).
7. Prevailing attitudes and public policy about child abuse.
8. Lack of trust and confidence between personnel from one profession and colleagues from another.
9. Cultural isolation of professional personnel (white professionals to blacks, minority families, middle class social workers).

We can arrive at some axioms of child abuse management:

1. An injured or neglected child on diagnosis is at great risk for re-injury or continued neglect.
2. A principal goal of initial intervention is the protection of the child but a programme for help to the family is essential for the crisis and follow-up.
3. Traditional social work in itself cannot protect a battered, neglected or deprived child in the basic environment. Medical follow-up and other contracts are necessary to encourage a healthy mileu.
4. If the child is re-injured, the parents are likely to seek care at a different facility.
5. In social service agencies the number of adequately trained personnel, the quality of administrative and supervisory functions all militate against effective operations especially when carried out in isolation from other care providing agencies.
6. Prolonged search for the exact agents of the injury and the minutiae of the 'facts' can be done only at the expense of the relationship and therapy.
7. Lack of evidence of parental guilt is not a criterion for discharge of the patient or family.
8. With a young child, at major risk, hospitalization to allow time for assess-

ment is very appropriate especially in the case of fractures, burns, bruises, scalds, drowning (or near drowning), or failure to thrive[169].

Involvement with abusing families teaches that early childhood experiences can lead to psychopathic states leading to child abuse; the abused have personality traits, perhaps difficult to differentiate from those of people in general[170]. Emotionally abandoned children develop character traits and the psychologically abandoned develop poor control. The physical punishment itself may lead to neurological states, mental retardation and death[171,172].

Just as terrible, children who hate are the children of neglect, having been chronically traumatized[173].

The future

We need to set up programmes to educate the public as well as all relevant professionals to the existence and nature of the syndrome and how to act upon the knowledge. We need to use all available media and resources – television, radio and the print media.

Most of all, we need to see that we do not end with a procedure which is highly organized but therapeutic outcomes which are superficial, sterile and do more for the professionals with vested interests – doctors, social workers, teachers, nurses, lawyers and judges – than for the families in dire distress. We need not to dissipate our resources of money, professionals and perhaps most importantly of caring human beings. We need to share in 'a more optimistic approach to child abuse'[174]. We need to understand that the causal dimensions of child abuse include the dominant social philosophy and value premises of a society, the socio-economic and political institutions shaped by its philosophy and values and the quality of human relations to which these institutions, philosophy and values give rise. Other causal dimensions are the social construction of childhood and the social definitions of children's rights; the extent to which a society sanctions the use of force in general and more specifically in the child rearing context; stress and frustration resulting from poverty and from alienation in the work place which may trigger abusive acts and expression of intrapsychic conflict and psychopathology which in turn are rooted in the social fabric.

The primary prevention of child abuse would require fundamental changes in social philosophy and value premises, in societal institutions and in human relations. It would also require a reconceptualization of childhood, of children's rights and of child rearing. It would necessitate rejecting the use of force as a means of achieving societal ends, especially in dealing with children.

It would require the elimination of poverty and of alienating conditions of production, of major sources of stress and frustration which tend to trigger abusive acts towards children in adult/child interaction. It would necessitate the elimination of psychological illness.

References

1. Anthony, E. J. (1973). The Syndrome of the Psychologically Invulnerable Child, Lambie Dew Oration, Oct. 1973, University of Sydney, School of Medicine
2. Mulvihill, D. J., Tumin, M. and Curtis, L. A. (1969). The interpersonal relationship between victim and offender. *Crimes of Violence* Vol. 2, Washington D.C. Superintendent of Documents, US Government Printing Office
3. Orville, G. B., Jr. (1975). Macrostructural influences on child development and the need for childhood social indicators. *Am. J. Orthopsychiat.*, **45**, 516
4. Kempe, H. C. (1955). Family intervention, the right of all children. *Pediatrics*, **56**, 693
5. Freud, A. (1975). On Receiving the C. Anderson Aldrich Award. *Am. Acad. Pediatrics*, **56**, 332
6. Storr, A. (1977). Keynote Address, 2nd World Congress of the International Society on Family Law, 'Violence in the Family' Montreal, June 1977
7. Radhbill, Samuel X. (1968). A history of child abuse and infanticide. In: *The Battered Child*, C. H. Kempe and R. A. Helfer (ed.). (Chicago: University of Chicago Press)
8. Fontana, V. J. (1964). *The Maltreated Child, The Maltreatment Syndrome in Children.* (Springfield: Charles C. Thomas)
9. Langer, W. L. (1974). Infanticide – A historical survey. *Hist. Childh. Q.*, **1**, 353
10. Olmesdahl, M. C. J. (1977). The extent and limits of parental authority in Roman and African customary law, 2nd World Conference of the International Society on Family Law 'Violence in the Family'. Montreal, June 1977
11. Stern, E. S. (1948). The Medea Complex. *J. Ment. Sci.*, **94**, 324
12. Butler, S. (1612–1680). *Hudibras*, Pt. 1, Ch. 3, **1**, 844
13. Salk, L. and Kramer, R. (1973). *How to Raise a Human Being*, Paperback Library.
14. Gordon, T. (1970). *Parent Effectiveness Training, The No-lose Programme for Raising Responsible Children.* (New York: P. H. Wyden)
15. Spock, B. (1974). *Raising Children in a Difficult Time.* (New York: W. W. Norton and Co. Inc.)
16. Fleming, K. and Fleming, A. T. (1976). *The First Time Interview with Dr Benjamin Spock*, p. 254. (New York: Berkeley Medallion Books)
17. Shaw, G. B. (1945). *Everybody's Political What's What.* (London: Constable)
18. Homan, W. E. (1970). *Child Sense.* (Toronto: Bantam Books)
19. Steinmetz, S. K. and Strauss, M. A. (1974). *Society*, **10**, 50
20. Shaw, A. (1973). Dilemma of 'Informed Consent' in Children. *N. Engl. J. Med.*, 885
21. Ardrey, R. (1974). *The Social Contract.* (Dell)
22. Mead, M. A. (1962). A cultural anthropologist's approach to maternal deprivation, In: *Deprivation of Maternal Care: A Reassessment of its Effects.* (Geneva: World Health Organization)
23. Lystad, M. H. (1975). Violence at home – A review of the literature. *Am. J. Orthopsychiat.*, **45**, 328
24. Winnicott, D. W. (1957). *The Child and the Family.* (London: Tavistock Publications)
25. Winnicott, D. W. (1957). *The Child and the Outside World.* (London: Tavistock Publications)
26. Williams, C. D. and Jelliffe, D. B. (1972). *Mother and Child Health* (Oxford)
27. Royal Commission on Violence in the Communications Industry, Interim Report. (1976). Toronto, Ontario, Canada
28. *The Globe and Mail*, September 24th, 1977
29. Child Abuse and Neglect, Standing Committee on Health, Welfare and Social Affairs, First Session 30th Parliament, 1974–75–76, July 7, 1976
30. The Mondale Bill, Child Abuse Prevention and Treatment Act of 1973
31. Greenland, C. (1973). *Child Abuse in Ontario*, Ontario Ministry of Community and Social Services, Research and Planning Branch, November 1973

32. Kempe, C. H., Silverman, F. N., Steele, B. F., Droegemueller, W. and Silver, H. K. (1962). The Battered Child Syndrome. *J. Am. Med. Assoc.*, **181,** 17

33. Newberger, E. H. *et al.* (1973). 'Trauma X', *Ped.*, **51,** 840

34. The Battered Child, Annual Council Meeting of the National Society for the Prevention of Cruelty to Children (1968) London, UK

35. Kempe, C. H. (1971). Pediatric implications of the battered baby syndrome. *Arch. Dis. Childh,* **46,** 28

36. Kempe, C. H. (1969). The Battered child and the Hospital. *Hospital Practice,* **44,** 44

37. Kempe, C. H. (1973). A practical approach to the protection of the abused child and rehabilitation of the abusing parents. *Pediatrics,* **56,** Suppl. 804

38. Caffey, J. (1972). The parent–infant traumatic stress syndrome. *Am J. Roentgenol.,* **114,** 218

39. Kempe, C. H. and Helfer, R. E. (1972). *Helping the Battered Child and his Family.* (Philadelphia: J. B. Lippincott Co.)

40. Jacobs, J. (1976). Child abuse, neglect, deprivation and the family syndrome, Child AND Family Syndrome, Mental Health Committee, Canadian Pediatric Society

41. Gil, D. (1970). *Violence Against Children; Physical Child Abuse in the United States.* (Cambridge, Mass.: Harvard University Press)

42. Bullard, D. *et al.* (1976). Failure to thrive in the neglected child. *Am. J. Orthopsychiat.,* **37,** 680

43. Morris, M., Gould, R. and Matthews, P. (1964). Towards prevention of child abuse. *Children,* 55

44. Young, L. (1964). *Wednesday's Children; A Study of Child Neglect and Abuse.* (New York: McGraw-Hill)

45. Polsky, N. (1969). *Hustlers, Beats and Others.* (New York: Anchor Books)

46. Fontana, V. J., Donovan, D. and Wong, R. G. (1963). The maltreatment syndrome in children. *N. Engl. J. Med.,* **269,** 1389

47. Tabiban, Y. (1969). 'Les enfants victimes de s'evictes', *Med. Hyg.,* **27,** 272

48. Editorial (1973). Non-accidental injury in children. *Br. Med. J.,* **4,** 625

49. Franklin, A. W. (ed.) (1975). *Concerning Child Abuse.* (Edinburgh: Churchill Livingstone)

50. McCandless, B. R. and Strauss, A. A. (1943). Objective criteria (diagnostic of deviant personality, exploratory study of accident proneness). *Am. J. Ment. Def.,* **47,** 445

51. Harrison, L. L. (1976). Nursing intervention with failure to thrive. *Am. J. Mat. Nursing and Child,* 111

52. Fischoff, J., Whitten, C. P. and Pettit, M. G. (1971). A psychiatric study of mothers and infants with growth failure, secondary to maternal deprivation. *J. Pediatr.,* 209

53. MacKeith, R. (1974). Speculation on non-accidental injury as a cause of chronic brain disorder. *Devel. Med. Child Neuro.,* **6,** 216

54. Till, K. (1968). Subdural haematoma and effusion in infancy. *Br. Med. J.,* **3,** 400

55. Aicardi, J. and Goutiere, S. F. (1971). Les epanchements sous-duraux du nourrisson. *Arch. Francais Pediatr.,* **28,** 233

56. Thompson, G. (1976). A fifth step, a report on an interprofessional seminar on child abuse, Queen's Park, Ontario, The Ministry of Community and Social Services

57. Greenland, C. and Rosenblatt, E. (1974). The home accidents and injuries study (HAIS), Ministry of Community and Social Services

58. Newberger, E. and Bourne, R. (1977). The Medicalization and Legalization of Child Abuse, 2nd World Conference of the International Society on Family Law, 'Violence in the Family', Montreal, June 1977

59. Newberger, E. and Bourne, R. (1977). Juvenile Justice Standards Project

60. Chisholm, B. (1977). Should children have rights?, Canadian Council on Children and Youth, Monograph One

61. Hepworth, H. P. (1977). The rights of children. Advocacy for a national resource, March 12–14, British Columbia

62. Fromm, E., foreword to A. S. Neill, Summerhill (1960). *A Radical Approach to Child Rearing*. (New York: Hart Publishing Co.)

63. Greenland, C. (1970). Violence and dangerous behaviour associated with mental illness; Prospects for prevention, The Annual Meeting of the John Howard Society, Saskatoon

64. Oettinger, K. (1970). The Abused Child. *Sciences*, **10**: 5, and 29

65. Sanders, R. W. (1972). Resistance of dealing with parents of battered children. *Pediatrics*, **50**, 6, 852

66. Corbett, J. T. (1962). A psychiatrist reviews the battered child syndrome and mandatory reporting legislation. *Northwest Med.*, **63**, 920

67. LeBourdais, E. (1972). Look Again. *Canadian Hospital*, **49**, 1

68. Silver, L. B. *et al.* (1967). Child Abuse Laws – Are they enough? *J. Am. Med. Assoc.*, **199**, 101

69. Hepworth, H. P. (1977). Child abuse a national perspective, Child Welfare League of America, North West Region Conference, Calgary, Alberta

70. Tellier, J. (1976). La protection des enfants soumis a des mauvais traitements – une nouvelle legislation au Quebec, 10th Congress I.D.E.F., Paris

71. Department of Health and Social Security Home Office. (1976). Non-accidental injury to children; the police and case conferences, LASSL 1976, 25 A.C. 50 Home Office Circular, p. 179

72. Park, E. A. (1935). Preface to the first edition of Kanner, L. *Child Psychiatry* (Thomas)

73. Eisenberg, L. (1967). The relationship between psychiatry and pediatrics, a disputatious view. *Pediatrics*, **39**, 645

74. Moghadam, J. (1974). The rare and the plentiful – a dilemma in pediatric manpower. *Can. Med. Assoc. Mon.* (March 2, 1974)

75. Clinic Proceedings Children's Hospital Nat. Med. Center, **30**: 2, 46 (Feb. 1974)

76. Jacobs, J. (1976). A fifth step, a report on an interprofessional seminar on child abuse, Queen's Park, Ontario, The Ministry of Community and Social Services

77. Gelles, R. J. (1975). The social construction of child abuse. *Am. J. Orthopsychiat.*, **45**, 3, 363

78. *Canadian Newsletter*, September 1976

79. The Abused and Battered Child, Federation of Women's Teachers Association of Toronto (August 1976)

80. *Harvard Review*, **53**: 4, November 1973

81. Bell, G. (1972). Parents who Abuse their Children, Canadian Psychiatric Association, Banff, Alberta (October 1972)

82. McRae, K. N., Feguson, C. A. and Lederman, R. S. (1973). The Battered Child Syndrome. *Can. Med Assoc. J.*, **108**, 859

83. Reports of the Royal Commission of Family and Children's Law, Vancouver, B. C. (1975). Part 5, Protection of Children and Child Care

84. Fraser, F. M., Anderson, G. P. and Burns, K. (1973). Child Abuse in Nova Scotia, A Research Project about Battered and Maternally Deprived Children, Halifax, N.S.

85. Wilkerson, A. E. (1973). *Emergent Concepts in Law and Society*. (Philadelphia: Temple University Press)

86. Helfer, R. E. and Kempe, C. H. (1968). *The Battered Child*. (Cambridge, Mass.: University of Chicago Press)

87. Gardner, L. I. (1977). The Endocrinology of Abuse Dwarfism. *Am. J. Dis. Childh.*, **131**, 505

88. Pickel, S., Anderson, C. and Holliday, M. A. (1970). Thirsting and hypernatremic dehydration – a form of child abuse. *Pediatrics*, **45**, 54

89. Nixon, J. and Dearn, J. (1977). Non-accidental immersion in bath-water: another aspect of child abuse. *Br. Med. J.*, **271**, 172

90. Peterson, B. (1977). Morbidity of childhood near-drowning. *Pediatrics*, **59**: 3, 264

91. Sick Children's Hospital Toronto Report (1972)

92. Bates, R. (1976). The Pediatrician's Role, Newsletter to the Canadian Pediatric Society

93. Committee on Child Health Services. (1976). *Fit for the Future.* Vol. 1 (London: HMSO)
94. Sibert, R. (1973). Stress in families of children who have ingested poisons. *Br. Med. J.*, **1**, 87
95. Sobel, R. (1970). Psychiatric implications of accidental poisonings in childhood. *Pediatr. Clin. N. Am.*, **17**: 3, 653
96. Rogers, D., Tripp, J., Bentovin, A., Robinson, A., Berry, D. and Goudling, R. (1976). Non-accidental poisoning: an extended syndrome of child abuse. *Br. Med. J.*, **1**, 793
97. Calman, M. W. (1974). Accidental childhood poisoning. *Comm. Hlth*, **6**: 91
98. *The Globe and Mail* (July 1977)
99. Portier, P. C. (1976). *Relationship Therapy, Mental Health Counselling with Children.* (Boston: Little Brown and Co.)
100. Stephenson, P. S. (1976). Project Toddler, 10 000 miles to go. *Can. Ment. Hlth*, **24**: 4, 20
101. Goldstein, J., Freud, A. and Solnit, A. (1973). *Beyond the Best Interests of the Child* (New York: Free Press)
102. Court, J. and Kew, A. (1971). Battered child syndrome, a preventable disease. *Nursing Times*, 695
103. Epstein, N. B. (1961). Treatment of the pre-school child; A family approach. *Can. Med. Assoc. J.*, **85**, 937
104. Strauss, M. A. (1973). A general systems theory approach to a theory of violence between family members. *Soc. Sci. Inf.*, **12**: 3, 105
105. Steele, B. F. and Pollock, C. B. (1968). A psychiatric study of parents who abuse infants and small children, In: *The Battered Child*, p. 103. R. E. Helfer, and H. C. Kempe (eds.), (Cambridge, Mass.: University of Chicago Press)
106. Oliver, J. E. and Cox, J. (1973). A family kindred with ill used children – The burden on the community. *Br. J. Psychol.*, **123**, 81
107. Robertson, J. M. (1976). *Canada's Mental Health*, **24**: 4, 18
108. Blumberg, M. L. (1974). Psychopathology of the abusing parent. *Am. J. Psychother.*, **28**: 21
109. Lunch, M., Steinberg, D. and Ounstead, C. (1975). Family Unit in a Children's Psychiatric Hospital. *Br. Med. J.*, 127
110. Eisenberg, L. N. (1962). The Sins of the Fathers – Urban Decay and Social Pathology. *Am. J. Orthopsychol.*, **32**, 5
111. Wolins, M. (1969). Group Care – Friend or Foe? *Social Work*, **14**, 35
112. *The Hamilton Spectator,* Saturday, October 1, 1977
113. Cavanagh, W. E. (1975). A view from the courts. *R. Soc. Hlth J.*, **95**: 3, 153
114. Scerri, V. J. P. (1975). The Welfare of the Child. *R. Soc Hlth J.*, **95**: III, 156
115. Rubin, J. (1966). The need for intervention. *Public Welfare*, **24**: III, 230
116. Cameron, J. M., Johnson, H. R. M. and Camps, F. E. (1966). The battered child syndrome. Medicine, Science and the Law.
117. Lynch, M. A. (1977). The Follow up of Abused Children. A Researcher's Nightmare, Violence in the Family. 2nd World Conference of the International Society of Family Law, Montreal, June 1977
118. Birrell, R. G. and Birrell, J. H. W. (1968). The Maltreatment Syndrome in Children, A Hospital Survey. *Med. J. Austr.*, **2**: 1023
119. Friedman, S. B. and Morse, C. W. (1974). Child abuse: a 5 year follow up of early case findings in the Emergency Department. *Pediatrics*, **54**, 404
120. Gregg, E. E. (1967). Developmental characteristics of abused children. *Pediatrics*, **40**, 596
121. Smith, S. M. (1975). *The Battered Child Syndrome.* (London: Butterworths)
122. Morse, C. W., Sabler, O. K. Z. and Friedman, S. B. (1970). A 3-year follow up of abused and neglected children. *Am. J. Dis. Child.*, **120**, 439
123. Martin, H. P., Bezeley, P., Conway, E. S. and Kempe, C. H. (1974). The development of abused children. *Adv. Pediatr.*, **21**, 25
124. Martin, H. P. (ed.) (1976). *The Abused Child, A Multidisciplinary Approach to Developmental Issues and Treatment.* (Cambridge, Mass.: Ballinger)

125. Elmer, E. (1967). *Children in Jeopardy.* (University of Pittsburgh Press)

126. Berant, M., Aviad, I. and Jacobs, J. (1966). A 'pseudo' battered child. *Clin. Pediatr.*, **5**, 230

127. Farran, D. C. and Ramey, C. T. (1977). Infant day care and attachment behaviour toward mothers and teachers. *Chld. Devel.*, **48**: 3, 1112

128. Kempe, C. H. (1975). Predicting and preventing child abuse. Ambulatory, Pediatric Association Meeting (June 9th, 1975), Toronto, Ontario, Canada

129. Kempe, C. H. and Helfer, R. E. (1972). *Helping the Battered Child and the Family.* (Philadelphia: J. B. Lippincott Co.)

130. *The Toronto Star,* October 12th, 1977

131. Finbar, M. (1967). Family-Centered maternity program in a general hospital, Child and Family, St. Meinrad, Indiana, Summer (1967) **6**, 3

132. Klaus, M. H. and Kennell, J. H. (1970). Mothers separated from their newborn infants. *Ped. Clin. N. Am.*, **17**, 1015

133. Rich, A. (1976). *Motherhood Experience and Institution.* (McLeod)

134. Bishop, B. (1976). A guide to assessing parenting capabilities. *Am. J. Nursing*, 1784

135. Jacbos, J. (1977). Report to the Federal Government (unpublished)

136. Steele, B. F. and Hopkins, J. (1975). (quoted in C. H. Kempe, Armstrong Lecture 1975 see ref 128)

137. Lozoff, B., Brittenham, G., Traust, M. A., Kennell, J. H. and Klaus, M. H. (1977). The mother newborn relationships, limits of adaptability. *J. of Peds.*, **91**, 1

138. Spitz, O. R. (1945). Hospitalism, an enquiry into the Genesis of Psychiatric conditions in early childhood. *Psychoanalytic Study of the Child*, **1**, 53

139. Bowlby, J. (1952). *Maternal Care and Mental Health*, 2nd ed. Monograph Series 2. (Geneva: WHO)

140. Ainsworth, M. D. (1962). The effect of maternal deprivation, deprivation of maternal care, A reassessment of its effects, Public Health Papers No. 14, WHO (Geneva: WHO)

141. Jacobs, J. (1973). Children, People, and Attitudes. *Canad. J. Occupational Therapy*, **40**, 21

142. Salk, L. (1970). The critical nature of the post-partum period in the human for the establishment of the mother–infant bond. A controlled study. *Dis. Nerv. Syst.*, **31**, 110

143. Wolff, P. H. (1976). Current concepts–mother–infant interaction in the first year. *N. Engl. J. Med.*, **295**, 999

144. Harlow, H. F. (1973). Love in infant monkeys, the nature and nurture of behaviour. p. 94. *Scientific American.* (San Francisco: W. H. Freeman and Co.)

145. Brazelton, T. B. (1975). Anticipatory guidance. *Ped. Clin. N. Am.*, **22**, 533

146. Brazelton, T. B. (1976). The parent infant attachment. *Clin. Obstet. Gynecol.*, **19**, 373

147. *The Globe and Mail,* p. 18. November 9, 1977

148. Hepworth, H. P. (1977). Issues in adoption or foster care, the Canadian Council on Social Development, Child Welfare League of America, North West Region Conference (June 5–8th, 1977) Calgary, Alberta

149. The World of Dysfunctional Families, A.C.D.N., Statewide Workshop, Phoenix, Arizona (Jan. 18–19, 1977)

150. Cooper, I. (1977). Report at 'Violence in the Family' 2nd World Conference, International Society on Family Law (June 1977), Montreal

151. Manchester, A. H. (1977). Sexual Offenses within the Family, 'Violence in the Family' 2nd World Conference, International Society on Family Law (June 1977), Montreal

152. Bluglass, R. (1977). Family Crime, Incest and Psychiatry, 'Violence in the Family' 2nd World Conference, International Society on Family Law (June 1977), Montreal

153. Peters, J. J. (1976). Children who are victims of sexual assault and the psychology of offenders. *Am. J. Psychother.*, **30**: 3, 398

154. Duffy, J. P. (1977). *Sexual Abuse of Children, Child Abuse: Its Treatment and Prevention, an Interdisciplinary Approach,* M. Van Stolk (ed.). (McClelland and Stewart Ltd.)

155. Gil, D. G. (1975). A holistic perspective of child abuse and its prevention. *Am. J. Orthopsychol.*

156. Frommer, E. A. and O'Shea, G. (1973). Emphasizing the importance of childhood, Antenatal identification of women liable to have problems in managing their infants. *Br. J. Psychiat.*, **123,** 149

157. Paulson, M. G. *et al.* (1975). A discriminant function procedure for identifying abusing parents. *Suicide,* **5:** 2, 104

158. Clark, A. L. (1976). Mother child relationships. *Am. J. Mat. Child Nursing,* March–April p. 94

159.. Pavenstedt, E. (1973). An intervention program for infants from high risk homes. *Am. J. Publ. Health,* **63,** 393

160. Rubin, R. (1963). Maternal Touch. *Nurse Outlook,* **11,** 828

161. Carey, W. B. (1970). A simplified method for measuring infant temperament. *J. Pediatr.,* 188

162. Broussard, E. R. and Hartner, M. S. S. (1970). The primipara's perception of the neonate as compared to the average infant. *Child Psychiat. Human Devel.,* **1,** 60

163. Rothenberg, M. B. (1976). Opportunities for psychological prophylaxis in the neonatal period. *Clin. Pediatr.,* 53

164. Kempe, C. H. (1975). Family intervention, the rights of all children. *Pediatrics,* **56:** 5, 693

165. Savino, A. B. and Saunders, R. W. (1973). Working with abusive parents, group therapy and home visits. *Am. J. Nursing,* 482

166. Farran, D. C and Ramey, C. T. (1977). Infant day care and attachment behaviour towards mothers and teachers. *Child Devel.,* **48:** 3, 1112

167. Eberling, N. B. and Hill, D. A. (1975). *Child Abuse–Intervention and Treatment.* (Acton, Mass: Publishing Sciences Group Inc.)

168. Epstein, N. B., Sigal, J. J. and Rakoff, V. (1968). Family Categories Schema, Montreal

169. Trube-Becker, E. (1977). The death of children following negligence, social aspects. *Forensic Sci.,* **9,** 111

170. Levinson, A. (Personal) In-Service Centre, Rockville, Maryland, Anne Arundel, County Department of Social Services (1974)

171. Jacobs, J. (1978). Child and Family Syndrome, An Overview. *O.M.A.J.,* **45,** 1, 13

172. Jacobs, J. (1978). Child and Family Syndrome, Social Pediatric Emergencies, *Pediatrician* (In press).

173. Redl, F. and Wineman, D. (1952) *Children who Hate.* (Glenoe Ill.: The Free Press)

174. Cupoli, J. M. and Newberger, E. H. (1977). Toward a more optimistic approach to child abuse. *Pediatrics,* **59,** 312

11 Medical-legal and societal problems involving children– child prostitution, child pornography and drug- related abuse; recom- mended legislation

JUDIANNE DENSEN-GERBER and S. F. HUTCHINSON

The average American citizen, when called upon to describe the problems of child abuse and neglect, typically speaks about the battering or starving of a child by a parent who hates the child or is mentally deranged. There certainly are many child abuse and neglect cases which fall under such descriptions, but there are many more cases in which the parent or adult perpetrator is motivated by sexual, commercial, or drug-related concerns. The use of the child as an adjunct or tool in fulfilling the parent's aberrant personal desires or needs is a form of child abuse distinguishable from the traditional formulation, yet as devastating to the child.

For purposes of discussion in this chapter, exploitative abuse and neglect of children will be defined as physical or emotional harm to a child arising from (1) use of the child by the parent or someone in locus parentis for his or her own sexual needs, (2) the use of the child in explicit sexual performances, whether for the purposes of prostitution, sexual exhibition or the production of pornographic materials, and (3) maltreatment of the child by a drug or alcohol addicted parent.

Let us consider the second category first, because it raises the least controversy for the public at large, the majority of whom are definite in their lack of understanding or compassion for persons who sell their children sexually or for others who commercially sexually exploit children for economic gain but are confused and sympathetic in the area of incest or drug-related child abuse. The sexual use of children, ranging in age from 3 to 16, has become a multimillion dollar industry. We have documented some of this exploitation in a cooperative effort of the Odyssey Institute with attorney Anthony Simonetti of the National Obscenity Law Center in New York, Professor George E. Stevens of Purdue University, and Robin Lloyd of Los Angeles; also much of what follows on child prostitution and pornography is based on articles written originally by

Odyssey for inclusion in the *Encyclopedia of Human Problems,* being compiled by Ann Landers.

CHILD PROSTITUTION

Child prostitution is defined as: the use of or participation by children under the age of majority (or sometimes defined as under 16 years of age) in sexual acts with adults or other minors where no force is present. Prostitution differs from statutory rape and incest in that there is an element of payment, usually in money, but often in drugs, gifts, clothing, food or other items. Prostitution is an age-old occupation and a lifestyle for women, men, adolescents and now, sadly, children, some as young as 3. Occasionally, parents who are involved in the sex-for-sale industries sell their daughters who are too young to have an idea of right from wrong. Child prostitution is closely allied with child pornography, incest, drug addiction, child abuse, and generalized family disruption and juvenile delinquency.

How many children are involved? Experts in the field of juvenile delinquency have shown that in the United States there is a minimum of 300 000 active boy prostitutes under the age of 16. Approximately 30 000 of these are located in New York City, with at least 2000 concentrated in the Times Square area. The Los Angeles Police Department has identified 30 000 boys working as prostitutes within that city of whom 5000 are under 14 years of age, and several hundred are as young as 8. No one has counted the number of girls involved in sex-for-sale, but most authorities agree that there are probably as many girls involved as boys. In other words, there are more than one-half million children in the United States who are actively engaged in prostitution! Some experts estimate the number of children involved is easily twice that number – 1.2 million, and this includes only children under the age of 16. The number nearly doubles again if 16- and 17-year-olds are added.

Odyssey Institute consulted on this problem in Atlanta, Boston, Chicago, Detroit, Houston, Los Angeles, Milwaukee, New Orleans, New York and San Francisco to name but a few cities. It touches all the cities of our nation and all walks of life. It has occurred in church-affiliated boys homes (Tennessee); independent schools (Massachusetts); and Boy Scout troops (Louisiana). It has reared its ugly head in the Roman Polanski case (California); in the making of a major movie, *Pretty Baby* (Louisiana) whose storyline is legalized child prostitution at the turn of the century in Storyville; in the recent death of a 12-year-old prostitute (New York) who fell or was pushed from a window of a 'quick-turnover' hotel; and in the Ms and Mr Nude Teeny Bopper Contest, which was scheduled to be held at Naked City (Indiana). There, children were to be paid $10.00 each, as were their parents, to enter the contest naked and you and I, fully dressed, were to pay $15.00 to go photograph them. An unexpected visit in the summer of 1977 to one of the truckers' stops at Naked City by CBS Television, Chicago, uncovered 11- and 14-year-old girls waiting bar stark naked for 18-hour shifts for which they were paid only $15.00 a day. These circumstances were found to be violations of the minimum wage law, the child labour law and the liquor licensing regulations. There were no laws to address the matter of their nakedness. However, we are delighted that community and official action in the state of Indiana has halted many of these objectionable practices. But much still remains to be done.

An interesting sidelight is that in Victorian England, a group of concerned women organized to raise the ages of girls within the brothels from 9 to 13. They were successful.

Children engaged in prostitution often are recruited from rural areas or midwestern cities. There are more than one million runaway children each year, many of whom turn to prostitution for survival; others as rebellion. Many leave homes of violence and sexual abuse, others are lonely because of distant, neglectful, personally preoccupied families, and still others are overwhelmingly bored and unchallenged – a few are severely mentally ill but untreated. The longing for adventure and to be rid of parental abuses leads hundreds of thousands into the streets, brothels and bus terminals. Their common fervent needs are affection and attention. These needs make them vulnerable to smooth-talking pimps who woo them with protestations of love and promises of fun and big money. For some, drugs and alcohol are part of the enticement; for others, these habits follow. Most are involved in substance abuse sooner or later. The drug habit only insures their captivity in the lifestyle of domination by the pimps.

Many child prostitutes travel from city to city. In many cases, this travel is due to their being employed by organized prostitution rings which often carry the children's vital statistics on computers in order to efficiently meet customers' demands. Boston, Chicago, and New Orleans have eliminated such technologically advanced rings in recent months. Child prostitutes are rotated around the country like circuit riders because the men who desire children also desire variety. These men need the illusion of innocence and virginity. One child I have treated literally claimed to have sold her maidenhood 44 times. In other cases, the wandering is to avoid arrest or territorial disputes with local established prostitutes. Still others follow conventions of professional and business groups.

What happens to these children? The life of a child prostitute is generally far different from what may have been promised to or anticipated by the child victim. Besides the drug and alcohol abuse, there are frequent beatings by pimps, violence from customers, and conditions of slavery. If the girl has a child, her pimp often takes her baby from her; he sends the infant out of state to be cared for by one of his relatives whose name or whereabouts she does not know; thereby if the prostitute tries to leave his stable (the name for a pimp's group of girls) he threatens her with the reality that she may never see the child again. The youngest mother I personally delivered during my medical training was 9 years and 8 months old. She had been prostituted by her own mother from age three. When delivered of a son, she thanked God that it was not a female who would have to experience a life similar to what hers had been.

There is physical damage to the child arising from the premature and inappropriate sexuality of child prostitution. Nature did not intend for children to have sex with adults. In addition to lacerations of the genitals, venereal diseases, pregnancy etc. there are local infections of the genitals and a well-established correlation between precocious sexuality and cervical cancer in young women under 30 necessitating hysterectomies. When a child's normal physical development has been punctuated by extensive premature sexual activity a total disruption of emotional development usually occurs as well. How can we expect a child to trust an adult world which sexually exploits him or her?

What kind of people use children sexually? They are almost exclusively men. While occasionally we have treated mother–daughter incest and even more rarely, mother–son, when we have consulted on child-sex-for-pay, the buyer has always been male. The men come from all classes and races though there is a marked Caucasian preponderance. Many are married – even those primarily interested in boys, and a surprising number are middle or upper class. Many are men of prominence and power. Some are jaded and bored, but almost all feel inadequate and unable to meaningfully relate to peer sexual partners. They see sex as something one person does to another, not as a mutually reciprocal relationship. Sexual activity equals a performance, and they relish an inexperienced child as the judge. Persons who use children are called paedophiliacs. Paedophiliacs frequently feel disquieted with themselves and punish themselves with degrading sexual acts that the children have to perform – acts often sadomasochistic in nature or involving urine and faeces. We must never confuse healthy adult human sexuality and our own experiences with the activities these children must experience. Just the size discrepancy alone is cause for pain and fear.

Incredibly, during the British Psychiatric Society's meetings in Wales in May 1977, the first meeting of the International Paedophiliac Information Exchange was held. This is a group of persons who believe that sexual conduct between child and adult is perfectly permissible behaviour. This society is working for the rights of adults to so use 'consenting' children. Children, in my opinion, do not have the capacity to judge the consequences, or give consent in the true sense. There are many American sympathizers with this newest rights movement and indeed, one association, the René Giuon Society in California, claims to have 2500 members who have filed an affidavit that they have each deflowered a child under 8 (male or female). The motto of this group is 'Sex by 8 or it is too late'. I ask you: too late for what – to mutilate the spirit and body of a young developing life?

What can be done? First, we must recognize that a sexually permissive society without humanistic caring contributes to the defective values presently being developed in children. Children need structure; they need to learn that sex is more than just doing what mechanically feels good or earns them money. Sex is part of a relationship – a special kind of friendship which is not exploitive.

Second, children must be given attention and affection in the home. This includes loving, cuddling, warmth and concern – basic psychological needs devoid of genital sexual overtones. If these warm touching experiences are missing in the home, the child may seek them elsewhere, becoming vulnerable to sexual exploitation by others with their own agendas.

Third, we must develop and provide all children with thorough sex education, but not simply information on techniques and mechanics, but what to do with their feelings and honest information about human sexuality, including the preciousness of human relatedness, caring and commitment. Anatomy and warnings about masturbation are not a substitute for dealing with the very real concerns and frustrations of adolescence, but all information shared with our young must be appropriate for them, not for sophisticated adults.

Fourth, when a child gets involved in prostitution, authorities should recognize the behaviour as a symptom of more serious problems. The juvenile system or other strictly legalistic approaches can not alone prevent or stop the problem. We must take a comprehensive look at the child in trouble, including psychological, medical, educational, legal and intra-family issues.

Fifth, communities must recognize that child prostitution and paedophilia are very serious threats to all children in the community and to the community itself. Delivery of community resources must be organized to maximize the impact of appropriate skills and resources to return the victimized child to a happy, healthy and appropriate lifestyle. At the present writing there are no treatment centres specially designed to treat child sex abuse victims. Much remains to be done but at least we have begun by identifying that these problems exist; now we must create a society where children can enjoy love and affection without being subject to sexual abuse. All children should have an inalienable right to love and affection.

CHILD PORNOGRAPHY

Child pornography, also known as 'chicken porn' and 'kiddie porn', is defined as films, photographs, magazines, books and motion pictures which depict children under a certain age (usually 16) involved in sexually explicit acts, both heterosexual and homosexual. America's indifferent attitude toward its children manifests itself in many ways, including, unfortunately, a tolerance for child abuse and neglect in significant proportions and varieties. One form of mistreatment is the exploitation of children used in the production of sexually explicit films and magazines. By recent count, there are at least 264 different magazines being produced and sold each month in adult bookstores across the country dealing with sexual acts between children or between children and adults. These magazines – slickly produced – sell for prices averaging over

$7.00 each. This number of 264 does not include the vast number of films or other media. Until recently, it was incorrectly assumed that child pornography was produced mostly in Europe, but investigations have now revealed that much of it is produced in the United States – even some materials which are packaged in such a manner as to represent foreign origin.

Film makers and magazine photographers have little difficulty recruiting youngsters for these performances. Some simply use their own children, or buy the children of others; some rely on runaways. Recent findings of a US Senate Subcommittee on Juvenile Delinquency indicate that more than one million American children run away from home each year, often for good cause, having been victims of intolerable conditions, with physical and sexual abuse present. From this vast army of dispossessed children, exploiters select literally thousands of participants for their production needs and prostitution rings. Los Angeles police estimate that adults in that city alone sexually exploited over 30 000 children under 17 in 1976, and photographed many of them in the act. Five thousand of these children were under 12. In 1975, Houston police arrested a man after finding a warehouse full of pornography including 15 000 color slides of boys in homosexual acts, over 1000 magazines and paperback books plus a thousand reels of film. In New York City, Father Bruce Ritter of Covenant House, a group of shelters for runaway children, has reported that the first ten children who entered Covenant House had all been given money to appear in pornographic films. These children, in their early teens, could not return to their homes because of extreme conditions of abuse and neglect, and could not find jobs or take care of themselves other than in illegal ways. There is no other way for a child of 12 to support him or herself, and sadly, too few sheltering alternative environments are provided by our communities.

Many are not runaways, but come from broken homes. They can be induced to pose for $5.00 or a trip to Disneyland, or even a kind word. Sometimes the mothers are porn queens; often parents or guardians are addicts or alcoholics. Approximately 2.8 million of America's children are in the sole custody of substance abusers, and 2.2 million are with parents involved in sex for sale. In 1977, in New York's Times Square, we purchased *Lollitots* a magazine showing girls 8 to 14, and *Moppits*, children aged 3 to 12, as well as playing cards which pictured naked, spread-eagled children. We also looked at film depicting children violently deflowered on their communion day at the feet of a 'freshly crucified' priest replacing Jesus on the cross. Next, we saw a film showing an alleged father engaged in urolagnia with his 4-year-old daughter. Of 64 films able to be seen, 19 showed children, and an additional 16 involved incest.

Despite the highly secretive nature of the recruitment and sexploitation process, a growing body of information about the children involved confirms that psychological scarring and emotional distress which occur in the vast majority of these cases leads to significant other problems, many of which include the illicit use of drugs to deaden memories and desensitize present experiences.

Pre-pubescent sexual activity, especially under conditions of exploitation and coercion, is highly destructive to the child's psychological development and social maturation. Psychiatrists report that such inappropriate sexuality is highly destructive to children. It predisposes them to join society's deviant populations; drug addicts, prostitutes, criminals, the promiscuous and pre-adult precocious parents. Over 17 000 babies were born to mothers under 14 years of age in 1976. Venereal diseases in children have now reached epidemic figures. Although there may not be a proven link between adult pornography and sexual abuse, there is no doubt that this sexploitation of our young in order to produce child pornography often scars the children so used for life. This opinion is not based purely on intelligent conjecture, for a number of children and young adults who had been involved in posing and/or performing for sexually explicit films and magazines have surfaced. These children are now or have been in treatment programmes for substance abuse, delinquency or other aberrant behaviour. Some of these children have voluntarily recounted their experiences to law enforcement, mental health workers and news media people who are attempting to learn more about the recruitment process, the type of activities involved, the treatment needs, and the long-term effects upon the victims. Psychiatry has not yet developed a treatment design for these youngsters any more than it has for child prostitutes or incest victims, all of whom are on the spectrum of sexual abuse of children and all of whom understandably show a more marked inability than other patients to trust any adult or establish the therapeutic rapport which is so necessary for rehabilitation. Other children who are abuse victims hunger for affection and caring, and are immediately or shortly thereafter responsive to any adult who shares affection and warmth. This is far from the case with children who have been sexually used. They, better than almost anybody else, know when such exploitation and abuse masquerades as 'love'. It is 'love' and its closeness as defined previously in their lives that they most fear.

Many previously were victimized in a most brutal fashion. Los Angeles Police Investigator Jackie Howell rejects the commonly stated belief that nude posing is harmless to the children. 'We have found that the child pornographer is also often the molester. Photography is only a part of it, a sideline more often than not to prostitution, sexual abuse and drugs.' It is important to note that the victimization in the child pornography process goes beyond the child actor. For example, authorities in Rockingham County, New Hampshire, reported recently that, in 1977, every one of the 27 cases of incest reported in their jurisdiction included child pornography preceding and accompanying the assaults on the children. Many more such cases are beginning to surface, with recent reports from Ohio and California. Dr Henry Giarretto, one of the nation's leading experts in incest, who works directly with the Probation Department in Santa Clara County, California reports that he saw 50 cases of incest in 1975, had over 350 in 1976, and predicts that 800-plus will be referred in 1977. This increase he directly attributes in large measure to the burgeoning 'kiddie porn' industry[1].

The men who support this billion-dollar industry do so because they are seeking justification and rationalization for their deviant behaviour. Indeed, one magazine in the Odyssey Institute files, *Lust for Children*, is a primer for the sex molester, teaching him how to go to the park and pick up two little girls, what games to play to induce them to cooperate and what acts to perform which will have the least evidence for the police should the children report him. Another, entitled *Schoolgirls*, instructs a father in text and photographs as to those positions for intercourse best used with pre-pubescent girls (in this instance a girl of 9) and still another shows in serial photographs how to affix a lock to one's daughter's labia so that no other man may 'get to her'. Such sadomasochistic and snuff activities are an integral part of the 'kiddie porn' market.

Furthermore, not only are these activities harmful emotionally, developmentally and psychologically to the child actors and children subsequently sexually abused, but physically, as many suffer lacerations of the vagina and rectum. Additionally, the research of Dr Malcom Coppleson, one of the leading gynaecologists in Sydney, Australia has shown the vaginal pH of the pre-pubescent is not sufficient to neutralize infections that come with intercourse, so that she is subject not only to vaginitis, but early onset of cervical cancer often necessitating hysterectomies prior to attaining 30 years of age. It is obvious that children were not meant to satisfy the sexual needs of adults, and such use of them is like rape, a crime of power and abuse.

There are many parts to the solution of this problem. This menace will not be removed by simple changes in law or harsh penalties, although these are essential components of the complete strategy. There must be a public awareness in each community that child porn exists, that it is very big business, in large part run by organized crime, that it victimizes children in every community, that it can be stopped and that it will only be stopped by a commitment to the children of the community manifested in explicit actions:

1. Amendment of child abuse and neglect statutes to include sexual exploitation, and to prescribe harsh criminal penalties for offenders.

2. Amend the Civil Code to provide for licensing of all children used in commercial modelling or performing, with carefully worded proscriptions and substantial sanctions against the use of such children in sexually explicit activities.

3. Extend criminal liability to promoters and distributors of child pornography, without whose promotion and marketing of the finished product there would be no financial motive for the sexploitation of children in the first place.

4. Develop intervention and treatment models for children victimized by this process, to mend their emotional and psychological injuries and to return them to the mainstream of society.

There is evidence to show similarity in the psychological scarring between child porn and incest victims. Their common feelings of betrayal, guilt, worthlessness and rage can be expected to promote either inwardly, self-destructive behaviour – isolation, withdrawal, drug or alcohol abuse; or the child may turn outward in aberrant social behaviour, delinquency, promiscuity, prostitution or violence.

When Odyssey began its campaign in January, 1977, there was very little legislation on the federal or state level dealing with the use of children in sexually explicit materials or performances. On the federal level, five laws prohibit the distribution of 'obscene' materials. One prohibits any mailing of such material[2]; another prohibits the importation of obscene materials[3]; a third prohibits the broadcast of obscenity[4]; and two others prohibit the interstate transportation of obscene materials or the use of common carriers to transport such materials[5]. In addition, the Anti-Pandering Act of 1968[6] authorizes postal patrons to request that there be no further delivery of unsolicited mailings or advertisements that are sexually offensive. No federal statute specifically regulates the distribution of sexual materials to children. Likewise, no federal statute specifically regulates or restricts the production, distribution, or marketing of this material in interstate commerce. Laws pertaining to the dissemination of obscene material to minors have been enacted in 47 states and the District of Columbia. In early 1977 only six states, however, specifically prohibited the participation of minors in an obscene performance that could be harmful to them[7]. Enforcement of the then-existing statutes did not seem likely to significantly curtail the activity.

State criminal statutes dealing with sex crimes often are not helpful. The physical activity involved in sexploitation of minors in pornography may not meet the criteria of the statute, e.g. rape, sodomy, sexual abuse. Or the statutes may be so broadly worded as to discourage courts from applying them in terms of significant sanctions. Many states have child welfare provisions within their education laws that regulate the employment of children in commercial activities. Unfortunately, these same laws either abdicate control when the child is working for a parent[8] or the sanctions are so limited as to pose no deterrent[9].

Given the paucity of legislation specifically relating to this activity, there can be little wonder at the relatively scarce previous attempts at law enforcement. The problems of case-finding and evidence are compounded by a confusion between sexploitation as a form of child abuse and adult obscenity matters. These problems and the attitudes of many judges discourage and actually thwart the few criminal investigations attempted. In New York City, for example, police, after a year's investigation, seized 1200 pornographic films and magazines, many showing children. A major wholesaler was convicted. He could have been sentenced to 7 years incarceration. He got 6 months of 'weekends' in jail[10].

Today, 1 year later, in early 1978, Congress has virtually completed work on a significant federal statute, and more than 30 state legislatures have introduced or passed child porn legislation. Such legislation can achieve maximum success by prohibiting specific sexual acts when performed by minors for the purpose of producing a film or magazine. The production, distribution and sale is forbidden as a crime of sexual exploitation of children as opposed to obscenity which focuses on the reader or viewer. Thus, the preferred view is to legislate against the exploitation as a form of child abuse, and the material as a contraband product of the exploitation. There is ample historical precedent for this in the child labour law area.

Secondly, if the lawmakers insist on classifying the material as obscene, then an excellent argument can be made. The Supreme Court has already upheld restrictions against sales of obscene materials to minors. If states can constitutionally protect the minors' welfare by restricting materials available to them, it must at the same time possess the constitutional authority to protect minors from having to participate in the production of the materials. The legislation that the Law and Medicine Division of Odyssey Institute proposes is designed to address the sexual conduct and its related activities – from soliciting the child to marketing the product. The printed product cannot be isolated or removed from the process. The protections inherent in the First Amendment provisions regarding freedom of speech are not without some limit. Such guarantees cannot rationally be interpreted to include a right to abuse and exploit young children.

We are not going to produce mentally healthy and happy children by issuing an executive order that all children must be loved. But we can enact and enforce legislation to protect them and give them a fighting chance in this world. As Erik Erikson wrote: 'Someday, maybe, there will exist a well-informed, well-considered, and yet fervent public conviction that the most deadly of all possible sins is the mutilation of a child's spirit; for such mutilation undercuts the life principle of trust, without which every human act, may it feel ever so good, and seem ever so right, is prone to perversion by destructive forms of consciousness.'

The last section on the role the law must play in the protection of children at risk deals with the problems of sexual abuse confined within the family constellation (incest) and drug related child abuse together, because they are similar in that no outside factors such as financial gain or the role of unrelated third parties are present. Therefore, here society must choose to act and intervene in family matters, not matters of the commercial marketplace; such regulatory actions on society's part necessitate a much greater break with the tradition that a man's home is his castle and his wife and children his to do with whatever he will, even more so than his horse or dog. The latter animals are perhaps historically better protected under animal protection laws than the former humans. The first court opinion protecting a child was rendered in 1874 in upstate New York; an innovative and creative judge, faced with a horrendous situation involving child abuse and no laws or precedents, declared the child a dumb animal so that she could be protected within the dictates of the cruelty to animal statutes. Child neglect is the *sine qua non* of parental drug addiction, and abuse is a frequent occurrence. Of the states studied, only New York recognizes this relationship, and codifies it as a criterion for mandated intervention.*

The official New York City Department of Health statistics for 1975 indicate that in the 5-year period 1970–1975 there was an increase of 38% of drug-related child abuse cases.†

This section discusses the efficacy of the legal and medical professions in selected states (Massachusetts, New York, New Jersey, Utah, and Michigan) in responding to the incidence of such drug-related child abuse, including sexual abuse and incest. This review is based upon case histories of patients in the Odyssey House Parents' Program‡ as well as the various Odyssey House

---

* The New York provision states that a neglected child is one '. . . whose physical, mental or emotional condition has been impaired or *is in imminent danger of becoming impaired* as a result of the failure of his parent or other person legally responsible for his care to exercise a minimum degree of care . . . in providing the child with the proper supervision or guardianship . . . by using a drug or drugs; or by using alcoholic beverages to the extent that he loses self-control of his actions'. *Italics added*, New York Family Court Act §1021 (f) (i) (B) (C.L.S. 1971). Such a child must be reported by the designated persons to the Central Registry for Abused and Maltreated Children.

Cf. The Massachusetts statute requires only the reporting of infants 'who [are] determined to be physically dependent upon an addictive drug at birth . . .' Mass. Public Welfare, ch. 119 §51A (*Mass. Gen. L. Ann.*, Supp. 1976). Children born to drug or alcohol abusing parents, but who are not themselves determined to be addicted to the substance at birth are not reported. There is no Massachusetts provision equivalent to the New York one providing for the reporting of children in imminent danger of being harmed. Under the Massachusetts statute the reporter must have reasonable cause to believe that [the] child . . . *is suffering* serious physical or emotional injury resulting from abuse . . .' *Italics added*, Mass. Public Welfare, ch. 119 §51A (*Mass. Gen. L. Ann.*, Supp. 1976)

† As reported in Charts, Odyssey Institute, 1976. See Appendix III

‡ The Odyssey House Parents Program (OHPP), a federally funded research-demonstration project, provides treatment services, in the context of its research, to pregnant addicts, addicted parents with small children and women in distress who have histories similar to the former groups. These patients represent over 25 states with dissimilar systems for the delivery of child protective services.

Odyssey House, Inc. is a psychiatrically oriented therapeutic community for the treatment and rehabilitation of drug abusers. The Odyssey method was developed by Dr Judianne Densen-Gerber and a group of 17 ex-addicts starting in 1966. Central to the organization and philosophy at Odyssey are awareness of new problems in addiction-related fields, meaningful confrontation of these problems, expert and professional demonstration projects which identify the appropriate questions and test alternative treatment techniques, and comprehensive evaluation procedures for assessment of problems and successes within the programme.

In the OHPP, pregnant addicts are admitted to treatment, to be given appropriate detoxification and pre-natal services, to change the anti-social attitudes and behaviour in the mother, and, post-partum, to allow the parent and child to remain together within the therapeutic setting and undergo the resocialization process together. In addition to the proven value of the therapeutic community in rehabilitation of the mother, this modality allows parent and child to live together during the early formative years, under the observation and supervision of the treatment staff. Parents more advanced in the therapeutic process can teach others less mature the qualities and skills of good parenting. The infant can hopefully develop without deprivation of a proper nurturing parent. In short, the OHPP is confronting second-generation addiction at its source, the child-rearing practices of these antisocial parents

therapeutic communities. Within the past several years, child protective laws have been adopted and/or strengthened in all the 50 states. Unless otherwise indicated, this section will analyse the various case histories as though they had occurred under the present version of the respective state's child protective law. This approach is valid because the areas of weakness in the former and present laws are substantially similar. These weaknesses, as the cases will illustrate, occur predominantly in three areas: enforcement of mandated reporting of suspected cases of abuse and neglect; evidentiary limitations as to the acceptability of uncorroborated testimony by abused children, especially concerning sexual assault; and protection of the child from retributive acts by the respondent custodian pending investigation of the complaint, and during the processing of any orders of termination of the custodial rights.

First to be studied is the service system of the State of Michigan. The governmental agency responsible for child protective services is the Child Protective Services Division of the Michigan Department of Social Services[11]. The division is charged with investigating and responding to reports of abuse, neglect, cruelty, and abandonment and with assuring the provision of appropriate social services to both child and parents. Services provided include day care, medical, psychological and psychiatric counselling, foster care, placement, and family and marital counselling. The intake of new cases occurs in each county's local office of the Department of Social Services. The statute applicable is mainly the recently enacted Child Protection Law. Its purpose is both 'to provide for the protection of children who are abused or neglected'[12], and to safeguard and enhance the welfare of children and preserve family life[13].

The law[14] requires the filing of a mandatory accusatory report by any 'physician, coroner, dentist, medical examiner, nurse, school administrator, school counselor or teacher, law enforcement officer or duly regulated child care provider who has reasonable cause to suspect child abuse* or neglect'†[15]. Failure to report as required makes one civilly liable for the damages proximately caused by such failure[16]; there are no criminal sanctions for such failure to report. Any other person suspecting abuse or neglect may also file a report with the appropriate persons with the protection of anonymity if he or she so requests[17]. Any reporter acting in good faith is immune from criminal and civil liability; and there is a presumption of good faith[18]. The report of abuse or neglect is filed with the county department of Social Services of the county in which the child is living[19]. Although the Department of Social Services is charged with 'cooperat(ing) with law enforcement officials, courts of competent, jurisdiction and appropriate state agencies providing human ser-

* 'Child abuse' means harm or threatened harm to a child's health or welfare by a person responsible for the child's health or welfare which occurs through non-accidental physical or mental injury, sexual abuse or maltreatment. Mich. C.L. §722.622 (b) Supp. 1975)

† 'Child neglect' means harm to a child's health or welfare by a person responsible for the child's health or welfare which occurs through negligent treatment, including the failure to provide adequate food, clothing, shelter or medical care. Mich. C.L. §722.622 (1) (Supp. 1975)

vices in relation to preventing, identifying and treating child abuse and neglect[20], it is not required to provide copies of reports of suspected child abuse and neglect to the prosecuting attorney and the Probate Court of the county in which the report was filed, although it 'may'[21] do so.

Case History No. 1

Joanie (fictitious name)* a Black Catholic female, was born in Pittsburgh in 1958 to an addicted prostitute. No social agency intervened at this time. Shortly thereafter, the mother left, abandoning the child to her present lover (not the child's father) who was an alcoholic and an unemployed unskilled labourer. Again, no social agency intervened. He was unable to meet the child's or his needs alone, so he returned to his mother's home in Saginaw, Michigan. The baby was subsequently cared for until age 5 or 6 by this, her paternal grandmother, a 66-year-old, deaf and blind, bilateral amputee in Michigan. No social agency intervened, though the grandmother's welfare worker on a routine visit noted that the housekeeping standards were poor.

When Joanie was 6, her grandmother returned to her own birth place in the South for permanent nursing care and to die. Joanie was then left once again in the sole custody of her alcoholic foster father. It is reported that the father would get food from the neighbours under the pretence of giving it to Joanie, only to eat it himself, leaving her to survive on no more than one meal each day. It was not until she was in the fourth grade that Joanie came to the attention of the school social worker whose attention was drawn by the complaint of Joanie's classmates of her 'strong body odour, filthy clothing and behavioural problems such as stealing food and lying'. No record exists of any of Joanie's teachers having notified the appropriate persons that Joanie was potentially a neglected child. The investigation of Joanie's home prompted by her classmates' complaints led to a determination that she was not receiving proper guardianship and that her father was beating her.

At age 10 she was made a ward of the state and placed in a series of foster homes and children's shelters. This custody resulted in nine placements in 2 years, including foster homes in which Joanie alleges sexual abuse by the foster parents occurred. Joanie became involved in drug usage and shoplifting. She was caught by the police twice and returned to the children's home. At age 14, Joanie was living in the streets and supporting her drug habit by prostitution. At $14\frac{1}{2}$, she voluntarily returned to the Juvenile Center and requested placement. The Center officials promptly discovered that she was pregnant. Contrary to initial recommendations by the court, Joanie was given permission by yet another judge to marry a 19-year-old known psychotic heroin addict pimp,

* Joanie's history is more fully discussed at R. Wathey, M.A. and J. Densen-Gerber, J.D., M.D., F.C.L.M., 'Preliminary Report on the Sociological Autopsy in Child Abuse Deaths' (presented at the 27th Meeting of the American Academy of Forensic Sciences, February 20, 1975) (Odyssey House, Inc., New York)

not the father of the baby, in order that she be able to keep the baby.

Two months after the birth of baby Anne, Joanie informed her caseworker that she wanted the marriage annulled because her husband beat her. The baby was admitted to the Children's Receiving Home for custody until Joanie, who had been living with her husband and mother-in-law, could make new living arrangements. Medical records from the Receiving Home indicate that while there, baby Anne was 'quite relaxed when being held by anyone but her mother'; when her mother held her she began to 'scream in terror'. Examination of the baby's admission record reveals that the infant had a black eye, and several bruises about both arms. No mention was made whether a report of these injuries was filed with the legal authorities.

Joanie, at 15, moved into a new apartment, and was visited by her case worker who reported that there were adequate 'provisions to care for the child's needs', and that she found Joanie 'most anxious to have the infant Anne home'. The day after the baby was released to Joanie, the 4-month-old baby was brought to the hospital and pronounced dead on arrival. The attending physician noted that the baby had several fractured ribs resulting from having been held very tightly, and a fractured skull from being hit on the head at least three times with a heavy object. He further noted 'that both parents seemed very unaware of what (had) happened, and appear(ed) to be high on drugs'. After 3 months of intensive investigation, Joanie was charged with homicide. She was deemed competent to stand trial by several psychiatrists and psychologists. During the trial, testimony was entered that Joanie had attempted to kill herself by drinking turpentine and taking pills early in her adolescence, and that later, on at least one occasion, she had tried to get the baby to do the same. A polygraph test administered pre-trial indicated that Joanie was responsible for the baby's death. On February 17, 1974, after 2 days of testimony prior to the commencement of the defence, a motion to dismiss for lack of sufficient evidence was granted. Under court order, within 6 months and still less than 16 years old, Joanie, again pregnant, entered the Odyssey Parents' Program in order to be evaluated by the Institute's psychiatric staff as to whether or not she was dangerous to the unborn infant, and whether or not once the child was born Joanie would be fit to care for it. Before our evaluation was complete, but after she had been delivered of a baby boy, she and her legal counsel, who was from the federally-funded legal services of Saginaw, paid for by our taxes, and who claimed to be advocating her civil rights not to be incarcerated against her wishes, kidnapped the newborn by force from the Odyssey Parents' Program. Fortunately, prompt legal action on the part of our attorneys in Michigan secured a legal order placing the child in protective foster care. The alleged protection of Joanie's civil rights did no more than allow her once again to become addicted and ply her trade on the streets of Michigan – and all before she turned 17.

There is little indication that Joanie's story would have had a more satisfactory ending today under the present Michigan statute but there is some hope.

Had Joanie's initial living situation been reported to the authorities before Joanie was ten, her foster father's guardianship probably would have been terminated at the earlier date. A more successful initial placement might have resulted. But the failure of the grandmother's caseworker or Joanie's first-through-fourth-grade teachers to report her as a suspected neglected child, although they were mandated to do so by law, resulted in no punishment or civil action against them. In Michigan, legal sanctions for failure to report are limited to *civil liability* for damages proximately caused by such failure[22]. Who is going to bring suit? Joanie?

In the second generation, the initial release of baby Anne to Joanie was apparently not preventable under the newly drafted law since there is no indication on the record whether an investigation was ever conducted prior to the baby's initial release to her mother, to determine if she faced potential abuse within the statutory meaning of 'threatened harm to health or welfare by a person responsible (for the same) which occurs through non-accidental physical or mental injury, sexual abuse or maltreatment'[23]. *Under Michigan law, Joanie's status as a drug abusing, teenaged prostitute married to a criminally insane heroin-addict pimp did not establish a presumption that the child would be abused or neglected.* Contrast this with the situation in New York where the parent's status as a drug abuser raises a statutory presumption that the child will be neglected.

Baby Anne's second release from the custody of the receiving home was apparently also not preventable under the new law. Even assuming that the examining physician had made a proper report and had also determined that release of the baby would have endangered its health and welfare and had so notified the head of his department as required by law[24], the department head still had the option to discharge the child to the mother, rather than to detail it in protective custody[25]. Even with the authorities in possession of all the knowledge reported above, Baby Anne would have died without the law establishing any institutional liability.

New York has a multi-agency approach to the care of its children which is wasteful and duplicative at its best and shifting of responsibility at its worst. The New York State Department of Social Services, Emergency Children's Services places children on an emergency basis through crisis intervention. The New York Foundling Hospital has a comprehensive programme using a multi-disciplinary approach to prevention of further abuse within a family setting. The New York City Bureau of Child Welfare functions as the City's family protective services agency. It provides services for children that are supplemental to or substitutes for parental care. The Bureau is charged with investigating reported cases of suspected child abuse and neglect and with providing adequate care, in foster homes and other child-caring institutions for children in need of such service. Various Societies for Prevention of Cruelty to Children receive complaints and offer services for maltreated children.

The stated purpose of the New York Child Protective Act is 'to encourage more complete reporting of suspected child abuse and maltreatment and to establish in each county of the state a child protective service capable of investigating such reports swiftly and competently, and capable of providing protection for the child or children from further abuse or maltreatment and rehabilitative services for the child or children and parents involved'[26]. The statute[27] requires mandatory, non-accusatory reporting by enumerated health care practitioners* school officials, social service workers, all child care or foster workers and peace and law enforcement officials who have reasonable cause to suspect that a child coming before them in their professional or official capacity is an abused or maltreated child.

'Abused child' means a child less than 16 years of age whose parents or other person legally responsible for his care:

(i) inflicts or allows to be inflicted upon such child physical injury by other than accidental means which causes or creates a substantial risk of death, or serious or protracted disfigurement, or protracted impairment of physical or emotional health or protracted loss or impairment of the function of any bodily organ; or

(ii) creates or allows to be created a substantial risk of physical injury to such child by other than accidental means . . .

(iii) Commits, or allows to be committed an act of sexual abuse against such child as defined in the penal law . . . Family Court Act §1012 (e) (McKinney, 1976).

A 'maltreated child' includes a child under 18 years of age:

(a) defined as a neglected child by the Family Court Act; or

(b) who has had serious physical injury inflicted upon him by other than accidental means; Soc. Serv. Law §412 (2) (McKinney, 1976).

'Neglected child' means a child less than 18 years of age:

(i) whose physical, mental or emotional condition has been impaired or is in imminent danger of becoming impaired as a result of the failure of his parent or other person legally responsible for his care to exercise a minimum degree of care:

(a) in supplying the child with adequate food, clothing, shelter or education in accordance with the provisions of part one of article 65 of the education law, or medical, dental, optometrical, or surgical care, though financially able to do so or offered financial or other means to do so; or

(b) in providing the child with proper supervision or guardianship, by unreasonably inflicting or allowing to be inflicted harm, or a substantial risk thereof, including the infliction of excessive corporal punishment; or by using a drug or drugs or by using alcoholic beverages to the extent that he loses self-control of his actions; or by any other acts of a similarly serious nature requiring the aid of the court; or

(ii) who has been abandoned by his parents or other person legally responsible for his care. Family Court Act §1012 (f) (McKinney, 1976)

---

* Any physician, surgeon, medical examiner, coroner, dentist, osteopath, optometrist, chiropractor, podiatrist, resident, intern, registered nurse, hospital personnel engaged in the admission, examination, care or treatment of persons, a Christian Science practitioner . . .' (New York Social Services Law §413 (McKinney, 1976))

Supplementing the Child Protective Act, the Family Court Act states that the child of a parent who utilizes drugs is by definition a 'neglected' child[28]. Although the statute does not identify the child of a drug abuser as an 'abused' child, case law states that such a child is 'abused' by the narcotics addicted parent by reason at least of the abandonment caused by that addiction[29]. Wilful failure to report an abused or maltreated child constitutes a Class A misdemeanour[30] punishable by not less than 15 days nor more than 1 year imprisonment. Failure to file a mandatory report also subjects one to civil liability for the dangers proximately caused by such failure[31]. The statute also provides for the voluntary reporting by any other person who has reasonable cause to believe that a child is abused or maltreated[32], with immunity from suit for reporting in good faith[33]. The Family Court Act also empowers designated individuals including representatives of the Social Service Department, agents of the duly incorporated Society for the Prevention of Cruelty to Children and treating physicians to take a child into protective custody without a court order and without consent of the guardian where releasing the child presents imminent danger to its life or health[34]. New York's statutes are excellent and comprehensive, and could well be copied by the rest of the nation. However, good law is only the first step, it must be followed by adequate and swift law enforcement; able, foresighted, progressive, caring, non-overburdened judges with sufficient staff both within the court system *per se*, and social agencies to do the investigative and evaluative reports vital to the trial and best disposition of the case; and last, by treatment options available to the court to support the family when rehabilitation is indicated, and viable better alternatives for placement than the brutalizing family in which the child is living. Sadly, this is far from the case in financially borderline New York, which should receive 'A's' for understanding and formulating legal solutions to the child abuse-neglect problems (particularly in the area of drug-related child abuse) but 'F's' in implementation. For within New York it would seem that some bureaucrats have polished to an excellence matched almost nowhere else, except possibly Washington, the skill of pushing paper, maintaining their jobs, covering each other's back, carving out small fiefdoms, nourishing their own turfdom paranoia, and crippling everyone else from meaningful activity through repetitive time-consuming accountability that does not ensure a minimum level of competence, but rather, sets a maximum of performance in order that no one else can accomplish anything which would embarrass everyone else. Somewhere in the above long list of the goals and priorities of bureaucracy, the concept of caring for and about children seems in danger of being forgotten. I would advise the rest of the States to do as New York says – not as New York does.

Case History No. 2

Carol, a 16-year-old Baptist Black, lives in New York. At age 7, she was molested by three of her alcoholic mother's boy-friends. At age 8 she was molested by her older brother, a practice he continued to engage in whenever the two of them were alone together. At age 8, her father, who had just been released from an institution, returned to live in the family home. The father had been jailed previously for molesting his 8-year-old nephew, but no social agency intervened to evaluate whether he presented any danger to the children in the home, or whether there was any other adult who could or would protect the children if he did act out. He did; and so at the age of 9 Carol ran away from home and went to live with her older sister and her sister's two children. Carol had been cared for by her sister on previous occasions when her mother was jailed for operating a gambling house. She remained with her sister until she was 14, even though her sister beat her on several occasions, necessitating visits to the local hospital's emergency room where no reports were ever filed. At age 15, her mother brought Carol to court on charges of incorrigibility and truancy. On disposition, Carol was sent to the Correctional Facility, where it was discovered that she was pregnant. This was Carol's third pregnancy. The first two, at ages 14 and 15, ended in abortions performed in hospitals, without reports filed that here was a child (the mother) in difficulty. Carol delivered the last time in a home for unwed mothers. She then came to Odyssey House. Her sister is now caring for her child.

Despite the statutory mandate, the school teachers, social workers, physicians and other health care professionals who had contact with Carol failed to report her to the authorities as an abused or neglected child. When Carol's mother took her to court, the judicial system failed to recognize that Carol's parental relationship should be evaluated and probably terminated. It was easier to blame and punish the child, particularly since she was now a terrible teenager. It appears as if the system neglects to aid a child of 7 or 8 who is at risk and by the time the child is old enough to rebel our attitude is punitive rather than protective toward that child. One would hope that we would have a second chance with the second generation, but there is no record that Carol's child, now a bright 2-year toddler, has even been evaluated as a potentially neglected child although such an evaluation is certainly indicated from facts on record.* Instead, the child has been released into the custody of the sister whom Carol reports as having severely beaten her. Similar to the case of Joanie in Michigan, the primary breakdown of the child protective system here is the initial failure by the designated persons to report the suspected case of abuse and neglect. Although failure to so report is punishable as a misdemeanour, there is no indication of enforcement of this penalty and in our opinion enforcement of a fine without loss of licence will not be effective against the medical professions. However, differing from Michigan, once Carol's case would have gotten into the system, the ability and opportunity to take responsive action is much greater in New York than in Michigan†.

---

* There were approximately 10 000 addicted adolescent parents in the New York area during this time

† Such an evaluation would be possible under Family Court Act §1012 (f) (i) (B), *supra* note 43

Case History No. 3

Edith is a 16-year-old Black female raised in Brooklyn. Until she was 13, Edith
lived with her grandparents, who collected welfare. When they died, she was
cared for by her alcoholic and drug-abusing mother and her mother's paramour.
They lived with their three younger children as a family group. The mother
was brought to court by a physician who reported that she beat the youngest
child. The child was first placed in foster care, then returned to the mother.
Meanwhile, the mother began to beat Edith in place of the younger sibling.
When Edith struck her mother back, occasioning the need for hospitalization,
the mother began to abuse the younger brothers again. Finally, Edith and her
siblings ran away to an aunt who successfully petitioned to have the children
removed from the mother's care. The younger children were placed in foster
care. Edith came to Odyssey House to be treated for her violent rages and intermittent drug use.

Although this case is the most successful of those reviewed so far, the
response of the agencies involved was limited. There is no record that the
physical condition of the other siblings was ascertained at the time of the
original decision to remove the youngest boy. Nor are there any reasons found
on the record as to why the child was subsequently returned to the home,
although no change in the home environment had occurred.

A look at Massachusetts reveals that the State Department of Welfare is the
agency which receives reports of suspected child abuse and neglect. The
Department provides necessary child protective services by purchasing these
from private agencies. The Judge Baker Guidance Clinic in Boston is one of
these private service providers. It follows the model but has a multi-discipline
psychiatric approach. It is excellent, but that is by its own choice;
Massachusetts does little monitoring of its private subcontractors and indeed
many services are bought outside of the state. Occasionally, purchase of out-of-
state service may be more economical, as in the instance of Odyssey New
Hampshire (where the cost of living is less) which provides contract services on
a fee-for-service basis to Massachusetts for delinquent youths in lieu of incarceration; but such economy is rare. Usually, purchase of services for states
with sufficient population to support the state facilities cost more, but the
states continue to do so because it meets the need: 'out of sight out of mind'. It
is easy to deny a problem once you send it away and it is no longer visible; then
officialdom can claim to have solved both the prevention and rehabilitation
aspects. Also, it is easier to send these difficult children (our abused, our
neglected, our emotionally crippled. our blind, our deaf, our dumb, our
delinquent, our less than perfect) to someone else's neighbourhood for them to
have to see and for their property values to decline. Unfortunately, it makes
good political sense to bow to these crass attitudes of one's constituents rather
than to lead in righteousness.

The stated purposes of the Massachusetts statute for the protection of
children is to insure that they are 'protected against the harmful effects

resulting from the absence, inability, inadequacy or destructive behavior of parents, of parent substitutes, and to assure good substitute parental care in the event of absence, temporary or permanent inability or unfitness of parents to provide care and protection for their children'[35]. Designated persons* who see children† in their professional capacity and have a reasonable cause to believe that a child is suffering serious physical or emotional injury resulting from abuse or neglect or 'who is determined to be physically dependent upon an addictive drug at birth'[36] shall immediately report the condition to the Department of Social Services. As noted earlier, this definition of drug related child abuse, based on a finding of withdrawal in the newborn, is nowhere as efficacious as one which uses the mother's addiction or potential addiction. Many children-at-risk will be missed under the Massachusetts test, and a few erroneously included when the mother, for instance, is on medically-prescribed barbiturates. Such reporting is mandatory, but no sanctions or penalties for failure to report are included. Any other person suspecting abuse or neglect may report the same[37]. The non-designated reporter is given immunity from suit for reporting in good faith, while the designated reporter is given immunity in all situations[38]. The Department may take a child into immediate temporary custody, without a court order, if it has reasonable cause to believe that the removal of the child is necessary to protect him or her from further abuse or neglect, with a filing for a court order to be made on the next court day[39]. Additionally, a treating physician or a hospital may obtain authorization from the presiding judge of the juvenile court to refuse to release a child to a respondent custodian if the judge believes such release would be detrimental to the child's health or safety[40].

Case History No. 4

Donna‡ is a 28-year-old White Irish Catholic female. When Donna was 8 years old her mother began to beat her, largely as a reaction to her situation as a battered wife, i.e. her own physical abuse by Donna's father, a chronic alcoholic, a not uncommon situation. Her mother never beat Donna in front of her father. Donna's older brother intervened whenever he was present. When Donna was 10 years old, she received a particularly violent beating from her mother. She ran away to her paternal aunt, who reported the abuse to the police. For reasons unknown to Donna, the case was dropped. Subsequently, the aunt returned her to her parents upon parental assurances that the violent

---

* These persons are: physicians, medical interns, medical examiners, dentists, nurses, public or private school teachers, educational administrators, guidance or family counselors, probation officers, social workers and policemen. Mass. Pub. Welfare, ch. 119 §51A (*Mass. Gen. L. Ann.*, Supp. 1976)

† A child is one who is under the age of 18. Mass. Pub. Welfare, ch. 119 §51A (*Mass. Gen. L. Ann.*, Supp. 1976)

‡ This case is discussed in detail at David Sanberg, Draft Manuscript on Donna M. (Odyssey House, 1976)

abuse would stop. The abuse continued. Donna states that a maternal aunt knew of the family beatings but did nothing. Early in the fourth grade Donna, a child of normal intelligence, but who by now had emotional problems, often withdrawing into the corner of the classroom or hiding in the coat closet, was misdiagnosed as slow, and was removed from the regular class and placed in a class for 'disturbed children' (most of whom in reality were retarded children, 14- 15- and 16-years-old). She remained in this class for the entire year. In neither the initial assignment to the special class nor the subsequent reassignment to the regular fifth grade was Donna seen by any professionals other than her regular teacher and the school principal.

When Donna was 9, she began sexually servicing her father two or three times per week. This activity occurred with her mother's active consent, as the mother felt she had had more pregnancies and children than she could adequately cope with, and she felt (misinterpreted) that as a devout Catholic she was prohibited from practising either birth control or sterilization and therefore it was better to meet her brutal husband's drunken demands by offering him the use of her prepubescent daughters, first of whom was Donna, at age 9. These happenings occurred before abortion was legalized, but even if there had been an alternative, it would not have been acceptable to this mother. The servicing continued until Donna's menses (at 14) at which time her younger sister replaced her. Donna's psychiatrist interprets that the severity of the beatings Donna received from her mother increased when she began to sexually service her father as a result of her mother's ambivalence in approving this activity and her jealousy. When Donna was 12, her father was hospitalized for a complete mental breakdown. When he returned to the home under intensive psychiatric care, no one came to investigate the home. When Donna was 14, her brother was arrested for numerous burglaries. At 18, he was out of control, enraged, having been a witness throughout the years to the violence and incest. Subsequently, he has often stated his guilt over his desire to kill both his parents, but particularly the father. He had begun to use heroin to quiet his anger and forget his guilt. As part of his probation report, the court social worker heard many stories of the family violence from one of the aunts. Still no intervention or home evaluation occurred. The boy was released but shortly thereafter engaged in a near-homicidal fight in a bar for which he was imprisoned.

Donna left home at age 15, living with a woman who had babysat for her, and for whom she now babysat, caring for that woman's children. At 17, she married a 19-year-old boy from an equally destructive childhood. The marriage was a poor one; she, though pregnant at the time, separated from him immediately upon discovering that her husband had exposed himself to her sister; Donna had long before vowed that she would not repeat the passive–aggressive misery of her mother's marriage. To protect herself from her violent estranged husband and to help with the children, Donna invited her recently-released-from-jail heroin-addicted brother to move in with her. At this point she, too, began to use drugs, to help her forget and cope with her problems. Although she suspended her drug usage temporarily during her pregnancy because she wanted to bear a healthy child, she resumed using drugs soon after the child was born. By age 24, Donna was working but receiving supplementary welfare assistance, about which she was embarrassed, for in this too she had vowed not to repeat her parents' pattern. She became more involved with drugs and had to quit her job now, receiving full welfare assistance. Her situation markedly deteriorated and though she had repeatedly vowed never to beat her children as often happens in child abuse, she, like her mother, began to beat her children, ages 4 years and 18 months. Child abuse victims frequently as parents become second generation child abusers because they have minimum resources to cope with stress and because they respond to learned behaviour. To quiet her children, and therefore not be driven to beat them, she resorted to what she analysed as the lesser of two evils, Donna taught her oldest son to smoke marijuana, and blew smoke into the face of the younger one who, at 10–14 months, was too small to smoke for himself, but who would be quieted by the contact high which resulted. Donna was well known to the local police of her small town outside of Boston. The police also knew about the children, but no report of her children as potential abuse or neglect victims was ever filed with the authorities. At the time she entered Odyssey House, Donna was pregnant with her third child by an unknown father. After treatment at Odyssey she realized how difficult it would be for her to care adequately for all three children and so she subsequently placed this daugher for adoption. She, like all of the previous cases, has been successfully rehabilitated. Presently she is a drug research consultant to one of Harvard's major drug treatment programmes, is successfully rearing her sons, and is engaged to be married to a fine young man.

As in the other cases, the Massachusetts system failed to respond initially when a person mandated by statute to report suspected abuse failed to do so. No penalty or sanction for such a failure to report is provided under the Massachusetts statute. Secondly, Massachusetts law does not provide for the circumstance where there is a substantial certainty that a child who is not suffering presently, will in the future suffer from abuse or neglect. The concept of protection of at-risk children is not sufficiently addressed within this state's system. Since Donna did not use drugs during her first pregnancy, and stopped early in her second, both children born of those pregnancies were precluded from being reported as one 'who is determined to be physically dependent upon an addictive drug at birth'[41]. Even though Donna returned to drugs within days of being discharged from the hospital after the birth of her second child, there was no way for that child to be protected when he returned home with his mother who was soon to quiet him with marijuana. As indicated previously, this would have been preventable under the New York statute[42].

In New Jersey, under a recently developed system, the Division of Youth and Family Services purchases child welfare services from various private agencies. No particular agency is identified as expert in the child abuse field, and none really functions as one. New Jersey ranks behind almost every other state in the union in its concern for its children. The New Jersey statute proposes 'to provide for the protection of children under 18 years of age who have had serious injury inflicted upon them by other than accidental means. It is the intent of this legislation to assure that the lives of innocent children are immediately safeguarded from further injury and possible death and that the legal rights of such children are fully protected'[43]. The statute requires that any person having reasonable cause to believe that a child has been subjected to child abuse or acts of child abuse report the same to the Division of Youth and Family Services. The reporter is given immunity from both civil and criminal liability[44]. Knowingly violating the provisions of the act causes the person to be classified as a disorderly person, a misdemeanour.

Case History No. 5

Grace is a 29-year-old White Italian Catholic female. Both her parents were alcoholics. Her mother was a prostitute. Before the time Grace was 12, her maternal uncle had sexually molested her in front of her younger brother. The uncle had a history of sexually abusing girls, and had spent time in jail for this activity. This was known to Grace's mother; but once again neither family nor society attempted to safeguard this child. From 6 years of age, Grace frequently came to school beaten. She was referred always to the same school nurse, who performed first aid but never reported her to the authorities, nor did her teachers or principal. Grace first came to the attention of the Children's Bureau at age 15; she was referred to them by the school after she had been so badly beaten by her mother that hospital care was required. Her first social worker assured her that if she was a good girl, did the dishes, etc. for her alcoholic prostitute mother (her father had long before left before Grace was 9) cared for her six smaller siblings, and obtained good grades (all of which seemed possible to the social worker) things at home would improve. When she continued to be beaten with marks that could no longer be ignored, and when she became so depressed that she attempted suicide with an overdose of pills, the social worker saw the light, relented, and placed Grace at 16 in temporary foster care. This reprieve was short lived because Grace was soon to return to her mother who was now so ill with cirrhosis that Grace was needed to care for the younger children. Certainly placement of these younger children or a visiting homemaker would have been a more rational approach than once again sacrificing Grace who was marginally coping at best.

Grace's contacts with other persons capable of reporting her abused status were similarly unfruitful. On the occasions that welfare workers visited the home, Grace's mother made certain that she was sober, the house clean, and no physical evidence of child abuse was present. Grace's family doctor magnanimously volunteered to help her if she developed unwanted pregnancies. I can only assume this was an offer to perform an abortion for remuneration, as this was prior to abortion on demand, rather than an offer to help Grace initial-ly avoid such a situation. The same doctor had hospitalized her previously to protect her from her mother's or uncle's abuse, but he had failed to report the situation to the authorities. His strongest action was to tell them to stop beating Grace, which they did for a short period of time, until they found a new family physician. The beatings then resumed.

At the end of her sixteenth year Grace was removed from school by her mother in order to work to support the family. When Grace protested this ac-tion, the school responded by writing her mother a letter that Grace was a good student with good potential and therefore they hoped she would be allowed to finish her education in night school. Little choice was left to Grace except to run away, for by now there was no way for her to imagine that any adult in-tended to help her out of this unfair suffocating situation. Later that same year, Grace finally ran away with her boyfriend. Using common sense, the local police refused to look for her because they felt that her situation with her boyfriend must be an improvement over her family life. Grace and her siblings were well known to the police, as the family lived across the street from the police station. Furthermore, at those frequent times when left unattended by the mother and without food, all the children would go for the day to the sta-tion where it was warm to be fed by the police. In spite of this the police had never actually intervened in this family situation, but they passively refused to bring her home. Grace says that her parents were themselves abused children. She further indicates that when her common-law husband deserted her and their two children, she went on welfare, began to drink, prostituted, and shifted the respon-sibility of caring for the children to her landlady, who lived in the same building. She knew she was repeating her mother's pattern, but she felt she was 'good for nothing' and 'predestined to fail' – certainly her mother had told her so enough times! Grace's children did not come to the attention of the authorities until later when they were reported to child welfare by Grace's mother who by then was caring for them because Grace had voluntarily entered a therapeutic community in New Jersey, in an effort to obtain psychiatric help for herself. This reporting was a retributive act by Grace's mother against Grace, rather than an action taken on behalf of the children. The basis for her mother's hatred of Grace originated in the fact that she had been the out-of-wedlock baby born to her mother when she was only 15. Though the mother had married the father several years later, she never forgave Grace for 'supposedly ruining her life'; she had been pretty enough to be sophomore cheerleader in high school before her belly enlarged.

As in other cases discussed, the breakdown in the system in the case of Grace and Grace's children was the failure of all those persons who initially observed the abusive and neglectful treatment, the police, the school teachers, the school nurse, the physician, the welfare case workers, the child welfare worker, and finally the landlady to report this maltreatment of the children as the law man-dated. The record of this case fails to indicate any investigation or follow-up by social service workers at the time of the changes in Grace's custody arrangements. Grace related that her mother abused her younger brother, but no investigation was made on his behalf either. There are many Graces and Grace's children in New Jersey, but its archaic Department of Hospitals and Institutions with everything subsumed within it, from prisons to foster homes, from the aged to the newborn, from licensing to direct service, from welfare to purchase of private service, from hospitals to adoptive homes, is unable to meet any needs adequately in a rational structured approach, particularly the needs of children. I suppose New Jersey is best understood by characterizing state government as divided into two branches: Gaming and Everything Else. The Everything Else branch just doesn't make it for children, for they can only cry out in tiny voices.

As a Mormon state, one would anticipate that Utah would be deeply committed to seeing that every child was protected within the family, but the basic nature and the wholesomeness of most of Utah families limits the realization of many of the problems within their communities. After working for many years in Utah, I believe that once the facts are known, corrective change will occur, for here differing from New Jersey, there is commitment to people. The Divisions of Family Services and Social Services within Utah provide some child welfare services, but neither agency is identified as expert in child abuse. Similarly, none of the other resources to whom child abuse cases are referred, including community mental health clinics and foster care agencies, are expert in child abuse. The development of such expertise is essential. The Utah statute requires the mandatory reporting of all known or suspected instances of child abuse or neglect* by any person having such suspicions[45]. Any person making a good-faith report is immune from liability therefor[46]. A knowing and wilful violation of the statute constitutes a misdemeanour. In cases of child abuse and neglect, 'it is the intent of the legislature that protective social services shall be made available in an effort to prevent further abuse or neglect and to safeguard and enhance the health and welfare of such children and to preserve family life whenever possible[47]. Reports are filed with the local city police or county sheriff or the office of the Division of Family Services[48]. The filing of a report of child abuse or child neglect is the sole criterion for the involvement of the child-protective service. There is no provision for or even contemplation of the entity drug related child abuse.

Case History No. 6

Linda was a 28-year-old White Mormon female from Utah. She had been conceived in the Utah mental hospital where her mother is still hospitalized. Her father is unknown, but it is rumoured that he was a staff attendant at the

---

* (1) 'Child abuse and neglect' means harm or threatened harm to a child's health or welfare by a person responsible for the child's health or welfare.
  (2) 'Harm or threatened harm' means any non-accidental physical or mental injury, sexual abuse, negligent treatment or maltreatment including the failure to provide adequate food, clothing or shelter . . . Utah C.L.A. §55–16–1.5 (Supp. 1975)

hospital caring for the mother. Linda was born in the insane asylum (a fact that haunted her the rest of her life) but was adopted when she was one month old by her maternal aunt and uncle. The uncle was an alcoholic, who often assaulted the aunt in Linda's presence. At age $5\frac{1}{2}$, Linda was molested by her uncle; he raped her and deflowered her the next year before she was 7. Sexual relations continued three or four times a month from then on until Linda was 13 and was old enough to run away to get married. Once married she bore her first child shortly after she was 14. She desperately wanted someone to hold and love for when Linda was but 8 or 9 she was so severely beaten by her aunt that she could not go to school for two weeks. Beatings continued approximately once every 3 months for the next 5 years. Linda believed that her aunt knew about the sexual contact between Linda and her husband, but was too afraid of losing him, so remained silent and punished Linda, having blamed the child instead. Linda, with her Mormon upbringing accepted the blame, felt she was crazy garbage similar to her mother, and attempted suicide in her late teens when her husband (who was also an alcoholic) learned of her incestuous past after questioning her about her never wanting sex and her frigidity. After she told him the truth, desperately needing his understanding and comfort, he turned on her, by now the mother of his three children, and not yet 20, calling her a whore and telling her she belonged on Second South (Salt Lake's redlight district). He left her that day and Linda attempted suicide. She was subsequently hospitalized for 1 year for a nervous breakdown. Two months after release, she was readmitted for another 9 months.

Between the ages of 9 and 13 Linda, who had begun using various drugs, made several suicide attempts. Each time she was hospitalized, then returned home. During this period she also saw several psychiatrists. But she missed many appointments scheduled for those times when she was severely beaten by her adopted mother. No inquiries as to why she missed the appointments were ever made. Linda also ran away from home several times during this period. Each time the police found her, sent her to the youth detention home, which sent her to the hospital which sent her home. Never was an inquiry made as to why she ran away and no information as to the beatings or incest was ever uncovered. Each time, Linda was later to relate, that she was found and incarcerated, she was made to feel 'what could you expect from a child who had been born within the confines of the state mental hospital to a hopelessly insane mother'. Subsequently, Linda left school at the end of the sixth grade. The school made no inquiries as to why this occurred. At 14, Linda married the 20-year-old alcoholic as mentioned earlier; she believed it was the only way to escape her father's sexual advances. During the first year of marriage, she was raped by her husband's father. During her 22nd and 23rd year, Linda was released once again from the hospital and she attempted to care for her three children. She related that she would routinely burn them with cigarettes in order to make them cry so that in turn she would be able to comfort them. Linda's children were removed from her care by court order when she was 26 after a series of arrests for heroin possession; the courts placed the children in her aunt's custody, who by now had divorced her husband, the incestuous uncle.

During most of Linda's hospitalizations, she was diagnosed as schizophrenic and placed on extraordinary dosages of Thorazine and other phenothiazines. It was felt that these large amounts were necessary because she was also a drug addict; but she never received any special treatment nor after-care for her addiction, and her children were always returned to her after all but the last hospitalization when Linda herself requested they be placed because she feared for their safety when she returned to live and work on Second South. At least, her cry for help regarding the placement of her children – now teenagers – was heeded then. During Linda's court-ordered 2½-year stay at Odyssey when for the first time she was psychologically tested, neither the psychologist nor the attending psychiatrist found any evidence that she was psychotic or suffered from a thought disorder. At Odyssey, she never required medication, nor was she out of control. And who is to say that the tear that she had tattooed below her right eye during one prison term because that was how she saw the world, 'through tears' was inappropriate? To me, who faced her many times in therapy, it was an eloquent summation of her life.

At 29, Linda committed suicide because she found herself unable to bear the pain of getting well; but first she wrote me and Odyssey a thank-you letter for having afforded her the only two and one-half happy years of her life. She killed herself because she felt no man other than her uncle would ever have her; and the only way she knew to resist his proposition, contained within a letter of the week before her suicide, was to withdraw into death. She asked all the Odyssey family to remember her with good feelings, and to consider this last act a happy happening for she wished to join her recently deceased beloved grandmother in heaven where she knew she would be protected and safe. Linda committed suicide in a hotel after having removed from her person all traces of her relationship with Odyssey because, as she wrote, she did not want to bring any criticism upon us. Thoughtful and solicitous to the end, I cannot help but wonder why someone could not have cared better for Linda as a child.

The school system, the hospital, the psychiatrist, the youth detention centre, and the police all had ample opportunity and evidence to suspect that Linda was an abused or neglected child. None so reported, nor was there any evidence that any person so failing to fulfil the mandate to report was questioned about their violation of the reporting statute – misdemeanour. The system failed to function because once again the initial report to the system was never made. Although Utah had a fairly sophisticated matrix of services for children and mandatory child abuse and neglect reporting system, the repeated failures of persons in that system to take the initial step of reporting completely prevented the engagement of the resources designed to intervene in this extreme case. It must be noted that when, in the instance of Linda's children, a report of their abused status was registered by the mother herself the system functioned well.

The social workers worked closely with Linda's treating psychiatrist at Odyssey, a thorough investigation of the aunt's fitness as custodian was performed, and the children were eventually removed from Linda's custody by court order. It must be further noted that the Odyssey House experience in this case showed that once a child was reported into the system, the Utah social service vigorously pursued the case until a satisfactory settlement was achieved.

CONCLUSIONS

Definitive statements, criticism or conclusions about the respective sample of state systems' response to drug-related child abuse, including sexual abuse, are difficult without further study (which we have proposed to New York State's Executive Branch).

Introduction

This memorandum is intended to serve as a preliminary sketch of an Office of Special Counsel to the Governor (or to the Legislature), preparatory to the creation of a Cabinet post, to be created either by Executive Order or by legislation. The Director of this Office will be reportable directly to the Governor and to a Senate Committee to be designated.

The mandate of the Office will be to identify the significant problems of children in New York State, and the availability and delivery of resources and services to meet their needs. The Office will operate on two approaches simultaneously: a component for survey and analysis of current legislation, delivery systems and service programmes; and a sociological autopsy component, tracing child abuse deaths. After a 12-month period, wherein data from both component studies will be assembled and analysed, the office will design and recommend policy and implementation of programmes and systems to more effectively and efficiently coordinate and administer the available expertise, resources and services on the state and local level.

SERVICES TO CHILDREN
SURVEY AND ANALYSIS COMPONENT
PROPOSED ACTIVITIES

1. Coordinate and direct a 12-month survey of all existing resources and services, including but not limited to health, social service, legal, education, juvenile justice and child protection legislation, programmes and systems on the state and local levels. This would include an evaluation and analysis of the legislation or implementing orders, the nature of services, the qualifications of service providers, eligibility requirements of recipients, criteria for intervention, scope of intervention, quality of services and impact on the designated problem areas, as well as the coordination with similar programmes or services from other sources, governmental or private.
2. Hold public hearings periodically in each county with state and local officials, service administrators and providers, community leaders, and private citizens to receive maximum input on needed changes and to help monitor the progress of and public response to legislative and/or programmatic developments. Transcripts and findings would be submitted to the Governor and to the designated Senate Committe.
3. Conduct a public education and awareness campaign to create a general understanding of the significance of children as the most valuable national resource; and of the numerous problems threatening the health, safety and development of children, individually and collectively. The campaign would present the public and its officials with facts and statistics which would facilitate and promote greater effectiveness and efficiency of the various components of the present system. Support will be sought for establishing the concerns of children as a priority of public services.
4. Organize and utilize an advisory board of citizens, private foundations, religious leaders, professional groups and service providers to meet regularly with the Director and to make recommendations on programmes and policy matters.

5. Submit a quarterly report to the designated Senate Committee by the Director on the activities, findings, recommendations, and problems of the Office. The Committee will be requested to take particular notice of any major issues raised which are of appropriate concern to the legislatire sector.
6. Examples of coordination of resources and efforts:
   a. Law enforcement monies and mental health monies should be coordinated in services and programmes to provide a comprehensive, effective effort at a reduced net cost to taxpayers.
   b. Develop mechanisms for local dissemination of information to the public of existing service programmes (such as the WIC programmes).
   c. Investigation of the problems of runaway children and abandoned children, and the coordination of resources allocated to their care and protection.
   d. Promulgation of guidelines for educational materials and courses on parenting for use in public school curriculae.
   e. Encourage the development and use of materials and courses in public schools with which to acquaint children with American values and traditions, and to update American history courses to reflect the participation of women and racial and ethnic minorities in the shaping of the development of the United States' position of world prominence.

This proposal was prepared for a state level position. A similar proposal for the creation of a national Cabinet post for the Concerns of Children has also been presented.

However, the evaluation of the application of the child protection laws in these case histories permits at least the following preliminary findings:

1. A comprehensive automatic child care delivery system similar to those operating in many Western European countries must be developed to replace the current delivery system, in which only the grossest incidents of child abuse and neglect are discovered.

2. The universal shortcoming encountered is the failure of the persons mandated to report suspected cases of child abuse and neglect to fulfil such obligation. To encourage reporting, a compulsory educational component, coupled with stronger penalties for failure to report these abuses, seems primary. It is evident from the non-reporting that a penalty of a misdemeanour is not a sufficient incentive. The Law and Medicine Division of Odyssey Institute suggests that failure to report by this class of persons be categorized as a felony, especially where non-intervention thereby results in death. Certainly those states which provide no penalty for failure to report, such as Michigan and Massachusetts, must prescribe a penalty. The imposition of such criminal penalties implies also. the loss of professional licensing, the threat of which always carries the most weight with doctors and other professionals.

3. Odyssey Institute approves the Massachusetts statement of purpose of the child protection law[49] which speaks to the interests of the child, with the parental interests and the goal of salvaging family life secondary. This approach vastly differs from the predominant approach of encouraging family life and parental interests even when this may be contrary to the best interests of the child. Towards this end of recognizing the interest of the child as paramount to the interest of the parent, the contents of the Michigan provision[50] requiring that in any action brought under the child protection law the child be appointed an attorney who will represent his best interests in that proceeding is insufficient. Even though the intent of this provision is to place

the child on an equal adversarial footing with all parties to such an action, the provision of a child's advocate produces only the illusion of such equality. Integral to the adversary system concept is the belief that the client is able to aid his attorney in the preparation of the litigation. Inability to aid one's advocate is a criterion for declaring incompetency to stand criminal prosecution. The ability to aid one's advocate is no less important in a child welfare determination proceeding. Yet one questions the quality of the aid, if any, that a 4-year-old client can give his attorney in developing a case that represents his best interests. For this reason, as well as many others, the adversary model is rejected as an appropriate model for the determination of child welfare questions. More lawyers certainly raise costs, but it is questionable whether the spending of more money produces a better result. There does not appear to me to be two sides to this issue – only one, protecting, preserving, fighting for – no, advocating for the child's well-being. The courts and the legal system have been no more stellar than the doctors and the other helping professions. Society as a whole has failed too many of its helpless children. It is time to hear the words of Jesus loud and clear, 'Suffer unto ye, little children, for he who does unto them, does unto me'.

An administrative hearing forum, subject to judicial review should be adopted instead of the traditional adversary model. Such a forum should and would not be bound by the traditional evidentiary rules. Moreover, such a forum should be charged with reaching a decision in the best interests of the child, regardless of the distribution of the weight of the evidence produced by the proponents of the various dispositional options. The issue is not that of affixing blame, but of protecting the child. The question is not *who did it?* but *what was done?* and *is there a reasonable certainty that unless an environmental change occurs, the harm is likely to recur?* The issue is not did the mother herself do it (or her husband, or her boyfriend or her) but is she capable of preventing another episode. This conceptual difference illustrates clearly the basic language difference and emphasizes the difference between the medical and legal professions. Lawyers must not and indeed cannot legislate good medical practice, for they are not trained to understand medical priorities and often inadvertently worsen situations with their legal mumbo-jumbo, such as debating the First Amendment protection of child pornography. Lawyers see facts on paper; doctors see suffering in people. In child abuse and neglect, the injury to the child speaks for itself (*res ipsa loquiter*) and raises a presumption by its very presence on examination alone that sustained intervention must be provided. Doctors must insist that they receive from the legislature the tools with which to successfully treat societal ills; so far, the doctors have remained too silent, and perhaps are even fearful of the legal process, to the detriment of us all.

In the area of children-at-risk and active child abuse and neglect the medical emphasis on the consequences of the act or risk and its predictability of reoccurrence rather than certainty must prevail over the lawyer's obsessive need to assess blame and to compulsively ensure against a possible reasonable doubt. I plead for leaving the age of the Socratic method and endless debate and entering an age of common-sense and commitments to our children – all of them.

Are we as a nation up to thinking new thoughts, accepting new data and trying new models? If we are not, then we shall surely perish.

4. A strengthening of the provisions allowing a physician without a previous court order to detain a child who he believes will be harmed if returned to his parent or guardian is necessary. The Michigan provision requiring a physician to report such a situation to his superior is only a half-way measure as it is discretionary with the supervisor whether custody over the child will be retained. Similarly, the Massachusetts requirement that a court order be obtained before the child may be retained is not sufficient. In both cases the discretion involved with deciding whether or not to seek a court order and/or detail the child will too frequently be resolved in favour of the least time-consuming alternative, the release of the child, or will fail because the medical realities will not be accorded their full weight by the non-medical professionals who make the ultimate decision concerning retaining custody over the child. It is recommended that health institutions with custody over abused children be mandated to retain that custody until alternative child care provisions can be made.

Moreover, the dicta in *Landeros v. Flood* is specifically rejected as detrimental to the child's interest. In that case it was recommended that the standard for civil liability of a physician for releasing a child to its parents when the child was possibly battered should be the same as the criminal standard adopted therein, whether it can be shown that it actually appeared to the physician that the injuries were inflicted on the child[51]. A reasonable belief that the injury could have been sustained accidentally would be sufficient to negate the physician's liability. This standard is rejected as a dangerous interpretation of the threshold at which child protective activities should attach. The concept of suspicion of abuse is mandatory if lives are to be saved and children not scarred for life.

Additionally, it is recommended that the Department of Child Welfare be given the right to remove a child from his or her present living situation when a complaint of abuse has been filed, pending a court evaluation of that complaint. Such removal may combat in part the fear of retribution by the guardian, resulting in the child's decision not to testify in a termination of custody proceeding, as noted in the above cases. This is particularly necessary in instances of an older child able to testify in cases of sexual abuse.

5. Finally, addressing the evidentiary problems, the New York approach wherein the standard rules of evidence are inapplicable to hearings under the child protective provisions is recommended to all states[52]. Under traditional evidentiary statutes such as in Massachusetts, severe evidentiary limitations handicap resolution of cases. These limitations are threefold. First, that in many jurisdictions a child under the age of seven is *non sui juris*. A recent

study conducted at the Odyssey House facilities resulted in a finding that 18% of the incest victim population had had their initial cross-generational incest experience under the age of 7. Incest is a crime that generally occurs in the home environment, with no witnesses present other than the participants in the act. The *non sui juris* rule automatically eliminates much of the ability to aid that portion of the population which is most in need of protection by the social institutions. Second, in all jurisdictions studied children between the ages of 7 and 12 routinely may give unsworn testimony. Such unsworn testimony is insufficient grounds upon which to base a conviction in a sexual abuse case. Again, given the nature of the act, it is improbable that such corroboration is available. Finally, in all states studied, with the exception of New York, the evidentiary rules requiring corroboration of charges of sexual misconduct again serve to severely restrict the probability of success of prosecution for sexual abuse. A survey of the case law reveals only one case discussing sexual abuse of the child, *In Re Hawkins*[53]. In that case a finding of abuse by the Family Court was made possible only because the act was corroborated by the victim's 13-year-old brother. The victim's unsworn statement that the act occurred would have been insufficient, standing alone, to support a finding of abuse and thereby protecting her.

These are but a few initial thoughts on the part of the Law and Medicine Division of Odyssey Institute, as well as myself. We ourselves have only recently begun to face the horrendous realities which face so many American children, crippling them from ever entering the mainstream of our way of life as full functionary citizens. Around us, we see many dedicated hard-working sincere people who struggle against overwhelming odds to provide service to children but few if any have had the experience or time to look beyond the instant presenting case to the issues that have made the disease of children-at-risk in a non-responsive society possible – no, probable. We, at Odyssey, have pledged ourselves not to be afraid to ask the questions for which as yet there do not appear to be answers, for only by articulating the questions can we perhaps together begin to communicate on the search for solutions.

SUMMARY

There exists adequate evidence of the causative relationship between substance abuse and child abuse to support a legal presumption of abuse and/or neglect where the parent or guardian is a substance abuser. This presumption should be integrated into all child protective systems.

The reporting provisions of the state child abuse and neglect statutes must be revised to include a felony penalty for noncompliance by the mandatory reporting source.

The child protective systems for insuring the physical safety of the child during the fact finding and adjudicative processes are of limited value. The lack of social services staff, placement services, follow-up and training often make intervention meaningless. The professionals who consistently release children back to such parents as discussed herein have some awareness of the problem but are not motivated to affirmatively act in the child's behalf. This lack of motivation may stem from frustration with the unwieldy and hostile adjudication process, or from apathy in the absence of meaningful tools.

The children of America deserve better. The legal and medical professions must accept the challenge of developing new tools and systems to significantly impact on the plight of the children of substance abusing parents. Detection, protective intervention and placement should involve a multi-disciplinary procedure. The court or decision-maker must assume the function of protector of the child above all others.

The welfare of American children must become a priority of government, as well as of the professions. The children's needs are different from those of adults whose voices are heard by policymakers and legislators.

At the national cabinet level these concerns should be formally represented, with the input and active contribution of the legal and medical professions.

ACKNOWLEDGMENTS

The research in this chapter was in large part supported by NIDA Grant H81–Da 01798–02 through the funding of Odyssey Institute's Parents' Program and written with the able assistance of Stephen F. Hutchinson, J.D., and Ruth Levine, J.D., General Counsel and Associate Counsel respectively of Odyssey Institute, Inc.

References

1. Private conversation between Dr Henry Giaretto and Judianne Densen-Gerber, June, 1977
2. 18 U.S.C. § 1461
3. 19 U.S.C. § 1305
4. 18 U.S.C. § 1464
5. 18 U.S.C. § 1462 and § 1465
6. 39 U.S.C. § 3008
7. Conn. Gen. Stat. Ann. § 53–25; N.C. Gen. Stat. § 14–190.1, *et seq.* N.D. Cent. Code § 12.1–27, 1–03; S.C. Code Ann. § 16–414.1 *et seq.*; Tenn. Code Ann. § 39–3013; Tex. Code Ann. § 43.24
8. Mich. Act 157, Public Acts of 1947 (as amended) § 409.14
9. N.Y. Educ. Law § 3231(a), (c)
10. Macpherson (1977). Children: The Limits of Porn, *Washington Post*, Jan. 30, 1977, § c, at 1
11. Public Acts of 1975, Act No. 238, Mich. C.L. § 722.621–722.636
12. Acts. No. 238, Preamble (1975)
13. Acts. No. 238, Preamble (1975)
14. Mich. C.L. § 22.621–722.636 (Supp. 1975)

15. Mich. C.L. § 722.623 (1) (Supp. 1975)
16. Mich. C.L. § 722.633 (1) (Supp. 1975)
17. Mich. C.L. § 722.624 (Supp. 1975)
18. Mich. C.L. § 722.625 (Supp. 1975)
19. Mich. C.L. § 722.623 (5) (Supp. 1975)
20. Mich. C.L. § 722.628 (2) (Supp. 1975)
21. Mich. C.L. § 722.623 (5) (Supp. 1975)
22. Mich. C.L. § 722.633 (1) (Supp. 1975)
23. Mich. C.L. § 722.622 (b) (Supp. 1975)
24. Mich. C.L. § 722.626 (1) (Supp. 1975)
25. Mich. C.L. xx § 722.626 (1) (Supp. 1975)
26. New York Social Services Law xx § 411 (McKinney, 1976)
27. New York Social Services Law § 411–428 (McKinnery, 1976)
28. New York Family Court Act § 1012 (f) (i) (B) (McKinney, 1976)
29. In re John Children, 61 Misc. 2d 347, 306 N.Y.S. 2d 797, 807 (1969)
30. New York Social Services Law § 420 (1) (McKinney, 1976)
31. New York Social Services Law § 420 (2) (McKinney, 1976)
32. New York Social Services Law § 414 (McKinney, 1976)
33. New York Services Law § 419 (McKinney, 1976)
34. New York Family Court Act § 1024 (McKinney, 1976)
35. Mass. Pub. Welfare, ch. 119 § 1 (*Mass. Gen. L. Ann.*, 1969)
36. Mass. Pub. Welfare, ch. 119 § 51A § 51A (*Mass. Gen. L. Ann.*, Supp. 1976)
37. Mass. Pub. Welfare, ch. 119 § 51A (*Mass. Gen. L. Ann.*, Supp. 1976)
38. Mass. Pub. Welfare, ch. 119 § 51A (*Mass. Gen. L. Ann.*, Supp. 1976)
39. Mass. Pub. Welfare, ch. 119 § 51B (3) (*Mass. Gen. L. Ann.*, Supp. 1976)
40. Mass. Pub. Welfare, ch. 119 § 51C (*Mass. Gen. L. Ann.*, Supp. 1976)
41. Mass. Pub. Welfare, ch. 119 § 51A (*Mass. Gen. L. Ann.*, Supp. 1976)
42. Cf. New York Family Court Act § 1012 (f) (i) (B) (C.L.S. 1971)
43. *New Jersey Rev. Stat. Ann.* § 9:6–8.8 (Cum. Supp. 197)
44. *New Jersey Rev. Stat. Ann.* § 9:6–8.13 (Cum. Supp. 197)
45. Utah C.L.A. § 55–16–2 (Supp. 1975)
46. Utah C.L.A. § 55–16–4 (Supp. 1975)
47. Utah C.L.A. § 55–16–1 (Supp. 1975)
48. Utah C.L.A. § 55–16–3 (Supp. 1975)
49. Mass. Public Welfare, ch. 119 § (*Mass. Gen. L. Ann.* 1969)
50. Michigan C. L. § 722.630 (Supp. 1975)
51. 131 Cal. R. Supp. 69 (S. Ct. 1976)
52. New York Family Court Act § 1046 (McKinney, 1976)
53. 351 N.Y.S. 2d 574 (New York County Family Court, 1974)

12 The contributions of the social agencies and the social worker

SHEILA M. NOBLE

HISTORICAL DEVELOPMENT OF SOCIAL AGENCIES

Concern for the rights of children based on humanitarian principles is chiefly a twentieth century development. It is true that in the past, children have been cherished and esteemed by their parents, yet they have also in other circumstances been exploited and misused to serve the need and greed of the adult world, whether it might be child marriages forced upon minors in sixteenth century England to secure the proper transfer of property between wealthy families or the use of child labour in the factories of England[1] during the Industrial Revolution, when the prosperity of the nation was thought to depend upon the exertions of young children working long hours in deplorable conditions. It is possible to trace little change historically towards the phenomenon of child injury until attitudes in society changed, leading to the establishment of the preventive social agencies.

We may discern the elements of savage cruelty in several surviving Greek tragedies: poetic fiction based on myth and magic this may be, but in Euripides' tragedy, the witch Medea is a woman of formidable dimensions. When Jason carried her off with the Golden Fleece, they were pursued by her father by sea. She then dismembered the body of her younger brother, taken as a hostage, and adroitly cast his limbs into the wake of their ship for his father, following hard, to find and retrieve from the sea, thus delaying his pursuit. Later, when Jason forsook her, she murdered their children, as an act of revenge against him and his new consort. Here we may see the forerunner of Lady Macbeth, who also represents dramatically a woman's irrational impulse to maim or kill her offspring: she would have 'dash'd the brains out'[2] even while her child was feeding at the breast. The threats and actions of these two theatrical figures are not so very far removed from those of contemporary

351

parents whose real and bizarre acts of barbarity towards their children have lately been accorded much coverage by the press.

The Old Testament contains vivid accounts of massacres and individual acts of savagery against children. In the prolonged strife between Israel and Egypt, Pharaoh commanded the midwives to kill at birth all male Hebrew children and it was under the threat of this edict that the infant Moses was exposed in an ark in the bulrushes. Abraham[3] was required by Jehovah to offer 'as a burnt offering', his only son Isaac 'whom thou lovest'. There are numerous references to the burning of children by fire, censured on the Book of Chronicles[4] as one among many heathen practices. Perhaps the modern counterpart is the deliberate act of burning, perpetuated by parents against young children and documented in research[5]. We may read that 'Rachel weeping for her children refused to be comforted, because they were not'[6]. Esther's[7] mission to king Ahasuerus was to intercede against the royal edict 'to destroy, to kill and cause to perish all Jews, both young and old, little children and women in one day'.

Under Roman law, 'potestas patria', the power of life and death was conferred on a father, if a Roman citizen, and he might kill his offspring without appeal. The sense of shame associated with illegitimacy gradually developed in association with the advent of Christianity but bastardy was in general not thought to be socially unacceptable up to the time of the Reformation. With the decline of the Catholic Church and the later advent of the Puritans, great emphasis was laid on a moral code which stigmatized adultery, illegitimacy and the child born out of wedlock. Unmarried mothers were, as a consequence, forced to procure the death of their children, to conceal them and when discovered, were often put to death themselves with appalling severity by a hypocritical society. Exceptionally a compassionate jury, sitting with a Coroner, refused to bring in a verdict of guilty, as we read in the entry on the pregnant cook-maid in Parson Woodforde's diary in September 30, 1765[8].

Darwin in the early part of the nineteenth century commented on infanticide and abortion as early, if crude, methods of population control, widely prevailing where it was impossible to support more children[9]. This view is supported by Bakan[10] who considers the main cause of child abuse 'the burdensomeness of children' and expounds on the basis of evolutionary theory, saying this 'depends on the resources for living and the availability of resources'.

In England, where the social evils of overcrowding and sweated labour started early with the momentum of the Industrial Revolution, there was little evidence of any social conscience at work on behalf of illegitimate children, if they were abandoned by their mothers. Victorian hypocrisy wore the mask of respectability and only in the latter part of the nineteenth century did concern show itself in the provision of charitable orphanages for such children, through agencies such as Dr Barnardo's Homes.

There was much scope for cruelty and severe neglect, resulting in death for some children at the hands of people taking care of them for gain. It is only just over a century ago in 1870 that much publicity was given to a notorious example of baby farming. Margaret Waters was executed, following trial, upon evidence that 16 babies within a month were found dead within close proximity to her home in Brixton. These children had been put in her care in response to advertisements offering 'a good home and a mother's love and care'. She was to receive £5 in payment with no questions asked. The fathers of these children were no less culpable: by their very absence they had left the mother and child unsupported in a world indifferent to their need. In the same year, 270 bodies of babies, mostly less than a week old, were found in London alone[11]. This led, as a result of political pressure, to legislation in child welfare passed in 1872, requiring the registration with the Local Authorities of anyone caring for two or more infants for 'reward or hire'. This first infant life protection Act led to a series of other Acts including the Children Act of 1908, known as the Children's Charter, which gradually eliminated the practice of baby farming. There developed a growing concern in legislation for the welfare of the child, the need for which was made plain by the mortality figures for infants under one year of age per 1000 live births in England and Wales[12].

| 1914 | Legitimate 100 | Illegitimate 207 |
| 1918 | Legitimate 91 | Illegitimate 186 |

Historically this brief survey of child abuse can be considered from several points of view. Society could and can look with tolerance upon the wholesale and deliberate slaughter of young children by edict or default and view with calmness their death from starvation or deliberate neglect. Parents acting under intense pressures of religious belief or the emotion of jealousy are prepared themselves violently to do away with their own child. Furthermore, where there are equally intense social or economic stresses they may make it possible for others for gain to allow their child to die from deliberate neglect. Yet again acts of violence against children may be undertaken on the part of a primitive community, hard-pressed to survive on limited resources. Similarly in industrialized communities of the present day, the deliberate injury of their own children by parents is no new phenomenon but only lately has it been openly acknowledged to exist as a problem at all and a matter of concern to everyone.

THE THEORY OF MATERNAL DEPRIVATION AND ITS INFLUENCE ON SOCIAL WORK PRACTICE.
AN OVERVIEW AND CRITIQUE OF BOWLBY'S THEORIES

At the end of the war in Europe in 1945, deliberations at the third session of the Social Commission of the United Nations were centred upon the needs of homeless young children. In 1948 Dr John Bowlby was invited to take charge of a study for the World Health Organisation. He published a monograph in 1951, *Maternal Care and Mental Health,* as a contribution to the welfare of children, homeless in their native country. His theories produced considerable interest, discussion and eventually controversy among people professionally concerned with child care and subsequently with child-rearing techniques. The controversy led on to criticism about the basic hypothesis as well as a reappraisal by the author and his colleagues ten years later but not before the original precept had made a profound and seemingly indelible imprint on social work theory as taught at this time.

Bowlby defines his theory of mental health by saying it is essential 'that the infant and young child should experience a warm, intimate and continuous relationship with his mother or permanent mother substitute in which both find satisfaction and enjoyment'[13]. Without this complex, rich and rewarding relationship with the mother in early years, a state of maternal deprivation will exist. On page 13 of the monograph he includes a reference to fathers, saying the relationship with the mother may be varied by contact with the father and siblings but this is not elaborated and later he makes it plain that the father is of secondary importance, as he is to act as emotional and economic support to the mother.

Having stated that there is a high measure of agreement among child guidance workers in Europe and America on the approach to cases, diagnostic criteria and therapeutic aims, he includes child psychiatrists among his adherents in the belief that the young child has an essential need for his mother's exclusive attention and ministrations during these first formative years. He further says 'there is no room for doubt regarding the general proposition that the prolonged deprivation of a young child of maternal care may have grave and far-reaching effects on his character and so on the whole of his future life'[14]. He considers that there is abundant evidence that deprivation can have adverse effects upon the development of children, during the period of separation, immediately after restoration to maternal care and with permanent effect in at least a small proportion of cases. He dismisses as 'of no consequence' the fact that some children seem to escape these predictions.

Deprivation, he says, can on the evidence produce an 'affectionless' and delinquent character in some children. This can arise from lack of opportunity to form an attachment to a mother figure during the first three years, from deprivation for a limited period during the first three to four years and, thirdly, from changes between one mother figure to another during the same period. He predicts that nothing but prolonged residence with an adult having the skill, insight and unlimited time to devote to the child is likely to reverse these results. These resources would be costly and scarce, so he considers it would be practical and less expensive to arrange the kind of care for infants and toddlers that would prevent such conditions developing[14]. We may see here the seeds of thought that later perhaps led in America to the management of families with abused children by means of intensive care from one social worker on perpetual call to a restricted number of families[15]. It seems important that these methods are fully evaluated before being universally applied.

It is interesting to observe that Bowlby in his research into maternal deprivation did not contemplate the idea that parents might actively maltreat their
children. In this he does not differ from his contemporaries but he goes further
and seems to imply that there never can be a home bad enough to drive a child
away or make it necessary for him to be removed from his parents' roof. In
developing his thoughts on the purpose of the family, he says 'It must never be
forgotten that even a bad parent who neglects her child is nonetheless providing
much for him. Except in the worst cases, she is giving him food and shelter . . . he
may be ill-fed and ill-sheltered . . . he may be ill-treated but unless his parents have
wholly rejected him, he is secure in the knowledge that there is someone to whom
he is of value and who will strive, even though inadequately, to provide for him
. . .'[14]. He goes on to find on these grounds reasons why young children thrive better
in bad homes than in good institutions and why children with bad parents are, apparently without reason, so attached to them. He describes this unreasoning loyalty as a never-failing source of wonder and accounts for it, almost ingenuously it
seems, as the result of gratitude on the part of the child.

The basis of Bowlby's research into the effects of maternal separation consisted of a group of forty-four known delinquent children, with a corresponding
control group[13]. They were described as being incapable of forming lasting
relationships with others and Bowlby concluded on the basis of research on this
modest scale that 'there is a very strong case indeed for believing that
prolonged separation of a child from his mother, during the first five years of
life, stands foremost among the causes of delinquent character development', a
condition which he later came to regard as irreversible.

Before approaching the critical literature, it is worth contemplating the
reception accorded to these writings at the time of their publication. In the
United Kingdom, there had been considerable disruption to children's lives,
caused by their wholesale evacuation during the war from the main industrial
areas of the country. Mothers had mainly accompanied young children but
school children had left their families behind and there was evidence in research,
such as Susan Isaacs' survey, that for 700 children, evacuated to Cambridge,
human relationships had taken second place to administration[16] and that
evacuated children were often disturbed and without a constant mother figure.

There followed the events that led to the enquiry and publication of the Curtis Report in 1946, namely the manslaughter of one child and maltreatment of
another in foster care, for whom the Local Authority was responsible. A lack of
trained staff was noted and a need was urged for 'a greater sense of personal interest and responsibility at Local Authority headquarters and far more
specialist staff here'[17]. There was a perpetual conflict and therefore divided
responsibility between Public Assistance and Education Committees and little
concern was shown for family ties. The appointment of a Children's Officer with
senior rank and status within the Local Authority was enacted and this was
followed by the setting up of Children's Departments. Courses of training were established for Child Care Officers who were relative late-comers to social work.

This was taking effect in the 1950s while trained staff were seeking a body of knowledge with which they could identify and support their newly formed professionalism.

Child Care gradually developed as an expanding branch of social work, and much emphasis was laid on preventive work with families. It is interesting to remember that the development of child care was evoked by compassion: other aspects of social work such as the needs of the mentally and physically ill and handicapped seldom arouse the same degree of sympathy and emotion. With trained staff looking for an identity, we may see how this new teaching was welcomed, for it must have seemed to fit their new role exactly, and to give an importance and urgency to their work. Regrettably much of what Bowlby wrote has been disregarded and his own modifications have been ignored, as well as those of subsequent research workers. The belief that the mother–child bond is not to be dissolved at any cost, can result in disastrous consequences for abused children. The Maria Colwell case is, after all, a more notorious one of a series before public attention.

A further WHO publication in 1962 included criticisms and assessments of Bowlby's work by a variety of contributors, several of whom dissent from his writings. The preface praises his contribution to a 'change of outlook and widespread improvement in the institutional care of children' but admits that after 10 years Bowlby had himself revised his position and incorporated theories from ethology in his views on child development[18].

Prugh and Harlow[18], writers from the disciplines of psychiatry and psychology, quote Bowlby's[13] statements that 'prolonged breaks in the mother–child relationship during the first three years of life, leave a characteristic impression on the child's personality. Clinically, such children appear emotionally withdrawn and isolated' and 'there is a specific connection between prolonged deprivation in the early years and the development of an affectionless psychopathic character, given to persistent delinquent conduct and extremely difficult to trust'. While not questioning the importance of Bowlby's contribution, they consider that unfortunately some of the implications of his statements have been accepted by certain professional workers so completely and without criticism that they have interpreted any separation of the infant or young child as necessarily resulting in serious emotional deprivation. Additionally there have been errors by them in concluding that all children entering institutional care at an early age inevitably develop into 'affectionless' characters and by inference they conclude that only children undergoing this extreme privation develop these personality characteristics. However on the basis of other studies[19,20], Prugh and Harlow would doubt that development of such personality characteristics are inevitable or permanent. Furthermore it has sometimes been concluded that any home setting is better than any institutional placement. Case studies by the authors and others underline the fact that the emotional satisfaction of the child is not guaranteed by the physical presence of the parent or foster parent, especially if that parent shows an inability to tolerate disturbed behaviour on the part of the child.

It is too easy to conclude that any child is better off in his own home than in any other placement, whether it be hospital, institution or foster home. We may say most children are happier with their own parents even if relationships between them are disturbed and lack satisfaction, but we may also see children admitted to nurseries and to hospital, coming from intact but very disturbed families, who are evidently so distraught that we may rightly conclude such homes do not provide the most suitable environment for their normal development. They go further and say 'on the contrary it is sometimes seen that only when the child is removed from home, is he able to begin to mature and develop'[18].

In 'masked deprivation'[20], where the effect of insufficient warmth and stimulation on the part of the mother is observed in relation to the intellectual development of some children, an appearance of mental retardation without an obvious cause such as brain damage is often seen. The provision of satisfying mother-substitute relationships and/or direct psychotherapy with the mother has shown that such subtle retardation can be reversed.

Studies by Orlansky[21], Rank[22] and others seem to indicate that the quality of mother–child relationships in the 'emotional climate' has more effect than the learning of any single child-rearing technique. The effect of separation must include consideration of such factors as its nature and duration, the age of the child and stage of his development, his physical health and the quality of mothering both before and after the event. Careful consideration of all these factors is essential for making good decisions about the best arrangements for the child. 'The conclusion ... that the child should continue to stay in its own home or foster home under all conditions does not seem warranted[18].' They quote Maenchen's[23] statement 'a child may never have been separated from his mother, yet have been deprived of much more than if he had been placed in an institution with small groups and good nurses'.

Prugh and Harlow consider that where 'masked deprivation' takes place, the best choice for the child may be in a carefully selected institution, 'especially if the planning includes sufficient preparation of both parent and child'. In this context, Court procedure is not envisaged but, when this takes effect in cases of severe injury to the child, removal to a place of safety may include an institution and here again advance planning and preparation must be attempted.

R. G. Andry[24] has also questioned Bowlby's concepts that maternal deprivation is the main cause of defects in personality development. He considers child development to be so complex that maternal deprivation can be seen as only one among several aspects of relationships between mother and child. He highlights the concomitant role of fathers, which he considers to be much neglected by maternal deprivation theorists who also ignore the importance of deprivation by both parents.

In his research[24] with delinquent boys and their parents, he found that both parents and especially fathers admitted not only deficiencies in their relationships with their sons but also an inability to improve matters. From this he deduces that Child Guidance programmes should also include work with fathers, pointing out his own successful work in Australia. Perhaps one might tentatively infer from the context of his work, that in families where child battering was admitted, and help was sought, emphasis on treatment should include the needs of the father as well as the mother, thus underlining what he calls the subtle and basic triangularity existing, as the child sees it, between himself and his parents.

More recently Bowlby has substantially modified his original views and incorporated many scientific principles from ethology, cognitive psychology and control theory as a way of conceptualizing the propensity of human beings to make affectional bonds to their caretakers. One awaits with interest further challenges to these views.

Further criticisms

Barbara Wootton[26] has led the vanguard of the attack against Bowlby's theory. As a corrective to Bowlby's views, she cites the work of Hilda Lewis[27] who found in a study of 500 children admitted to a Reception Centre that 'unless separation of the child from the mother had occurred before the age of two years and had been lasting, it bore no statistically significant relation to the normality or otherwise of the child's mental state at the time of admission. No clear connection was evident between separation from the mother and a particular pattern of disturbed behaviour. Neither delinquency nor incapacity for affectionate relationships was significantly more frequent in the separated children.'

Lewis herself has also commented that 'the mere physical presence or absence of the child's own mother is no true index of the quality of mothering which the child may have enjoyed' and points out that 'unduly dogmatic statements about the ill-effects of maternal deprivation often leave out of account the emotional hazards and harm children may suffer from bad mothers and indifferent mother substitutes, as well as the variety of sources, including the father, from whom children may draw the love and support necessary for their happiness'. The equal importance of the father's contribution has been stressed by Holman[28].

In a study of 277 children from one-parent families, Rowntree found that 'the great majority of the children from broken homes were as well and as normal in behaviour as those living in more stable circumstances'[29]. Too much emphasis is laid upon the experience of separation itself, not upon the condition of the home whence the child came, nor the institution to which it was sent. What is chiefly to be learnt from the studies of children in institutions is that they have not only a need to find love on which they can depend but that this is more likely to be found in a family than an institution.

The emphasis on separation from the mother obscures the significance of

Margaret Mead's observations where she suggests that a child may find the best opportunity for stability, if a number of warmly disposed, caring people share the responsibility of looking after him[30]. Little evidence has been produced to support the assertion that the damage brought about by maternal deprivation cannot be reversed. It may be asked whether as a corollary, one can accept the point of view that no change in personality can be achieved after adolescence or early adult life at the latest. In any case no such statement can be validated unless the children thus deprived are assessed throughout their lives and few research projects have such resources.

In considering the effect on a child of life in an institution, relative to his deprivation, it is not easy to prove whether it is the fact of separation from his parents, or the way the institution is run or even the quality of the diet that may cause the damage. The definition becomes less exact. In Bowlby's work, the stress placed upon the warm, intimate and continuous relationship with the mother, becomes a matter of dependence on the mother or mother-substitute. There is a shift of emphasis between physical separation and emotional rejection. It is important for the social worker to decide whether it is more significant to the child to live under his mother's roof or to be loved consistently by her or by some figure acting as a substitute. If we believe consistent affection is more important to a child than mere physical presence, then this will oblige us to reconsider our attitudes towards the break-up of the family, if such affection is not forthcoming.

We must also look at the implications of early separation between mother and child, not in isolation but seeing it perhaps as a precursor to a mother's rejection of her child; this in turn will have a harmful effect upon the growth of a child's personality. When we consider the effect of maternal deprivation upon anti-social behaviour and delinquency, there is a scarcity of published literature to support the belief that early deprivation promotes subsequent bad behaviour. Bowlby, while accepting certain elements of inexactitude, was prepared to support what he called 'the concordance of the whole'. Wootton considers more prudent a belief that did not go beyond Bowlby's alternative statement that 'relatively few studies, taken by themselves, are more than suggestive'[13]. She sees the discovery that a child has a need of dependable love and that without it, he becomes frightened or unhappy or mentally retarded, as a 'homely truth' arrived at after costly research but already familiar to many humane and kindly people. Most people would admit that there can be deprived children living in families and emotionally fulfilled children in institutions, that some children are more tough than others and that this toughness enables them to endure and survive without sign of change.

Research has demonstrated that children under present circumstances are more likely to find dependable love and affection in families than in institutions but this in itself is a comment on how institutions are run, namely that children may find no chance there of a 'warm continuous relationship with a mother-substitute' and this may be the cause of retardation rather than any inherently superior value in family life over life in an institution. Wootton expressly says 'as much good may be done by running institutions better as by leaving children in their homes', adding that this fact is explicitly appreciated by more careful investigators[26]. She indicates that the point is not always taken by those who make a crude comparison between home and institution, who deplore the separation of parent and child but who disregard the quality of family life or the regime in practice at the institution. She comments ironically that a misplacement of emphasis has caused research workers to obscure the genuine discoveries by placing significance on what is virtually self-evident. The cause of physical separation will preoccupy research workers rather than those of deprivation, which is a far more complex subject. Wootton has succinctly expressed her criticism: 'That the damage is life-long or irreversible, that maternal deprivation is a major factor in criminal behaviour, or that the younger the child, the greater the risk – all these must be regarded as quite unproven hypotheses'[26].

Other writers have made reassessments and further criticisms of Bowlby's original hypothesis. Mary Ainsworth, an early colleague, was in no doubt that maternal deprivation had an adverse effect upon a child's development, both during and after the experience and that this could lead to serious consequences for the child that might subsequently resist reversal[18]. However, she considered that misunderstandings had arisen because the original definition had become over-simplified. Research has indicated that the adverse effects of maternal deprivation differ in nature, severity and duration, and that they are related to qualitative differences in the experience suffered. The definition of maternal deprivation was used to cover every kind of mother–child reaction, such as rejection, hostility, cruelty and over-indulgence etc.

Michael Rutter[31] also comments on Ainsworth's 'excellent and thoughtful reappraisal of maternal deprivation' but he makes the point that it includes multiple aspects of stress and covers a wide range of different experiences: to use the single phrase 'maternal deprivation' has had the 'most unfortunate consequence of implying one specific syndrome of unitary causation'. Since even 10 years ago other causes have been suggested within the child's experience, such as the disruption or failure of the bonding process, lack of perceptual or linguistic experience, inadequate diet, early stress and discord in the family. Rutter himself considers the actual term 'maternal deprivation' to be misleading, because the adverse effects are not specifically related to the mother, nor due to deprivation[32]. He refers to the lack of or distortion of care, rather than to direct loss. While he agrees with Bowlby's claim that mother love in infancy equated for mental health with vitamins for physical health, he yet regretted that this view had induced 'some people mistakenly to place an almost mystical importance on the mother and to regard love as the only important element in child-rearing. This is a nonsense and it has always been a mis-interpretation of what was said in the 1951 report. Nevertheless the view has come to be wide-spread among those involved in child care.' In this regard it is interesting that Ainsworth[33] has recently commented that babies become more responsive and communicative if their crying signals evoke an immediate response rather than indifference as in the case with battering parents.

Morgan[34] attributes to the fragmentation of the family and the reluctance of people in authority to interfere, the fact that many children lead hopelessly deprived lives with no prospect of change, where children are regarded as possessions, not held in trust for their own future. She considers it important that a child's development should be shared with skilled people outside the family, who have natural contact with the parents through nursery schools attached to nursing developments and who are available as an acceptable source of help in an emergency.

Rutter makes two further points with regard to the mother, that differ from Bowlby's theory. First, he disagrees with the view that the mother has a special importance and that the bonds developed with her differ in kind from those made with others. Most children develop bonds with several different people and such bonds are likely to be similar in quality. Second, the child is not necessarily most attached to the mother, even though she does most for him: the person with whom the child establishes his chief bond need not be the biological parent, or the chief caretaker, nor even female. Furthermore this person does not necessarily feature as the most important figure to the child. Other figures making impact include father, siblings, friends, teachers, all influencing different aspects of development: 'a less exclusive focus on the mother is required: children also have fathers'.

The consequences for social work of unquestioning adherence to the theory of maternal deprivation

It is worth considering what happens when social workers put into practice their belief in the need to keep mothers and children inseparably together. Kempe[15] makes it very clear that where such a decision is made with regard to the abused child, casework and follow-up must be intensive and carried out under the direction of a psychiatrist, with a view to preventing a repetition of the abuse and improving the emotional climate in the home by changing attitudes and inducing emotional growth in the parent. He warns expressly that 'intermittent and occasional casework that is not intensive, nor highly skilled and which is not closely supervised, or the use of routine casework in the face of very major psychopathology, including frank psychiatric states, is specifically contra-indicated'.

One may sometimes discern reluctance on the part of some social workers to seek skilled help from an outside source. This is evident in the report on Maria Colwell where[35] neither the social worker directly concerned nor her Senior felt that the independent view of a psychiatrist would have assisted in understanding the disturbed behaviour of this little girl once her mother had reclaimed her. The social worker said she was prepared to make an intelligent guess 'at the child's true feelings under tension and stress' but the Committee of Enquiry felt unable to accept that 'in a case such as this, a child should be subjected to the degree of stress shown by Maria'. Furthermore while stating that they appreciated that social work training covered child psychology, they nevertheless expected 'such training should enable social workers to turn readily for specialist help when severe trauma presents, so that medical skill can supplement their own casework skill'. The author of the minority report explicitly supports the social worker in her rejection of psychiatric assessment. Furthermore she goes on to say 'I reject the view that qualified social workers are not competent to make an assessment of children's or adults' behaviour and to place an interpretation upon it. I would go further and say it is an integral part of their job.' She cites the effects of separation and deprivation upon children as a subject of special relevance to social workers and from this, puts the view that the social worker involved had therefore the right and duty to consider and interpret Maria's feelings at the time.

While not denying this, we may ask whether an independent assessment might perhaps have produced an answer that would have spurred on the social workers to become less tolerant of the stress this child was undergoing. They were at that moment able to consider 'Maria's reactions, distressing as they were, to be normal rather than pathological given the stress to which she was subjected'. We know that psychiatric help often is not available to social workers when they seek to assess such problems on an everyday basis, for instance when injury is threatened. However where liaison is made a reality with medical and psychiatric services and where mutual communication and understanding are effective, skilled and informed help from the medical field can be a considerable resource to the social worker in making decisions based on the child's best interest.

In the Birmingham Child Abuse Study 134 hospitalized children were examined[36]. Full psychiatric and social reports and recommendations were forwarded to Social Service Departments following diagnostic evaluation. In most cases the abused children were not brought before the Juvenile Court, voluntary supervision being mostly relied upon. Of the 24 cases where legal proceedings were taken, 21 received Care Orders and 3 received Supervision Orders. In 21 cases, no arrangement was made for supervision and this was seen to be a surprisingly high figure, in relation to the high mortality and morbidity reported and the number of occasions when the children were re-battered.

Although the specialist research team made it known that they were available for further consultation, this offer was rarely made use of and then only (with one exception) by unsupported junior members of staff. The research concluded that Local Authorities were failing in their statutory role of protecting the child by their reluctance to institute care proceedings[37]. Kempe[15] criticizes social workers for undertaking casework 'at the risk of further damage to the child', in the mistaken belief that 'there is no such thing as a person we cannot help'. Where the child remains in the house as a source of irritation, and so liable to further injury, casework alone can at best be precarious and at worst a dangerous method of management. The social worker undertakes a grave responsibility in leaving the child in a position of hazard in the home, relying upon the possible development of a relationship between the parents and himself. The child can become a kind of yardstick of success or failure, depending upon whether re-injury takes place. The developments of such casework relationships depends very much upon the ability of the parents to enter upon them and to sustain them, yet such parents may well be unable to develop any kind of lasting relationship with another individual either within or outside their family.

Social workers have become reluctant to use authority, failing to make a distinction between its personal and professional use. In commenting on this, Young[38] sees it to be governed by responsibility and accountability, in the context of child abuse. 'In casework it is authority used to protect those unable to protect themselves. To relinquish it can be only to cripple that power to protect.'

We have heard that social workers concentrate undue attention upon the needs of the parents and ignore the fact that grave injustice has in some cases already been perpetrated against the child. They forget they have a prime duty to defend the child against further outrage. Davoren[15] has some controversial recommendations to make about the social worker's contribution and one may question whom she sees as most in need of her help, parent or child, when she describes her reluctance to intervene while she witnessed a child being sadistically injured by the parent. She gives as the reason her belief that if she had tried to restrain the cruelty, the child would be treated even more harshly when she had gone. So she remained silent while a mother twisted her boy's arm and hit him till he fell to the ground, later blandly denying that she had hurt him. The social worker reserved 'her real efforts at protection in helping the mother to tolerate her own feelings (about separation anxiety) enough to allow them conscious acceptance'. She claimed here some success in changed behaviour by the mother but one may surmise at what cost in physical and mental trauma to her child.

Davoren further adds that in terms of treatment her research team felt able to give help on a 24-hour basis to the families in their care. This was offered in the belief that this service gained for them an intensive knowledge of the family's day-to-day living habits and their behaviour in times of crisis. Most of their work involved leaving the threatened child in the home. It was admitted that these methods might not be universally feasible but nevertheless they were adopted with enthusiasm by certain social work agencies in the United Kingdom as a means of meeting the problem and perhaps of assuaging social workers' anxieties about their relationships with the parents. Necessarily the consumption of scarce resources in the form of trained staff devoted to a small number of families is costly in terms of time and effort, resources and money. The outcome of this method of intensive management of such families has not yet been evaluated in depth. It is a matter of interest to know whether the results will justify the input of such resources.

THE RELATIONSHIP BETWEEN SOCIAL WORKERS, POLICE, TEACHERS AND VOLUNTARY AGENCIES

The police

It has been shown[39] that only a third of child abuse cases are referred for police investigation. It may be that the difference of approach between the doctors and social workers on the one hand and the police service on the other can arise because possibly there is a difference of objective. These differences will now be briefly examined.

In the USA, the police are leading advocates of the reporting system with complaints made to them direct[15]. They argue that the police are on duty 24 hours a day, that criminal matters should be brought first to their attention and that Child Welfare Agencies have neither the staff nor the training to put in hand the kind of enquiries necessary to bring the matter to court. Furthermore, they would like to see a development of cooperation between police and social agencies, each pursuing its own role in mutual confidence. Kempe in the same publication, while agreeing with much of this, has stated that he and his colleagues could not accept such forthright advocacy of invariable prosecution as it would exclude opportunities for reconciling the family by the less drastic means of psychiatry, psychotherapy and social casework.

In the United Kingdom, Collie on behalf of the police has laid emphasis on the primary need to protect the child from serious injury and death, to provide redress before the courts and to emphasize the function of the police as professional interrogators in the matter of crime[40]. He urges early referral, as delay may result in insufficient or inadequate evidence being made available for court proceedings, as lengthy enquiries by doctors or social workers may alert the perpetrator. In fairness it has to be said that some doctors consider that this may well cause some parents to hesitate in seeking medical aid, perhaps with disastrous consequences to the child in extreme cases, and some social workers contend that police enquiries, especially when there is finally insufficient evidence for prosecution or where the charge is not upheld, may antagonize the parents to the extent that they will not tolerate subsequent intervention on the part of any person representing the interest and concern of society. Collie also observes that delay may be as unfair to the parent who remains too long under suspicion as to the child who remains without redress. He emphasizes that the courts are as concerned with rehabilitative procedures once the facts are established as the social services are themselves. Such serious cases are handled by experienced staff advised by senior police or the Director of Public Prosecutions. He also calls for better communications between all agencies concerned and police representation on review committees.

If the police are designated as the agency to enquire into an allegation it does not necessarily follow that the case will be mismanaged, if the objectives of the law are clearly seen to be the prevention of further abuse and the preservation where possible of family life, not solely the punishment and retribution against the abuser. The police have a right to exercise discretion and indeed in an emergency the public may well call upon them for help rather than the less well known social services departments.

The NSPCC[41] takes the view that since their own main emphasis was to be on treatment and rehabilitation they would prefer the police not to be involved with their families, 'as we did not believe that they had a therapeutic role to play in battered baby cases'. The opinion of the American Judge Delaney[42] is entirely endorsed, namely that 'the criminal process as a solution to child abuse is totally ineffective'.

Some attempt at the start of the NSPCC research project was made to establish contact with the police but not wholeheartedly followed up. The writers concede that probably 'there is some deterrent effect on the parent capable of controlling his conduct, but its chief value lies in satisfying the conscience of the community that the wrong to the child has been revenged'. There is perhaps some inconsistency in the further comment that 'it is clear that social workers and police must learn to communicate and trust one another' in what is admittedly a confused and unsatisfactory situation.

Others hold different views. The Select Committee on Violence in the Family[43] makes a recommendation that 'the police be fully involved in the management of non-accidental injury and particularly that they be invited to all case conferences'. The evidence showed 'a thread of optimism based upon the results which have been achieved when suspicion, mistrust and ignorance of role and motive are replaced by a close working relationship'. A team based on Derbyshire Children's Hospital[44] were in no doubt 'that through our cooperation with the police our management of cases has improved without loss of humanity'.

The Review Panel on the case of Wayne Brewer[45] thought the police should be invited to case conferences where non-accidental injury is suspected and furthermore should be asked for direct intervention where their skills of investigation could provide important evidence not otherwise obtainable. Perhaps the answer lies in greater involvement of the police in the joint training schemes devised by the Area Review Committees[46], for other agencies, with a view to furthering better understanding of each other's function. This is recognized on some training courses for social workers and is an established feature incorporated in the teaching of legal studies on the CQSW course at Birmingham Polytechnic.

There has been some pressure coming from local authorities upon the Home Office requesting confidential information on past criminal records to be made available to social services departments by the police in connection with stepfathers who may have entered the family of the child after parental rights have been transferred to the local authority[46]. It is thought that in this respect the step-father should be regarded in the same way as prospective, adoptive and foster parents, about whom such information can be made available under a Home Office ruling. Where this kind of information about the adults in such a family is not shared between the police and social service agencies, no decision, reached on the child's behalf, can truly be based on all the existing information, and certainly past crimes of violence can be said to be very relevant to such decisions. There is, of course, a most urgent need for maintaining complete discretion over the exchange of such information between responsible staff, for the right to privacy is an important personal liberty and it seems proper to insist that the record is checked with the individual concerned to prevent mistaken identity. Subject to this, social workers should welcome such help in identifying children at risk.

By April 1975 over a hundred local authorities had complied with the request of the Social Services Secretary to submit plans for co-ordinated action in cases of child abuse, stressing the need for better communication. The predominating pattern[47] to develop took the shape of a case conference of the professionals concerned, to be convened by a Senior Social Worker or a paediatrician. Other members might include a Senior Nursing Officer, general practitioner, health visitor, representative of NSPCC, psychiatrist and day nursery matron. Some have felt that this would form too large and diverse a body to be able to act quickly and effectively in the child's interest in an emergency[37]. A smaller review committee might, where possible, be based on a university department so that serious research and evaluation of the methods of treatment could be undertaken over a period of time.

It is true that some schemes nominate a 'key worker' to ensure decisions are carried out as to the best place for a child to be cared for and whether the police are to be informed. There seems to be some reluctance about involving the police automatically in every case conference, especially among doctors and to some extent social workers, who are concerned about the consequences if in discussion the police decided it was necessary to prosecute the parents and other members of the case conference were opposed[48]. Other local authorities have sought to involve the police from the beginning in an effort to resolve any jealousy or suspicion between the two agencies. Representation would still come from a wide number of interested parties but there was some evidence of reconciling differences of approach to be seen in public statements from the police, showing appreciation of the other party's point of view.

It seems apparent that some impatience is felt by other participants towards social workers, who too readily protect from prosecution those parents who deliberately injure their children, believing that family unity must be preserved[49]. There have been statements also on behalf of the police[50], confirming that prosecution in such cases did not necessarily ensue when the police were involved in case conferences, as they had considerable powers of discretion in deciding what action should be taken.

It is perhaps appropriate here to quote from Boardman writing on the matter in the USA as early as 1962 and confronting this very problem of the respective roles played by social worker and police[51]: 'The solution is not for the social worker to absorb a law enforcement responsibility but to learn to work with law enforcement and to share its responsibilities'. In observing this the social worker will not fall into the fallacy of disregarding or setting his actions above the law.

Teachers and Educational Welfare Officers

In the American context, the problem of the abused school child is placed fairly on the shoulders of teaching staff with an expectation that an early report from them in suspicious cases will reach child welfare agencies[15]. Where this is followed by responsible action, good cooperation will result to the advantage of the family.

In the United Kingdom the close identification of social workers with a particular neighbourhood, that is desirable if their work is to be effective, must include direct association with the life of the schools. Teaching staff have special opportunities for informal talk with the children in their care during the school day, and can gain considerable insight and understanding. Social workers often have few such opportunities to get to know the children in care who are their special responsibility. They need to know how to get on terms with them as well as to concede that teaching staff may understand them even better and be more able to assess their problems. Students must be made aware of this aspect of care through school contact and visits during training and when in a permanent post they should endeavour to gain an exact knowledge of the staff, the organization and the structure of the schools attended by the children who are their responsibility in care, as well as by children on whom they may be called upon to make special reports in enquiries about child abuse. If a good relationship is cultivated by regular contact, the information is more easily obtained and likely to convey more insight and conviction.

This relationship between teaching staff and social worker can be developed through confidence and understanding of the respective role of each. It is important for the legal aspects of child care to be explained to the staff by the social worker as well as the significance of the different kinds of Court Order. The part played by the Education Welfare Officer should be important in any system that links staff who are interested in the same child, but responsible to different bodies of the same local authority. At field work level it is vital to establish the kind of contact and understanding on which information about any child observed to be at risk can be shared with confidence, so that the observations and actions of each worker are known to the other and communication maintained. This is a matter for comment in the Maria Colwell report which dwells precisely on this lack of communication and states 'we wonder whether there were problems which are not simply administrative, (but) which reflect a lack of confidence in an understanding of respective roles and responsibilities between professions'[35].

Voluntary agencies

It is common knowledge among social workers that voluntary agencies have often been successful because they can develop a greater flexibility in their policies. They are responsible to their management committees only and do not have to account for the use of public funds. Subject to the policy of the individual agencies, they are free to experiment with new ideas. We may remember that the voluntarily organized clinics for mothers and babies set up to combat the maternal and infant mortality figures between the wars, were later successfully adopted as the more familiar antenatal clinic of the Local Authority today.

Similarly, the establishment in the UK of the National Society for the Prevention of Cruelty to Children reflected concern on the part of people interested in the fate of children who were neglected or cruelly treated. The society has developed and increased the scope of its work since the start of this century, changing its character somewhat with time and receiving recognition through having the same powers conferred upon it with regard to child care, as are vested in the local authorities. The allocation of areas of responsibility between the two agencies must always be a delicate matter and while relations with departments of social service are generally cooperative and cordial it is no new problem for there to be differences of opinion about management. Nearly 20 years ago in an article on preventive work with children Easton[52] described work in a former Children's Department where there was conflict with NSPCC staff over a definition of responsibility for visiting. This is now past history and perhaps more staff on both sides receive better training nowadays. It might be dismissed but for the evidence in the Maria Colwell report which plainly indicates how the lines of demarcation of responsibility in this case were not made clear. In her record the Duty Officer indicates when she received a further complaint of ill-treatment of Maria, that it was definitely the responsibility of the NSPCC, 'if there was a suspicion of ill-treatment'[35].

There is a general requirement here to spell out roles, status and relationships between NSPCC and social services departments with other authorities such as schools, doctors and nurses. There is a need to decide who shall co-ordinate matters between them. It may be that the public generally makes an approach to NSPCC in cases of cruelty rather than to the less familiar social services departments. If so, the reasons arise largely from historical association in people's minds in that the NSPCC existed first as a preventive agency. It seems desirable that consultation at top level should take place between the two agencies, with written instructions issued to field workers as guidelines over the conduct of cases where there is a joint interest. Where this is done, they should be strictly adhered to by both sides. In connection with their family study this difference of approach is made plain in the NSPCC[41] report over the division of their work with the local social services department. It was proposed that the dual role of the social worker should be shared by agreement, so that the social worker in the Local Authority took on the 'bad role' of prosecution, leaving the NSPCC worker to continue in the therapeutic role. In practice the outcome was not successful, because it was thought the Local Authority staff were reluctant to consider action through the Juvenile Courts against the parents' wishes. It might be more helpful in the long run for one worker to assume both roles, explaining honestly in open discussion with the parents, that, with the best intentions, it is not possible to protect them from the consequences of their actions but, even so, the social worker is there to support and help both parents and child following the court's decision.

One might hope that in the teaching process certain aspects of the role of the NSPCC in modern society might be put before students. They might consider the continuing usefulness of a voluntary agency that functions beside a Local Authority department, fulfilling and perhaps duplicating some of the same purposes. They might ask whether a voluntary agency is now out of place in such a context and if not, what its special contribution might be. They may also consider what action has been taken to create a balance between the costs of fieldwork and of administration, to enable the former to function to best advantage[35].

Special units have been established for the study of parents and children by the NSPCC research team of social workers and psychologists. These were set up in 1975 in Manchester, Leeds, Newcastle, Northampton and Coventry. Some modest research has been published[41] on the basis of study of twenty-five families, where battering is known to have taken place and upon the study and examination of the special unit registers in 1975[53]. It focuses chiefly on mothers and children, as it proved difficult to interview fathers. Criticism is to some extent pre-empted by a declaration of bias on the part of the social workers who acted both as therapists and research workers. Difficulties arose when at interview there was conflict between the need to probe for further information yet for the same person to make expressions of supportive help as therapist. Much of the data can be accounted as 'soft' and impressionistic while the value of the hard data is limited by the small number of families involved and the absence of a suitable control group.

The special units developed by the NSPCC have as their main purpose the support of the parents as a preventive measure, and this has resulted in some evidence of less violence. The techniques adopted seem mostly to be based on the programmes of 'mothering' and other kindred methods outlined by Kempe and Helfer 1972[15], to which reference has already been made, on account of the risk of reinforcing dependent behaviour. The evaluation of a programme of social relearning by skilled therapists still calls for attention from research.

THE CONTRIBUTION OF THE SOCIAL WORKER

Expectations by society

There must first be established a framework for an active contribution by the social worker, who should primarily feel he or she has a right and a responsibility to intervene and to remain within a situation of child abuse or neglect. In this sense he acts overtly as the expression of the community's concern on behalf of the child. He must continue to offer help, even though it may be neither warranted nor accepted by the parents[54]. He has a duty to make clear to the parents that society cannot allow harm to the child to persist and he must also point out that he is willing to play his part in any treatment plan that is devised for the child and his parents if this could lead to a permanent reconciliation within the family. He must participate in decisions about when neglect or abuse has ceased and help can be terminated.

Finally he must, when necessary, initiate action to remove the child from his parents and find a place of care and security for him away from further assault, even if he must act without the co-operation and consent of the parents. Such actions take into account the two conflicting roles of giving help and holding authority, which by training and experience, the social worker must learn to resolve and reconcile for himself.

Social workers can be unrealistic in their expectations, persuading themselves that some kind of relationship still exists between a child and his natural parents, long after they have ceased to give any sign of genuine interest in their child. Sometimes it is evident that no real family life had ever existed, to which the child might be restored, as the parents have led such deprived lives as children that they can barely manage their own affairs and are totally unable in any sense to support a dependent child. They can be parents only in a biological sense. 'It is an unwarranted and almost arrogant assumption to suppose that a little case work support can cure this sort of deprivation or make up for a basic inadequacy to fulfil the parental role'[55]. This is not to say there are not other families whose children can be returned from care, where enough case work support is made available at the right time.

Society has a right to ask whether social workers are justified in insisting as often as they do upon reuniting the injured child with his family. In principle it is right to say that most children are better placed at home with their own parents than with other people, however well intentioned. This view has influenced thinking by hospital staff, for example, and has led in some cases to easier access at all times for mothers prepared to visit and devote time to a sick child in hospital. Social workers rightly apply this principle to the general management of families with problems, often going to great lengths to prevent family disintegration, for they know that it is very hard to reconstruct any family as an entity.

Parenthood carries rights, but also responsibilities, including the protection of the children of the family. Where these break down and the child is injured, or suffers neglect, it may not be in his best interest for parents to insist on their right to have him home again. Social workers may say that emotional problems ensue for a child removed from the care of his parents but we know from research[55] that the worst of such problems arise, not from the institutions, nor from the foster homes but from the loveless parental home where the child and his siblings may be re-injured or even killed. Here one may perhaps quote the aphorism of one experienced teacher of social work and say: 'Dead children, after all, have no emotional problems'.

The training of social workers relevant to the needs of the abused child

It is true that the problem of the battered child was not acknowledged by doctors until the last decade and that child abuse was only then incorporated in the *Index Medicus*. It is evident also from random inquiry that teaching at this time on social work courses did not regard the deliberate injury of children by their parents as a reality or even a possibility and little was included in the syllabus of probation officers or child care staff that was directly relevant. We may conjecture that the care of such families at fieldwork level was in the hands often of untrained staff. Great efforts are currently being made to expand the training of social workers in the UK[56-58].

This expansion of training for staff involving two years absence, combined with the recent revision of Local Authority boundaries, has made many difficulties for social service departments. There has on the other hand been criticism for expanding such courses in times of retrenchment. Yet we must remember the pressing needs of children at risk and the considerable powers vested in Local Authorities to be exercised on their behalf with knowledge and wisdom, as well as their many other statutory powers.

Momentous decisions, such as the removal of children from parents or the return of a previously injured child to his parents' home, call for positive and exact knowledge of legal powers and children's needs. Training enables social workers to be made aware of the special needs of people who are disturbed emotionally or withdrawn from society. It helps them to confront and control their own feelings when working under pressure and gives them opportunity to learn in detail the legal obligations under which they work, as well as the welfare rights that are due to the people whom they seek to help. It is important also that their training is broadly based; for example a knowledge of physical or mental illness and handicap is important to those who will work in probation and it is vital to facilitate better understanding between social workers whose work lies in different fields.

Morgan[34] in dismissing what she considers to be unnecessary theory from the training of social workers, comments on their lack of direct skills and advocates that such skills, e.g. in child care 'are best transmitted by learning from those in the immediate community, who do it well'. This must however be supported by sufficient understanding of the theories of child development in human growth and behaviour. Social work without a basis in theory depends only on intuition.

The needs of social work students in understanding this problem

Students have been known to approach child abuse problems with attitudes ready made, sometimes seeing their role as not designed for the overt action of recommending to the courts that families are divided or children removed to institutions, even for the best of reasons. They look on such action as incompatible with the beliefs of social workers, whose work is seen to be an attempt to remove the handicap that prevents an individual from measuring up to the standards of the community, not to punish him for his defeat through personal inadequacy or hostile environment.

Their sympathies tend to lie with the family as a whole, whose entity they believe must be maintained, or with the parents, however indifferent they may be, only seldom with the child itself, the infant who is without speech and without defence in situations within the home that are fraught with the greatest hazard. Often there is a failure to see the child as the person most in need of help, especially where the parents are but ill-equipped to care for his physical and emotional needs, because they are of low intelligence, or have received little instruction in parenthood at home or at school; or have themselves a history of violence in their background. It is unlikely these parents will quickly respond to overtures of casework, based on a warm personal relationship with the social worker, yet prolonged delay will increase the risk to the child.

The consequences are described almost daily in the press, which carries reports of children left to scavenge rabbit food, assaulted seriously enough to cause spasticity and cerebral damage, even sustaining fatal stomach injuries from a karate chop. Social service departments are invested with immense legal powers to protect children at risk, but the signs indicate that these powers are invoked too infrequently to protect the child, rather than that they are abused by precipitate or misguided action to separate children from violent parents. Management by Local Authorities is marred by acts of omission rather than commission.

Students must be encouraged to learn to communicate easily with children. It may be there is less opportunity for this, on account of generic training. They must realize there are problems connected with interviewing in privacy, that parents become defensive and may coach the children in their answers or inflict reprisals afterwards for 'wrong answers' that are too close to the truth. Through contact with the child guidance clinic, students may learn to use this service as another resource for communication taking place under easier circumstances. They must be encouraged to stand outside themselves and be made aware that even they may be seen possibly as a threat to parents because of their power to remove children. They have to learn to use authority in a constructive way for the family's benefit. For children subject to care orders, it is necessary to understand the importance of gaining the fullest possible knowledge of step-parents, especially a new step-father, invited into the home by the mother[59]. These men, whose background is often so little known, are often also least accessible to interview or assessment[51]. In seeking information to supplement interviews from official sources such as the police, general practitioners or social security records, it is important to remember the need to respect privacy, the risk of impairing the public's trust in the confidentiality of records and the understandable reluctance of the social worker to exchange information.

It is important to recognize and respect the fact that some men have a well developed antagonism against authority, as well as to assess its real effect within the family he has joined. Also children are more particularly at risk when they are returned home after prolonged separation to the care of an unknown parent. Health, employment and criminal records are important aids especially if any crime of violence is discovered in the record of the new step-parent. Social work skills can be made use of at interview with such new fathers, especially in any attempt to increase his awareness of the need for an emotional involvement with the new family. Training in social work must keep in step with present day thinking, where more attention is being paid to the role of the father in helping to rear the children.

From some points of view, child abuse can be seen as a problem to be met by the community[35]. Where there is some continuity and stability in appointment among social service staff, they may find a useful source of prevention in maintaining contact in the community with people of good-will who have its interests and well-being at heart. They can take part with local community workers, perhaps, in seeking early warning, or even come to see themselves as growing more involved with the community they seek to serve. In the same way, they can make liaison with the doctors in general practice as well as the Health Visitors on attachment, as this makes for better confidence between participants known already to each other when a crisis arises. It is important to point out ways of developing good relations with the public to whom social workers become known.

They must consider how best to handle tactfully complaints made against any vulnerable member of a neighbourhood or requests for help on their behalf. They must take the complaint seriously, keeping the complainant informed, but only in a general way. There are risks of victimization for the family reported and hazards also for the social worker, of being looked upon as a source of unwanted interference. Objectivity is a lesson to be learnt; that is not pre-judging any situation, yet at the same time showing concern and interest. Professional judgement must also be developed, to enable the social worker to make that most important decision of all, namely when it is right to risk breaking a relationship with a family for the sake of the risk to the child.

An essential ingredient for all decisions is good clear concise record-keeping, free from jargon and unsubstantiated conjecture. Such information can support a team approach, replacing the element of chance, based on one individual's point of view. There is a great need for simple accuracy, including exact sources of information, precise details of alleged incidents and injuries, dates of visits and names of interested parties. The record must show plainly the distinction between fact and impression. It is most important that the criteria for intervention, determined by the review committee, are made plain to the fieldworkers and followed. Students must be taught at an early stage that a full report on family circumstances and attitudes, based on personal observation, is of great assistance to the courts in reaching decisions about revoking Care Orders. Indeed there should be a high onus of proof in applications for revocation of Care Orders when it is unsupported by local authorities. In this respect, they must on no account pre-judge the court's decision, if for no other reason than that this can influence what is said in evidence at court, sometimes with disastrous consequences for the child. They must be warned that they will be called upon to fulfil a plurality of roles, including representing the local authority who will be respondents, acting as advocate for local authority policy in court as well as preparing the report, and finally carrying out the court's decisions fairly and without prejudice. It is useful to know that the court may order that a child shall receive visits at home from the social worker, thus ensuring that it must be produced on demand, if the social worker has any reason to suppose that such a child is still being abused or neglected.

There is evidence that the approach to the Juvenile Courts is seen in several different ways. Arthur[44] remarks that 'social workers sometimes think that a Court hearing upsets clients and damages the casework relationship, but we suggest that social workers should take clients into their confidence at the outset and explain to them that Care Proceedings, if undertaken, should be seen as a framework within which the child and often the family can be supported, and not as a punishment'.

While supporting, in principle, the setting up of family courts as soon as possible, the Parliamentary Select Committee[43] say that much could be done and is done by magistrates and their clerks to ensure that an atmosphere is created where both parties can present their cases effectively and excessive delay avoided.

While accepting that the Juvenile Court can be an experience of caring and understanding for parents the NSPCC[41] reports that 'all parents in their group found the experience distressing, shaming and felt alienated from the whole procedure'. Real endeavours are made by those responsible for Juvenile Courts to make them more informal and to enable parents as well as older children to know what is taking place. In some cases a simply worded leaflet is issued in advance to explain the procedure under English Law. Magistrates[60] make use of improved opportunities to learn about new thinking and research into these problems, with the intention of making better informed decisions in the interests of justice, towards parent and child alike. The child has rights before the law and these may not be overlooked out of mistaken consideration towards the parents.

The student must also be aware of the importance of keeping full statistics on children under supervision, on which to base plans. Consideration must be given to the proper deployment of time by staff when a case conference is called. Enthusiasm diminishes among the other participants if they see their own valuable time being wasted. While being seen[45] as a means of formulating plans of management, an experienced chair person is needed as a means of co-ordinating and exploiting the discussions. Records should be carefully kept and minutes circulated to include those unable to attend. Doctors are asked to look on their attendance as a means of making a positive contribution to the problem; perhaps more in the patient's interest at the time than further consultations.

The Select Committee[43] recommends they should be conducted speedily, efficiently and with the smallest number of members, conducive to effective case management. Three simple objectives should be envisaged: a. Assessment and diagnosis: b. Plan for treatment and management: c. Implementation. Police attendance was considered valuable and we are reminded that in terms of time the cost of case conferences can be £130–150.

The use of registers for names of families 'at risk' is not new but has been advocated by the NSPCC[41] as a useful tool for research. The Area Review Committees are seen as the means of setting them up to promote better co-operation between agencies. They also support the establishment of a national register with common terms of reference for statistical purposes. It is recognized that it may be difficult to agree upon common criteria for referral, as well as the problems of confidentiality and access. With so many different agencies having an interest it would take time to reach agreement.

One may ask who takes responsibility for entering the names of families and whether the parents are invariably told. It is important the names are kept under review and removed when advisable. It may even be that the registers are kept as a means of allaying the anxieties of social workers and others directly concerned. Elsewhere[45] it is remarked that Wayne Brewer's name was already on the Central At Risk Register but in this case its use was of no significance as the child's family was already known to the agencies involved. Registers are seen by the Select Committee[43] as a safeguard to the children and a means of locating mobile families. Individuals have the right to know about entries and criteria should be set up for removal of names.

Most important of all is knowledge by the student of the limits of disturbed behaviour shown by a child in transition between households and at what point the continuation of such behaviour becomes intolerable. It may be painful for social workers to relinquish their notions about the indivisibility of the family and to accept the fact that parents can and do cruelly abuse their children without being mentally ill. It will have been observed that most of the remedies canvassed are devised to meet the problem at a practical level, leaving the personality defects untreated. We may agree that by temperament and training the social worker prefers to help rather than to sit in judgement but it may be that the answer to this complex problem lies in reaching informed judicial decisions through the courts linked with more research into better means of psychiatric, psychological and casework help, as well as improved communication between all interested parties – a matter that cannot be too greatly emphasized.

THE PROBLEMS THAT CONFRONT THE SOCIAL AGENCIES IN THE FUTURE

Finance

Administrators of social services frequently complain that there is a lack of adequate resources to meet the special needs of the battered child among the many other problems that confront them. The Central Government seldom indicates the ways in which the costs of compulsory or permissive measures for the benefit of the unprotected members of the community are to be met.

Public opinion has a firm expectation from the social services that social workers will be aware of individual families where children are being mistreated and will act on society's behalf to prevent this from occurring, investing them with magical powers of prescience, resources and tested methods of solving the problem in all its degrees, from the parent who neglects or threatens injury to the one convicted by the courts.

Yet it is true that many other agencies rightly claim to have a direct contribution to make to this problem and in this sense, responsibility for the means of solving the problem must be shared. Before this can properly be debated, the matter of financial responsibility will have to be faced squarely. Interested parties, with a commitment to finding answers to the problem, over and above Social Services Departments, financed at Local Government level, will include the National Health Service and Social Security interests from Central Government, Education and Housing from a combination of both sources, while the police and the courts derive funds chiefly from Central Government through the Home Office.

In the matter of the cost of training social workers, important points of responsibility are raised in a leading article in the *County Councils' Gazette*, November 1975, which debated the consequences of finding funds through Central Government for developments in training. Hitherto the cost of training in social work has been borne by Local Authorities and there is difficulty in choosing between continuing thus with probable restrictions on numbers and accepting help from central funds with possible uncertainties about long term consequences, such as making a balance by restricting grants to Local Authorities.

One may ask where a common factor is to be found among all these concerned government agencies, that will provide an answer to this crucial problem of financial responsibility and its apportionment among the several bodies concerned. It is by no means clear at what common level a point of entry to the administrative structure can be effected, to enable these decisions to be reached. This must be done before deciding upon the kind of Review Committee that will be given power to guide the overall strategy, as well as the infra-structure that will be given tactical responsibility. Both will be powerless without adequate resources.

Existing facilities – statutory and voluntary

Both statutory and voluntary agencies, if taken together, already exist as considerable resources of help to be mobilized. The courts are empowered to provide legal sanction for the protection of abused children where need arises: to this end magistrates, especially those on Juvenile Court panels and clerks to the justices should be made aware of the extent of the problem and the powers within their hands. There are also the different arms of the Health Service, both hospital and community based. The former will include paediatric and other specialist facilities for overall physical assessment and treatment, psychiatric services with similar skills offered through hospital and child guidance clinic, where available. The latter, community based, will provide primary care from general practitioner, health visitor, paediatric and district nurse. The Local Authority can make available, through social services, a number of specialist facilities to help children in need: these include assessment centres, children's homes, foster parents and day nurseries.

Voluntary agencies make a positive contribution, perhaps by their very ability to be more flexible than statutory authorities. The National Children's Home, the Church of England Children's Society, Barnardo's, as well as the National Society for the Prevention of Cruelty to Children have all been established by people with the needs of children especially at heart, though their public image will have changed with time. These can be used as resources for shelter or for treatment, including homes, day nurseries and playgroups for observation. The National Children's Bureau, through its longitudinal studies of all aspects of children's behaviour, holds a special, not to say unique, position in the field of research.

The public in this and other countries cannot be said to remain indifferent or ignorant of this problem. Press reporting of cases of child cruelty has increased considerably in the last five years. The matter is constantly pressed upon public attention, provoking comment and correspondence as well as promoting changes in public opinion and attitudes to the problem.

The general availability of social services throughout the UK must be taken into account also, for properly deployed, they can provide coverage for every neighbourhood. The sequence of tragedies to young children at the hands of their parents reported over recent years, has focused attention unfavourably on the social services who are still a long way from having trained field work staff to help with these crucial problems[56,58]. The service is presently stretched to the utmost, especially since the advent of the generic approach, in that few social workers have a specialization but all are expected to meet with appropriate skills the diverse social problems that present themselves. The generic team, with each member having some special knowledge and skill in a single field, such as child and family care, mental or physical illness or handicap, or care of the elderly, would seem to provide better hope of more comprehensive social care. In view of all these agencies, it must be admitted that a substantial network of established sources of help already exists.

The Review Committee

It seems right that responsibility for decisions over this problem should be shared among the members of the Review Committee. Every case of child injury brought to light would be directed to a screening process laid down by this body, who would make an assessment on the facts and establish the broad principles for guidance in each case. Such a team of experts would need to have among them people who had the skill, the courage and the wisdom to take the lead, to make decisions, to be flexible where necessary and to know when to stand fast and adhere to their decisions. They would have to be people with the time and the patience to see the problem through and already be possessed of experience in all aspects of children's needs.

It is possible that such leadership might come from doctors in general practice, or in the hospital field: it might equally come from social workers with extensive knowledge and field work experience of family problems. The sources used for information would include, by prior arrangement, general practitioner, health visitor, the matron of the day nursery, social workers' reports on home visits. Where the child is of school age, there should be consultation with school staff. A relationship based on trust should be built up between the Review Committee and the police, so that they are always consulted in cases of injury, where they are not directly represented on the panel. For the full guidance of those taking decisions in the more serious cases, it may be considered desirable for accurate confidential information on any history of criminal or violent act on the part of either parent, to be made available where the return of the child to the parents is under consideration. It might, however, be more appropriate for this to take effect through the courts.

At this stage one could envisage social service staff acting as co-ordinators pending decisions, later presenting the case in court if it were decided to apply for a Care Order, and subsequently, acting alongside the parents from the first day that the child is removed to a place of safety.

Means of intervention

Programmes of education in personal relationships for school leavers

In some educational circles, the matter of contraceptive advice for adolescents was considered to be of sufficient importance to merit a two part survey in family planning and school leavers[61]. It was thought that they needed help and advice over the use of the contraceptive Pill, not least because of the loss of education by girls on account of pregnancy. It was found that while instruction and advice on specific problems of contraception was made available, there was little provision for counselling on the emotional problems involved. There had been recognition of this in a Health Service circular issued to regional and area Health Authorities and general practitioners in May 1974, when it was admitted that such opportunity might be welcomed by young school leavers. Recommendations were made to Local Authorities and area Health Authorities to consider these as part of a health education programme that would include a wider range of health and social problems and opportunities for discussion with doctors, nurses and social workers.

It recommends consultation with other public and voluntary bodies to exchange views and information about such counselling. The National Marriage Guidance Council is already very much involved in this field having a well established obligatory training programme for all its members engaged in schools to lead groups and discussions on problems related to the emotional aspects of sex. Considerable experience has also been built up by the MGC in conjunction with staff within schools, with the intention of developing responsible attitudes among adolescents in preparation for marriage and adult life. It has, however, to be recognized that many young people feel intensely rejecting towards such discussion and counselling, coming as it does from a different age group of older people. They deny that there can be any common ground of approach and feel they must meet these problems in their own way. However, some experienced workers in this field can successfully offer discussion on the important aspects of emotional problems of sex: these include expectations from partners, marriage itself, the roles of husband and wife, the choice of time to have a baby, whether wives and mothers should go out to work, the earning and spending of money and a father's place in child rearing. Often young people at school have considered these problems themselves and welcome a forum where responsible discussion can take place. Problems of truancy may keep others away and it may be that these are most in need of this kind of instruction.

Another aspect of this education comes from opportunities to learn normal expectations in growth, development of babies and young children, as well as methods of rearing them. With smaller families, there is less chance to learn at home through experience. Alvy[62] in an article directed specifically towards the prevention of child abuse in the USA, calls for programmes for school centres that will help towards positive expectations in parenthood and cancel the acceptance in American culture of physical force as a 'legitimate and appropriate educational and socializing technique'. He outlines positive participatory and observational experiences for such groups with young children in day care, nursery school and kindergarten. He describes classroom and fieldwork experience that would expose teenage groups to the stages and processes of normal human development, which it is hoped might help future parents to understand a young child's emotional and cognitive growth. At this stage they would usefully have contact with social workers directly associated with child and family care, who through experience and observation could make them aware of the needs of young children.

Cohen[63] writing on 'Meeting Adolescents' Needs' holds that this kind of practical experience can have the effect of making future parents 'sensitive to the central importance of parents in the child's life', as well as becoming aware of individual differences between children and the need for a broad range of conditions to enable a child to develop its full potential. Such programmes for school leavers would call for co-operation by many agencies, courage, imagination, a wise use of resources and adequate finance.

The social worker

In the last section of this chapter, discussion will focus on social workers, in order to consider three aspects of thought that have bearing on their contribution to this problem.

First there will be an attempt to define their rightful place against the background of the community in which they work and the general expectations of society. There will follow an examination of their relationship towards those whom they seek to help and finally an explanation of an experiment in social work combining casework with behaviour modification. These methods will be looked at to see what lessons may lie here for future exploration and research.

In contemplating their proper place, against the background of their work, social workers are always aware of a sense of tension within themselves, between the concern they feel for the needs of individual people and their families, as against the wider issues connected with the needs apparent within communities and society itself. This is seen by Rice[64] as a conflict between the social worker operating at an individual level, hoping thereby to improve society as a whole by relieving one family's needs (the microist) and the sociologist (the macroist) who sees the individual's problem as but a symptom of the wider ills of society, which call for revolutionary action to remedy them. He calls this the individual as against the global approach. The former focuses on the personal help the social worker offers to an individual, yet his contribution may be set aside in turn first by the group worker and later by the community worker until finally all aspects of the helping services seem to be superseded by those who call for revolution to solve society's problems on a global scale. To help an individual is seen as a halt in progress towards relieving the needs of the truly deprived, those living beyond the benefits of the Welfare State. The problem arises as to where intervention should come in a given issue. We find an interesting exposition of the idea 'that radical beliefs and progressive programmes are often conservative in effect because they express an unconscious wish for inaction'.

Choices in social work have constantly to be made between short and long term help, between groups and individuals, between what is more or less urgent, all of which may result in no help at all for the individual in need. Decisions in these fields are influenced by the temperament of each social worker whether he will respond to an immediate need or derive satisfaction from a long term approach in a broader front. These tensions continue within the individual, 'between the rights of the individual and the rights of the many'. We may see them in the context of the problem of the battered child, as between the child's immediate needs and the expectations of society relative to the parents and the long term solution to the problem.

Such tensions are part of human experience and always present. If we accept that life is a compromise, we must yet distinguish between what is moral and immoral in compromise and what is a realistic answer. We must also understand that this entails 'a willingness to accept the complexity of problems, the uncertainty of one's decisions, the pain of solutions' ... in short 'a degree of moral maturity much needed in the face of today's social and political problems'.

There are special difficulties that beset the social workers when seeking to establish a realistic relationship with the parents of a child who has received injuries at their hands. This is even less easy when a complaint has to be investigated at the stage when injury is threatened, suspected yet indeterminate. By visiting a home, by showing a direct interest in the problems both of child and parents, by seeking to observe the whole problem, the social worker offers the parents the kind of relationship that can be used as a means of help. The means by which this can be established is frequently under discussion in training when emphasis is laid upon those principles that include respect for people as individuals and an acceptance of each individual as different, unique and valuable in his own right.

These ideas are taken further by Jordan[65] when he asks whether social workers see the people whom they seek to help as members of the same community, as fellow citizens and whether this position is somehow diminished by the fact that clients receive the social worker's attention in the form of assistance or supervision. Since 1948 social workers have had powers to provide discretionary benefits and to supervise and try to control certain kinds of deviance. These powers might be regarded as a means of subtle social control and perhaps decisions were taken that limited the status of their clients and rendered them different.

Misapprehensions developed between the social worker and his client because politicians and administrators created special roles for both. A special group of 'welfare cases' grew up, whose multiple social problems needed certain kinds of help. In some way this actually deprived them of direct access to help through the major services, because social workers took these responsibilities upon themselves, to intervene over housing needs and social security benefits for children and the elderly, with some consequent loss of rights for those needing help. The quality of the service offered was further diluted by taking on additional and often unnecessary duties from other Local Authority Departments, rather than selecting situations for which social work skills were most appropriate. In this way services had to be rationed and standards have declined as the size of departments have grown.

An example of difficult decision-making involves the phenomenon of child abuse. There is a temptation to pre-judge such families as deprived or different in some way. The social worker is tempted to be imprecise about the nature of the complaint and the reason for his visit. If problems in child care come to light, they may be dealt with only at a superficial level, by offering help through the provision of day care, playgroups, etc. If the social worker becomes anxious on behalf of the children, the parents may receive no clarification but continue to receive supervision for ill defined purposes and chiefly to quieten the anxieties felt by the social worker: in fact this may only exacerbate existing anxiety in the parent and precipitate the child injury that is feared. It is significant that in some of the worst cases of child abuse the families were already known to social service departments.

Seen from the client's point of view, it must seem that there is failure by the visiting social worker, who keeps silent about the anxieties felt for the child, to enter upon the multitude of anxieties that beset young emotionally immature parents with sympathy and understanding. Here the social worker seems to be making decisions and assumptions without discussing them openly with the parents or giving them a chance to challenge their validity. Instead there is a predetermination to see them as people in difficulty, without resources and in need of support and supervision.

The question whether the child had been neglected or injured may seldom be expressed nor might the parents be told whether suspicion rested upon them. Instead it may seem that the matter is prejudiced by 'a judgmental classification of the person'. It is only by receiving a clear decision, based on the facts and observations of the social worker, that a parent can take action that has either meaning or effect. 'It takes a special kind of courage to help clients face the worst aspects of their situation and of their feelings about them, to share with them their testing of their own resources as they struggle to reach their own solutions to problems.' There is no place here for collusion. While parents may accept support, they may later work out their anger with us by violent acts against their children.

In the most difficult of family situations, where battering is threatened but the evidence is inconclusive, the first approach has much to recommend it. It lines up with the principle of respect for individuals, treating them as adults, able to make their own choices and decisions. They can choose to deny the evidence, refuse help and close the door. They may however surprise themselves and others by overcoming their fears and seeking help which can be the starting point of giving and receiving help on open terms.

Very little has yet been said about the practical methods that can tentatively be put forward as solutions to the problem. The reason is not far to seek. Much has been written about methods of alleviating external pressures, manipulating the environment to enable parents of battered children to live under less stressful circumstances. Far less has been published on the subject of effecting any change in attitudes or personality, for this is a far more intractable problem. There is little conclusive research published and while in a few experimental units promising results are being achieved, this is only a small part of what needs to be done. Dr Kellmer Pringle has succinctly stated 'No reliable let alone quick cure has yet been found nor is it reasonable to expect one'[66].

However, there is some value in looking at a case study recently published on closely committed work based on a good relationship with a woman described as inadequate, immature and unable to manage her family responsibilities. She was variously diagnosed by psychiatrists as suffering from reactive depression, hysteria and finally as having an inadequate personality. It must be emphasized, however, that there was no question in the account of child abuse. However, as will become evident, there were, apart from this, a number of similarities of diagnosis and circumstance with the mothers described in the Birmingham Child Abuse Research Study[39] and it may be that here is a starting point for learning about how to begin to help.

The case study by Hudson[67] is described as having a dynamic beginning and a behavioural ending. Treatment, given in a psychiatric setting, included support from a social worker who helped this mother with many of her problems. Even so she had difficulty in controlling her children, debts mounted, her home management was criticized, while neighbours and friends alike were unkind to her. The social worker started to establish a good working relationship, assured her of her good will and asserted her belief that she could learn to manage her problems herself.

In early life, the client suffered the loss of her father to whom she was attached. Her mother was indifferently disposed to her, expecting her to have charge of the younger children. She made an early marriage to a man earning low wages and had three unplanned pregnancies early in marriage. These parents had some similarity to one another, feeling isolated in their lives, resentful towards others and despairing towards the problems presented by a lack of home management skills, knowledge of child rearing and accumulation of debts.

Help was planned, based on her experience of worthlessness in herself, as a result of a lack of mothering in childhood. While these feelings prevented her from helping herself, yet she seemed able to care, to examine her own feelings and reactions and she had a good marriage. At first it was hoped that supportive help from the social worker would enable her to see herself as more acceptable and more competent to manage her own affairs, thereby gaining a new confidence. Methods at first depended upon a minute discussion of all the difficulties she daily encountered, including the landlord, the children, the housekeeping, money, her use of contraception. Responses were negative and accompanied by signs of withdrawal. In spite of some comfort from social work help, frequent visits and active help, there was no real change or improvement.

The social worker changed emphasis, leading her on to a deeper discussion of childhood memories, resentment against her mother and her self-esteem. Some positive factors were sought in her feelings towards her father. The client remained unhappy and lonely while the social problems remained unchanged. Only a good working relationship had been achieved.

Again the method of intervention was changed to one based on methods of behaviour modification. The rationale indicated that in order to meet her present problems, the client needed to learn new behaviour patterns, first in areas of housekeeping and money management, and secondly in personal relationships, learning to ask for help as well as to stand up to other people and her children. It was hoped her feelings of failure and despair would abate with external improvements.

The new approach began with a reassurance that she mattered and was able to meet her difficulties. Approval was shown of progress thus far: she was told that often people found it helpful to break down big tasks into smaller ones before starting and that further help would be forthcoming. The social worker would help her to rehearse these situations so this would give her confidence, and she would learn how to manage the tantrums shown by her youngest child. In detail she was asked to find a piece of good news for each visit. Tasks began at an easy level, such as small efforts of reorganization at home. On each visit praise was given for achievement; when there was no result, the visit was delayed or withheld. On some occasions the social worker had to try hard to keep within her agreed limits of help. Progress was rapid and by the end of the social worker's contact, the client was holding down a part-time job as well as keeping a better home and making herself more presentable.

The actual methods used are described in detail. Praise was not given in advance of achievement. The client was encouraged to separate the child in another room during tantrum attacks, in the hope that he would cease to be a trial and learn that his behaviour would not receive reinforcement. Role play was developed between client and social worker, to help to combat problems with bullying landlords, persuasive salesmen and to improve family relationships with her mother. In this family the husband provided an unsought source of help, as some of his problems were like hers. When she made a successful application for a job, she received full-hearted support from him. Also natural reinforcement improved the result as she got on better with other people and more easily persuaded them to help her. She managed the children better and felt better about herself. Six months later, improvement had been maintained, she had made friends in her own right and said her relatives seemed more kindly disposed.

Here we may find two aspects of social work, the dynamic and the behavioural. The first had continued for at least six months and was based on regular weekly visits lasting half an hour. Methods included the use of continuous reassurance and empathy, attempts were made to help the client to express her feelings easily, events were looked at from a cause and effect viewpoint and later an attempt was made to link her present conduct and emotion with past life experience. During the behavioural period, the chief method employed was operant conditioning. Main objectives were featured as a series of secondary goals, more easily gained and the desired behaviour was differentially reinforced. A method of control was developed for dealing with the children; Time Out (that is from any kind of positive reinforcement) produces results in children, in that when they cease their bad behaviour, they receive reinforcement, with a gradual learning that bad behaviour does not in the end achieve results. This method might well be considered in working with battering parents as one alternative in child rearing that has a positive result without doing harm. This second stage continued for about seven months, with a gradual reduction of visits.

In weighing up the contribution of each technique to solving the problem, it must be remembered that neither method should be looked upon as the only means of helping. Some flaws in detail became evident in both methods and it is openly acknowledged that there is no case for making general inferences from one particular success.

The following observations are tentatively offered from this approach. The behavioural approach achieved both change and improvement not found in the dynamic stage. While there is little evidence of published work on behaviour modification used to help the 'inadequate housewife', its effectiveness is known among a wide variety of people and problems. Time Out for coping with the child's tantrums, operant conditioning to help with the learning of new behaviour and assertive training for people with social anxiety, all seem to confirm the greater effectiveness of this kind of treatment over dynamic casework. At the first stage, the problems of home and child management, making friends and taking part in social activities, remained unchanged.

The author examines and rejects the idea that her enthusiasm for behaviour modification prevented her from making full use of the dynamic method because she became aware this was not helping about the time she came to learn behaviour techniques but before then she had felt convinced that her casework techniques were effective. She also considers the suggestion that in a more subtle way, the dynamic stage achieved more, as a result of insights gained by the client, so that good results due from this stage became evident later. This cannot be proved. When working with a client so closely, it is essential to have complete co-operation based on confidence in the helper and in the methods used and the assessment made. The client must also understand the process in hand, and must surely depend here upon the professional skill and certainty of the social worker. The quality of the relationship is essential to the success of using it for reinforcement and modelling techniques. So the first process based on dynamics was important for gaining good will: it was also necessary to study the client's past and present interaction with others in order to plan and share intervention. In short, if the definition of the problem had not been shared and the client had not responded to the approach of the social worker, the behaviour programme could not have been undertaken. However, in the author's opinion the time spent on the first stage could have been substantially reduced. She felt prompted to seek the client's opinion, as the consumer, as to when she had felt helped and was told 'It had all helped ... it was when she realized she was still acting like a child, while all the time having it in her to be an effective grown-up, that she began to feel and do better. But precisely when this realization took place, she could not say'.

Both approaches can be said to be helpful whether used separately or together. It may be that one method suits one person better but 'these questions deserve further consideration and more important they deserve early attention in social work research'.

The research initiated by Ounsted[68] into bonding failure has been developed and expanded by testing a variety of social work techniques at the Park Hospital for Children at Oxford. Lynch et al.[69] claim that at least 3% of all mothers delivered at a large modern maternity hospital have identifiable problems, likely to lead to bonding failure or child abuse. Fifty recent referrals, for child abuse, were born in the local maternity hospital. Of these, 29 had been known to the social worker there during pregnancy or the neonatal period. They could be distinguished from a typical group of social work referrals in three ways. The abused group were more likely to have been in special care nursery (59%: 24%). Concern over mothering was recorded in the Maternity Hospital records in proportion of 72%: 15%. Their family's social problems at delivery were described as diffuse rather than defined, i.e. 'Defined' represented isolated problems in otherwise stable families, e.g. Housing and miscellaneous practical problems. 'Diffuse' were those associated with severe relationship problems (90%: 27%). It was concluded that families 'at risk' can in practice be ascertained in the maternity hospital and preventive help offered early.

This was followed by a further experiment, Beswick et al.[70] linking the work with the primary health care team, in the belief that any programme for non-accidental injury should aim at prediction and prevention starting in the community. In a rural practice of 9250 patients there were 1841 children under 10 and between 1973–76, 12 cases of actual abuse occurred.

A preventive scheme was established with a good short-term outlook. No serious cases occurred among the children at risk. The major contribution of the primary health team was seen as the recognition of early warning signals in families with a high potential for abuse. The team was then in a unique position to help such families and work towards preventing actual abuse.

In March 1976, 30 children in 22 families were considered at risk. The family was treated as a whole, but separation of the child was not ruled out. Recognition and acknowledgement of the problem can be achieved at a surgery appointment. A diagnostic interview, with health visitor or social worker present, followed when problems were defined and a plan for treatment reached. Suggestions include 24 hour life-line, a therapeutic relationship, child care at home or at clinic, practical help and referral to other agencies. Each member of the team has a continuing contribution to make to the assessment and management. As a result, 2 out of 30 children subsequently had minor injuries inflicted but the children were all seen to make developmental progress. Mothers and children attending therapeutic groups especially benefited.

The syndrome must be seen as a continuing process, not as an isolated medical event. Medical symptoms can sometimes be seen as a way of seeking other help, but the primary health care team can treat the family in the community and work towards prevention.

As part of a wider management plan to test out measures that could help parents and children involved in cases of non-accidental injury, a joint project[71] was set up between the same general practice and research team at the Park Hospital. The aim was to provide help for families with child-rearing problems that could lead to abuse[72]. Two groups were set up on a weekly basis, one for mothers and the other for children, the former with the purpose of increasing the mother's self-esteem and confidence especially in the area of child-rearing and the latter to help mother and child, both as individuals and within their mutual relationship.

After three months it was found that demands made by their families on the local services were reduced. Both health visitors and social workers found work with these families easier and provoking less anxiety. In crisis they could accept help and use it constructively. As a result, staff in health and social services raised their own morale because a system of help was being developed and there was better hope of success.

The comparatively long-term treatment in a special residential setting for families at the Park Hospital is described elsewhere[73] as a different source of help. It is to be regarded as complementary to the other measures described, all of which demonstrate imaginative experimentation with recognized methods of social work, within a well defined medical setting. The co-operation and mutual acceptance of each others role by doctors and social workers is implicit in the several accounts and should encourage social workers elsewhere to explore similar lines of treatment for themselves.

Social workers are known to be very reluctant to admit battered children and others to residential care in time of crisis. This is not only because of the serious risk of breaking up the family, but because of the low proportion of trained residential staff[49] available to care for them in a stable and committed way.

It may be that fostering arrangements for such children could be devised as an extension, for example, of the special family placement project that receives support from Kent Social Services Department. Boys and girls over 15, subject to care orders, are placed with specially chosen foster parents who are paid a substantial sum for giving such adolescents an opportunity to live normal family lives within their homes. The foster parents make opportunity for the young person to develop an individual relationship with them and their family, committed to his well-being. Hazel *et al.*[74] who monitor the project, advocate that all parties, the adolescent and his family of origin, the placement family and the social worker, should negotiate together on equal terms towards voluntarily agreed objectives, capable of achievement.

While the objectives would be different for special foster parents working with young and abused children, who had become subject to care orders, it might be that, given the same kind of incentives and encouragement, such foster parents might be encouraged to receive a young battered child into their family, where it would effectively be removed from hazard. Then with the help of an experienced social worker, they could begin to develop a plan with the child's parents, to relearn the essentials of parenthood in an informal setting. It has to be said that those parents who admit to child abuse will be more likely to co-operate in such planned operations. When this was successfully negotiated, a reconciliation of the parents with the needs of the child might be achieved and perhaps eventually the restoration of the child to the home of origin. If this is not successful, nothing is lost and much experience has been gained upon which a realistic plan for the child's future could be built.

Concluding comments

It seems evident from past experience that new ideas relevant to the practice of social work have been absorbed without adaptation, with more enthusiasm than objectivity. This is especially true when one considers the influence of analytical thinking on social workers in the past. Its use was chiefly as an aid to understanding rather than as a direct means of helping but misuse of this method sometimes led to no help being given at all, when regarded from the client's point of view. Methods of help, contained within the idea of making a contract with the client and working on the basis of limited goals achieved within a fixed span of time, produce some success but do not altogether meet the needs of families where child injury takes place. The account outlined above of help given through behaviour modification, combined with the use of a good relationship between worker and client, may hold the elements of a new approach that will alleviate some of the negative personality traits evident in the parents. Its development through research to explore its usefulness in helping parents who injure their children seems to be one of the more hopeful possibilities for the future, because it comes close to the heart of the matter, namely the personality disorders of the parents, that remain unaffected by the well-meaning manipulation of external circumstances. There will be difficulties with parents of battered children who may be hostile to the worker and some will lack the motivation to act in partnership towards an objective, yet one may discern some chance of success with those parents who acknowledge a need for help.

References

1. Pinchbeck and Hewitt (1969). *Children in English Society.* p. 49
2. Shakespeare, *Macbeth* I: vii
3. Genesis 22: 2
4. Chronicles II, 20: 3
5. Smith, S. M. and Hanson, R. (1974). One Hundred and Thirty-four Battered Children: A Medical and Psychological Study. *Br. Med. J., 3,* 666
6. Jeremiah 31: 15
7. Esther 3: 13
8. Woodforde, J., *Diary of a Country Parson.* p. 34. (Oxford World Classics).
9. Darwin, C., (1936), *The Origin of Species and the Descent of Man.* p. 429
10. Bakan, (1971), *Slaughter of the Innocents.* p. 119. (London: Jossey Bass Inc.)
11. Hopkirk, Mary, (1948), *Nobody Wanted Sam.* p. 92. (London)
12. McWhinnie, A., (1967), *Adopted Children. How They Grow Up.* p. 4. (RKP)
13. Bowlby, J., (1952), *Maternal Care and Mental Health.* p. 11. (WHO)
14. Bowlby, J., (1953/65), *Child Care and the Growth of Love.* p. 53. (London: Pelican)
15. Helfer, R. E. and Kempe, C. H. (eds.), (1968), *The Battered Child.* p. 166. (Chicago: University of Chicago Press)
16. Isaacs, S., (1941), *The Cambridge Evacuation Survey.*
17. Middleton, Nigel, (1974), *When Family Failed.* p. 230. (London: Gollancz)
18. Prugh and Harlow, (1962), *Deprivation of Maternal Care, A Reassessment.* p. 9. (WHO)
19. O'Connor, (1956), Evidence for the Permanently Disturbing Effects of Mother–Child Separation. *Acta Psychol.,* 12: 174
20. Clarke and Clarke, (1959), Recovery From the Effects of Deprivation. *Acta Psychol.* 16: 137.
21. Orlansky, (1949), Infant Care and Personality. *Psychol. Bull.,* 46: 1.
22. Rank Pitnam and Rochlin, (1948), *Significance of Emotional Climate.*
23. Maenchen, (1953), *Notes on Early Ego Disturbances: The Psychoanalytic Study of the Child* **3,** p. 262. (New York: International University Press)
24. Andry, R. G., (1960). *Delinquency and Parental Pathology.* (London: Methuen)
25. Bowlby, J., (1977), The Making and Breaking of Affectional Bonds. Aetiology and Psychopathology in the Light of Attachment Theory. *Br. J. Psychiatry,* p. 130
26. Wootton, B., (1959), *Social Science and Social Pathology.* (Allen and Unwin)
27. Lewis, H., (1954), *Deprived Children. The Mersham Experiment. A Social and Clinical Study.* (London: OUP)
28. Holman, P., (1953), Some Factors in the Aetiology of Maladjusted Children. *Journal of Mental Science*
29. Rowntree, G., (1955), Early Childhood in Broken Families. *Population Studies.* **8,** 247
30. Mead, Margaret, (1954), Some Theoretical Considerations on the Problems of Mother–Child Separation. *Am. J. Orthopsychiat.,* **24,** 471
31. Rutter, M., (1972), *Maternal Deprivation Reassessed.* p. 122. (London: Penguin)
32. Rutter, M., (1972), Maternal Deprivation Reconsidered. *J. Psychosom Res.*

33. Ainsworth, M., (1974), Infant–Mother Attachment and Social Development, Socialization as a Product of Reciprocal Responsiveness to Signals. In: *The Integration of a Child into a Social World*. M. Richards; (ed.), (London: Oxford University Press)
34. Morgan, P. (1975), *Child Care, Sense and Fable*. (Temple Smith)
35. Report of Committee of Inquiry into the Care-Supervision Provided in Relation to Maria Colwell. (1974), (London: HMSO) paras. 59–61.
36. Smith, S. M., Hanson, R., and Noble, S., (1973), Parents of Battered Babies: A Controlled Study. *Br. Med. J.* **4,** 388
37. Smith, S. M., and Noble, S., (1973), Battered Children and Their Parents. *New Society,* **26,** 393
38. Young, Leontine (1964), *Wednesday's Children*. p. 126. (New York: McGraw Hill)
39. Smith, S. M., (1975), *The Battered Child Syndrome*. (London: Butterworths)
40. Collie, J., (1975), *The Police Role In Concerning Child Abuse*. Papers presented by the Tunbridge Wells Study Group on Non-Accidental Injury to Children. A. White Franklin; (ed.), (Edinburgh: Churchill Livingstone)
41. NSPCC Battered Child Research Team, (1976), *At Risk*. p. 106. (RKP)
42. Delaney, J. J., (1972), Helping the Battered Child and his Family. In: *The Battered Child and the Law*. Kempe and Helfer; (eds.)
43. First Report from the Select Committee on Violence in the Family, 1976–77. (1977) Vol. I. *Violence to Children*. (London: HMSO) para 119–121
44. Arthur, L. J. H., Moncrieff, M. W., Milburn, W., Bayliss, P. S. and Health, J. (1976). Non-Accidental Injury in Children. What we do in Derby. *Br. Med. J.,* **1,** 136
45. Report on Wayne Brewer, Somerset and Review Committee For Non-Accidental Injury to Children, (1977)
46. Report on Children at Risk–East Sussex County Council, 1975
47. Ealing, Hammersmith and Hounslow AHA and SSD Report (1975). *The Guardian,* April 8
48. *The Guardian* Report (1974). October 4
49. Turner, M., Chief Nursing Officer, Ealing. (1973). Report in *The Guardian,* November 21
50. Beck, S. C., Conference on the Battered Child, Police Representative Scotland Yard (1973). Report in *The Guardian,* November 21
51. Boardman, H. E., (1962), A Project to Rescue Children from Inflicted Injuries. *Social Work,* **7,** 43
52. Easton, (1959), *Case Conference,* **6,** 60.
53. Chreighton, S. J. and Owtram, P. J. (1977), *Child Victims of Physical Abuse* (NSPCC)
54. Paulsen, M. G., (1967), *Columbia Law Review,* **67,** 1
55. Rowe and Lambert, (1974), *Children Who Wait*. p. 106 (Association of British Adoption Agencies)
56. Manpower and Training for Social Services 1976. p. 39 (London: DHSS)
57. Report on Violence to Children. para. 153. (London: HMSO)
58. Survey by working party British Association of Social Workers on children at risk. 1977.
59. Scott. P. D., (1973), Fatal Battered Baby Cases, *Medicine, Science and the Law,* **13,** 197
60. *The Magistrate,* **33,** No. 6
61. *Times Educational Supplement* (1974) 1 and 8 November
62. Alvy, K. T., (1975), *American Psychologist,* **30,** 931
63. Cohen, D. J., (1973), Meeting Adolescents' Needs. *Children Today,* 29
64. Rice, D., (1975), Of Microists and Macroists. *Social Work Today,* **6,** 512
65. Jordan, B., (1975), Is the Client a Fellow Citizen? *Social Work Today,* **6,** 471
66. Correspondence (1975). *The Guardian,* May 16
67. Hudson, B., (1975), An Inadequate Personality. *Social Work Today,* **6,** 506
68. Ounsted, C. Ed., Oppenheimer, R. and Lindsay, J., (1975), The psycho-pathology and psychotherapy of the families: aspects of bonding failure. In: *Concerning Child Abuse*. A. W. Franklin; (ed.). (Edinburgh: Churchill-Livingstone)
69. Lynch, M. Roberts, J. and Gordon, M., (1976), Child Abuse. Early warning in the Maternity

Hospital. *Devel. Med. Child Neurology*, 759

70. Beswick, K. Lynch, M. and Roberts, S., (1976). Child Abuse and General Practice. *Br. Med. J.*, **4**, 800

71. Roberts, J. Beswick, K. Leverton, B. and Lynch, M., (1977) Prevention of Child Abuse –Group Therapy for mothers and children. *The Practitioner*, **219**

72. Lynch, M. (1976), *The Abused Child.* H. P. Martin; (ed.). (Cambridge Mass.: Ballinger)

73. Roberts, J. and Lynch, M. (1977), The Treatment of Abused Children and their Families. *Social Work Today*, **8**, 43

74. Hazel, N. Cox and R. Ashley–Mudie. (1977) Second report of the special family project. (Kent Social Services Dept. Maidstone)

13   The emergence of the child as a legal entity

D. FORD

The recognition of the separate individuality of the child is largely a phenomenon of the last hundred years, and the recognition of its legal identity in its own right has still not been accorded. For the purposes of law the child has, over millennia, been regarded as a possession of the parents (which they, but not the child, can dispute), and latterly, as an adjunct of a family group. Law has always had great difficulty in regarding the child as an entity. The child first assumed legal identity as a malefactor, when authority wished to control him or visit punishment upon him. The one possible exception to this rule was the child as an inheritor of a name or property (usually both, or the matter was not an issue), but the child was seen as the projection of adult concerns rather than as an individual possessed of any rights in himself.

In English law, with which I must be primarily concerned, the first mention of the rights of a child was in 1925, in the Guardianship of Infants Act: 'Where, in any proceedings before any court . . . the custody of upbringing of an infant is in question, the court, in deciding the question, shall regard the welfare of the infant as the first and paramount consideration'. Here, significantly, the fundamental argument is still about the possession of a child.

In trying to write about law in early times there is always the difficulty of determining where custom, attitude and usage cease and codification begins – usually the law is an attempt to regulate custom and usage through the codification of accumulated tradition. In the oldest such record we possess, the Code of Hammurabi, we learn of the punishment provided for a negligent wet nurse, but there is little else about children. In other codes the one matter dealt with is adoption – again where a child is treated as the possession of adults.

The child in many early legal systems seems of no great consequence. The individual steps into law in classical Greece with the acquisition of citizenship and the assumption of the duties and privileges accorded to the free citizen of a city state. It must always be remembered that slavery existed and that freedom was itself a privilege; on the whole children were regarded as slaves rather than as individuals possessing rights.

There is no reason to doubt that the normal feelings of love and concern were not operative over the larger part of the community then, even though life was short, and conditions could be harsh and brutal. But there was a degree of insensitivity towards children and their expectation of life which we find cold and, in part, incomprehensible.

In classical Greece infanticide was enjoined by both Aristotle and Plato, to limit the population of the city state and to eradicate weaknesses from the stock; the Laws of Solon and Lycurgus give sanction to this practice. This is an aspect of the rationality of the Greeks which we find repellent today, yet tales, myths, legends and drama demonstrate how widespread this attitude was and how acceptable to the thinking of the day.

The legal power of the Roman Paterfamilias over his family would seem to be tyranically complete, and there are many accounts of how these powers were exercised by the Roman father. On one or two occasions, which become subject to comment, these powers extended over members of his family who were well into adulthood and seemingly of independent existence. But then the Romans worshipped their ancestors and their regard was directed backwards to parents, and grandparents rather than given to the coming generation. Infanticide on the Greek model was well known, but there were differences which were, in the end, to prove critical. Early Roman law which, according to Lecky, was popularly ascribed to Romulus, restricted these rights 'enjoining the father to bring up all his male children and at least his eldest female child, forbidding him to destroy any well-formed child till it had completed its third year, when the affections of the parents might be supposed to be developed, but permitting the exposition of deformed or maimed children with the consent of their five nearest relations'.

The first significant detail is the discrimination in respect of sex; the second is the emphasis on the sound, healthy child and the exception of the deformed; most significant, however, is the fact that the child is looked at from an extended family, or clan, point of view, and judged in part from the point of view of its potential as a contributing member of that group. Whether the child was seen as a possible contributor to the life of a group, or as an immediate consumer of scarce resources is of great importance in any recorded history of the attitude to children. It determined attitudes in many primitive communities, and later found codification in law.

Historically this point establishes an important difference between the Greeks and Romans. The Greeks seemed from early times concerned with the limited resources of their city states; they, along with the Romans, shared a concern about the healthiness of the racial stock. The Roman attitude is different. They seemed concerned from early times with the growth of population and seemed to encourage such growth. Their territorial limits extended to provide for this growing population. This difference in attitude might be one part of the explanation of the differing historical roles of Athens and Sparta, and Rome. The Greek city state was always jealous of the privilege of citizenship and reacted with suspicion to the idea of wider dominion and power. The Roman Republic, while not aware of its future development into a vast imperial power, seemed always more inclined to look to the potential of its young people, and to be concerned with the growth of the number of its citizens.

Nevertheless there were anomalies in the Roman attitude. Exposure of children – Lecky's exposition – never received the same condemnation in Roman law as did infanticide until late in imperial history. In the early years of the Roman Republic, despite the decree attributed to Romulus, exposure was never made a punishable offence. Indeed there was a well-known and acceptable way of carrying out the process. Children were brought to the recognized and traditional spot, a column near the Velabrum, where women in milk offered themselves as wet-nurses, and there were left on display; once the child was left anyone could take possession of it. Usually such children were taken off by speculators, who were usually slave dealers, who fed the children and provided for them, and might educate them to be slaves or prostitutes. Some of those who were not deformed were mutilated to be used for begging.

As might be expected, there is no consistent attitude; the voices are confusing. References are scattered throughout Latin writing, and examples can be drawn from the time of the Republic, the pagan Empire and the Christian Empire. Most of the references show that whatever attitudes were enjoyed by thinkers and writers, practice did not much change. Nor did the passage of laws effect much change.

Juvenal could write: 'You owe the utmost reverence to a child'. Yet there is plenty of evidence that children continued to be abandoned, exposed, murdered, offered as pledges for debt, sold directly into slavery and abused in very large numbers and, except for the occasional voice raised in sorrow or rebuke, little concern was expressed and less done.

Probably one of the best known passages which deals with the potential of a child is that of Quintilian about A.D. 100. 'For there is absolutely no foundation for the complaint that but few men have the power to take in the knowledge that is imparted to them. ... Those who are dull and ineducable are as abnormal as prodigious births and monstrosities and are but few in number. A proof of what I say is to be found in the fact that boys commonly show promise of many accomplishments, and when such promise dies away as they grow up, this is plainly not due to the failure of natural gifts but to lack of requisite attention ...' It must always be remembered that this passage specifically refers to boys and is concerned with those who are free.

Concern for the potentiality of children leads on to considerations of education and their needs in this area. Augustus, the first Emperor, made a grant of corn, the common form of dole, to young children to provide for their education and upbringing. This seems an isolated first instance, although the empire was always concerned about the falling birth-rate of its citizens from the earliest times; indeed the problem had already caused a great deal of concern during the later years of the republic. Nerva, emperor from A.D. 96–98 tried to raise the population level through the first systematic scheme of child maintenance and Trajan, his successor, continued this policy and extended it beyond Rome and Italy. The imperial government assumed responsibility for some five thousand children in Rome alone during Trajan's reign. He was also responsible for the foundation of an institution to provide support for 270 children in Velleia; this may well be only one of a number of such places, known to us because references to it have survived. Trajan also decreed that no child who had been born free could be enslaved. Hadrian, who succeeded Trajan, increased the provision of corn for the maintenance of such children, and this policy was continued by his successors, the Antonines, whose dynasty lasted until A.D. 193.

During this period Christianity, although subject to persecution, was a yeast working in the whole empire. The Roman concern for the child was as a future citizen of the empire on this earth; the Christian Church was concerned with the child as a future inhabitant of heaven or hell. The fact that infanticide was still rife throughout the Empire is evidence by various decrees, and, ironically one of the shrillest complaints against the Christians was that they were infanticides. The Christian concern for the child, as it emerges, was not a matter of law or sentiment; it was a concern for the salvation of the soul, and the threat of eternal damnation which every child carried until he or she had been redeemed by baptism. The child was also a reminder of the Fall of Man; this was a concept introduced from Judaism, and is a new element in thinking in respect of children, and one which was to play an increasingly important part in forming attitudes to children in the Christian west.

The dichotomy of the pagan world was evident in its attitude to children; the Christian dichotomy was of another order, but in practical terms the formal adoption of Christianity as the religion of the empire by Constantine in the Edict of Milan in A.D. 333 made very little difference to the fate of children. Despite the condemnation of infanticide by both pagan and Christian authorities, it long continued, and the Christian authorities did little to prevent the exposure of children or their reduction to slavery because of the indebtedness of their parents.

Indeed, in legal terms, there was regression in some areas. The provision of dole which had begun with Nerva was continued by Constantine, and extended, possibly for the first time systematically to Africa and other parts of the empire. But the same decree of Constantine doomed children who had been exposed by their parents to slavery unless the father, when reclaiming the child, could pay the expenses of the person who had assumed responsibility for the rearing of the child. This went back on the previous edict of Trajan which had forbidden the enslavement of exposed children who had been born free.

This regression was not made good until A.D. 529 when the Emperor Justinian decreed that the father automatically forfeited all rights in the child the moment he allowed it to be exposed; Justinian also decreed that no freeborn child could be deprived of its freedom as a result of exposure. By this time, however, the empire had split in two; the law enacted by an emperor whose seat was in Constantinople applied only to the eastern empire. In the west, which was now nominally Christian, the old law prevailed, and children continued to pass into slavery through exposure, with consequential danger of mutilation, prostitution and death.

The sale of children in times of famine and distress also continued, although it was denounced by various Church Fathers, but no Christian emperor ever reenacted the decree of Diocletian which absolutely condemned the sale of children. The Theodosian Code in A.D. 322 had certain observations to make on the same subject: 'We have learned that provincials suffering from scarcity of food and lack of sustenance are selling or pledging their children. It is repugnant to our customs to allow any person to be destroyed by hunger or rush out to the commission of a shameful deed'. This was followed by a decree: 'A law shall be written on bronze or waxed tablets or on linen cloth to restrain the hands of parents from infanticide and turn their hopes to better things. If any parent should report that he is unable to rear a child there shall be no delay in issuing food and clothing since the rearing of a newborn infant cannot brook delay'.

Constantine did introduce one measure for the protection of children; it was a law to prevent the sacrifice of children in pagan rites, something which had been a commonplace in pagan times. But his concern seems to arise more from the need to suppress pagan religions in the empire rather than from any direct concern about the fate of children. Valentinian in A.D. 374 seems to be the first Christian emperor who made infanticide a capital offence, and also condemned the exposure of children, but these enactments did not mean that either practice ceased.

The attitude of the Church towards children, which was increasingly the determinant in the framing of law in this period, remained ambiguous. This derived from the Church's dichotomy about sexuality, which it has not resolved to this day. The early Church Fathers had seen this issue in stark terms, placing their emphasis on chastity. The radical asceticism of many of the Desert Fathers seemed to condemn all family concerns and cares as matters which came between the soul and the contemplation of God and aspirations to eternal salvation. The perfect state was chastity, and the birth of any child was a breach of that perfect condition and a reminder of the fallibility of man. But the Church had to compromise with Old Adam, and also recognize there was not much future for any institution without continuing recruits; there were some outright millennarists, like Origen, who had to be attacked because of their unyielding attitude on this matter. Jerome writes: 'To prefer chastity is not to disparage matrimony. ... Married ladies can be proud to come after nuns, for God Himself told them to be fruitful and multiply and replenish the earth. .... I praise matrimony. But only because it produces virgins.'

The Church was also conscious of a charitable duty towards the weak and poor and unprotected, but in respect of foundling and abandoned children its duality again became evident. The abandoned child was seen usually as a sign of sexual promiscuity, and the Church was concerned not to seem to offer encouragement or aid to the sinful. Where the child was not the result of sinful sexual behaviour and an object of shame it was the result of sexual improvidence, and in both cases the Church took the moralistic view that the sins of the fathers should be visited on the children.

Nevertheless the Church did make some provision. There is evidence that certain charitable institutions were in existence in Treves during the sixth century and Angers in the seventh; certainly there was a foundling hospital in Milan in the eighth century, founded by Datheus in A.D. 789 – this is known because records of the institution have survived. It is not likely to have been an isolated initiative.

There is no doubt that the monasteries and nunneries absorbed many children who were unwanted by their parents; some were abandoned and taken in, others were dedicated to the religious life and the service of God. But those that were abandoned, or rescued from abandonment, were often treated as slaves while slavery persisted in the west and many more, in later times, became the property of the Church through the mediaeval concept of serfdom. God could be served in many ways. The religious institutions did become important centres for the training of children, in preparation for the priesthood either in the monasteries themselves or in other fields.

This movement found its culmination with Brother Guy of Montepellier, who was responsible for the foundation of the Order of the Holy Ghost (Santo Spirito) in 1160, one of whose concerns was the care of orphaned and foundling children. Pope Innocent III, who had been appalled at the sight of 'countless infant bodies' floating in the Tiber, became Guy's patron and summoned him to Rome, where he founded two establishments, the foundling hospitals of Santo Spirito and Santa Maria in Saxia; subsequently the movement spread throughout Christendom. The first foundation, however, undertook only to provide for children, whether orphaned or destitute, whose parents had been married; later there is evidence that this rule was relaxed.

Much later St Vincent de Paul, who had been taken prisoner and enslaved by the Muslims, began a society to rescue others who had suffered in the same way. He also turned his attention to the children left destitute and homeless in France as a result of the Thirty Years War and the Fronde. There is need to scrutinize the motivation of the whole of this exercise, however, in the light of what he is reported to have said when appealing for funds to help him in his work. In the effort to quieten the conscience of some of those whose aid he sought he pointed out to his patrons in 1638 that scarcely one of the children had survived in the past fifty years. Contemporary evidence of the care provided in the Hotel de Dieu in Paris testifies to the fact that the babies 'being neither cleaned, nor cared for nor bedded as their young age requires, not a single one was found to have survived to adulthood'.

This casts a lurid and searching light backwards on the standards of care, and, indeed, the motives of many of these charitable institutions. The Church forbade the taking of life, but it seems possible that they had adopted anachronistically Clough's 'Latest Decalogue': 'Thou shalt not kill, but need'st not strive officiously to keep alive'. If an abandoned child died through inadvertence it was acceptable to both doctrinal teaching and the sensibility of the day; these institutions would seem to have embodied the dichotomy which ran through the whole issue for the Church.

There is other evidence of the concern of the Church in respect of infanticide. It is to be found in many of the penitentials which have survived. Charlemagne was one of the Christian kings who again decreed that infanticide was to be treated as homicide, and Henry I of England enacted 'that if anyone should kill or overlay a child entrusted to him to be reared or taught, the penalty shall be the same as for adult homicide'. The problem of overlaying is dealt with time and again in various church decrees and enactments throughout the late mediaeval period.

A French law punished voluntary infanticide by death by burning, but the distinction was maintained between voluntary and involuntary acts causing death. The involuntary act was to be dealt with by canonical law and within the purview of the ecclesiastical authorities and proper penances were decreed by way of expiation. But a law of St Louis of France made a distinction between the woman who was reponsible for one death, which could be treated as involuntary and dealt with by the church authorities through penances, which themselves could be quite severe; if a second death occurred and the same woman was involved, even though it was claimed that the death was involuntary, the woman was to be handed over to the secular arm of the law, where the consequences were likely to be death by burning at the stake.

In 1217 the Synod of Salisbury issued instructions that women were to be warned to nurse their children with proper care, and were forbidden to take them into bed with them in case, during the night, they 'overlay' them; they were also exhorted not to leave children alone in the house where there was a fire or near water without someone being instructed to watch over them, and 'this should be said to them every Sunday'. Warnings of this kind are given again and again in most places during this period, indicating the frequency of such deaths, and the concern they occasioned.

Many of these instructions may have been intended to regulate the wet-nurses into whose charge, through many centuries, children were entrusted. There was also concern that the natural children born to peasant women in the countryside were being disposed of in any number of ways in order that the mother could receive payment for the suckling of children of more prosperous families. The office of wet-nurse in royal and noble households was a position of some consequence and dignity. The practice of putting children out to nurse was widespread and extended far down the social scale.

There is also evidence of the suspicions of the church and secular authorities that the wet-nurses were, on occasion, in league with families where the birth of a child was likely to prove embarrassing, and that their chief service was to encompass the death of the child. The wet-nurse, the midwife and the lying-in woman are recognizable prototypes of the sinister witches who appear in folk tales and fairy stories which may embody deep hidden fears and folk memories; these women disposed of children by beating them to death, starving them, roasting them in ovens to eat, imprisoning them, slitting their throats and losing them in the depths of woods. The wise woman and midwife were objects of dread, often used to frighten children with.

In communities not directly affected by Roman and Christian tradition, or only coming late into that tradition, the recognition of the identity of the child follows another path. There is interesting evidence of how the Viking father acknowledged his child; he proffered the haft of his spear or the handle of his sword to the youngster, who, in effect, became a legal entity and the acknowledged child of the father at the moment when his grip closed upon spear or sword. A child who failed to seize the object or who was never offered it had no legal existence, was bastardized and, in some communities, was completely outside the law.

The mingled Viking/Anglo-Saxon tradition in England is seen in part of the legislation of Canute as King of England. It was part of Canute's adoption of the Anglo-Saxon method of law enforcement: 'And we will that every freeman be brought into a hundred and into a tything ... as soon as he is twelve years old'. The tything was a division of ten families, and the hundred was the larger division of a hundred families. The tythingman and the hundredman led these groups; it was their duty to muster the able-bodied to fight for the King, and also to raise the hue-and-cry for the apprehension of anyone who broke the King's Law or the King's Peace.

This was a late enactment dealing with a process which had come down from at least the time of King Alfred and from probably much earlier. Above the hundredman was the shire-reeve, whose authority was supreme under the King, and whose name still survives in our modern sheriff. The importance of this decree is the indication it gives of the termination of the period of childhood; childhood ended at the age of twelve when a young man had to be ready to go to war and take part in the pursuit of malefactors, and also to stand answerable for the delinquencies, either of omission or commission, of all the other members of the grouping.

Just as significant is the qualification 'freeman' which should serve to remind us once more of the existence both of slavery and serfdom. The child was born slave, serf or free depending upon the status of the parents, especially of the father. The newly born child was the possession of those who had ownership or overlordship of the parents. For those abandoned or left fatherless the likelihood was that they would revert to slavery or serfdom, if they survived. Children were regarded as appurtenances of an estate and belonged to the land on which they were born.

It is a reminder that children were put to work from a very early age. The Puritan work ethic is one of the clichés of history, but this is to ignore the fact that in mediaeval times there was an universal doctrine of the church: 'Laborare est orare' – to work is to pray or, more succinctly, work is worship – which justified the working of children in the fields both of feudal lords and monastic foundations and in the households of the rich and powerful. They were put to work at all sorts of tasks and in all sorts of conditions, and were sometimes less regarded than the cattle in the fields.

Idleness was a sin long before the modern doctrines of Puritanism were propounded; Satan was always ready to prompt idle hands to do his work. Children were often characterized as 'imps of Satan', and the term did not have the jocular overtones which might be attached to the phrase in any modern context; it was part of the expression of the fundamental dichotomy of the adult and church attitude towards children.

The concern of the monastic orders to supervise such children as came into their care, particularly in the dormitories at night, is an indication of the moral ambiguity and sexual unease which children could occasion. Various penitentials show that the use of children sexually, which had been notorious in classical Greece and Rome, had not vanished from Western experience after the coming of Christianity and its gradual triumph in the West.

In some penitentials the adult, especially when in Holy Orders, is treated with greater tolerance than the child, whose innocence is flawed by the original sin of Adam and who is seen on occasion as an agent of Satan, tempting the devout and bringing them to sin. A number of the temptations recorded in the biographies of the saints deal with this explicitly or hint at it and show the far-reaching nature of this problem in the human psyche.

This view of children was also the justification for the harshness with which they were disciplined; children were whipped regularly and often, sometimes for misdeeds, on other occasions for the good of their souls and because they were children. This derives partly from the mediaeval Christian siege mentality, for the Christian world saw itself as a beleaguered fortress surrounded by the Devil and all his minions, protected only by the walls of Faith. The child within the walls was often regarded as an ally of the Devil without.

This particular way of thinking culminated in the witch-hunting epidemics which periodically swept across Christendom in late mediaeval times, and continued down to the eighteenth century both in Catholic countries and the countries of the Reformation. The burning of witches is the dramatic manifestation which always comes to notice, but the suffering of children over centuries, partly as a result of this superstitious fear and hysteria should not be overlooked, even though it was so commonplace that it was not considered worthy of mention by most commentators at the time.

Yet there were sweeter, gentler and more sensitive voices throughout this whole period of history. The precepts or example of such figures as Anselm and St Hugh of Lincoln in the English tradition bespeak the growth of a kinder attitude towards children. Hugh of Lincoln serves to remind us of the emphasis in the lives of the saints, one of the most popular forms of reading of the mediaeval period, of the growth of an attitude which depicted the natural gentleness and mutual regard of parents and children at this time – though not all the young lives of the saints were marked by loving gentleness. The growth of the cult of the Virgin and Child throughout the mediaeval period also served to present an idealized picture of motherhood and the relationship between the ideal mother and the ideal son must have been potent exemplars, even if such an example only served to point the contrast during a period which was harsh and bitter for the majority of children. Tenderness and compassion towards children, and a growing attempt to understand them and their needs, become evident during the later Middle Ages, and emerges more strongly in both the false Renaissance of the period of Abelard, and the true Renaissance later.

The humanist heirs to this tradition in Northern Europe, especially Sir Thomas More in England, developed more gentle attitudes towards children and were concerned with their education. The Reformation in England, which resulted in the disappearance of the monasteries and other religious organizations which had provided for children and their education, in whatever form, made the Tudor governments re-think their attitudes towards children whether as part of the deserving poor or as in need of education. The secularization of education can be seen to begin in a formal way in the Protestant countries.

In England there were many new foundations for education, and the provision of hospitals for foundling and orphaned children proceeded apace. At the end of Elizabeth I's reign the Poor Law was instituted, and much of its work was concerned with provision for children of the parish. Though there was much harshness of attitude under this system, the general impulse was towards care of children and a growing insight into their needs; as a result a more sensitive understanding of the child, its nurture and education did begin to develop. The Poor Law was long-lasting in England, and the foundling and orphaned child remained primarily the responsibility of the modified Poor Law system right into this century.

Education of children is the area in which authority external to the family first begins to impinge upon, and to challenge in particular, the father's rights over the child. The new grammar schools devised curricula which demanded application from the child and commitment to work of a high order, but also allowed time for play. The first mention of a master to supervise games (a rudimentary type of football) appears in the writings of the High Master of St Paul's school, one of the more famous grammar school foundations of the Tudor period. Education, as part of the process of the training of gentlemen was reinforced by the impetus it could give to the upwardly mobile classes of

Tudor England. Three centuries later, as an echo of this first aspiration, at the beginning of the nineteenth century, Thelwall, a radical follower of Thomas Paine makes the claim of 'the right to education through which the labourer's child might rise to the highest station in society'. This is after the French Revolution, and all its consequences, but it serves to show how gradually the importance of education begins to be realized by class after class in the community, and assumes increasing importance in the thinking of succeeding generations about the role of the child.

In Catholic countries education remained very much a church concern, but the foundation of the Jesuits in response to the Lutheran and English Reformations was quickly followed by the Order's involvement in the education of the young. Despite these movements, on occasion because of them, there is good evidence that throughout this period the disciplining of children remained as harsh and as damaging as ever for the generality.

John Wesley, in the eighteenth century, has many interesting things to say about the bringing up of children: 'Break their wills betimes. Begin this work before they can run alone, before they can speak plain, perhaps before they can speak at all. Whatever pains its cost, break the will if you would not damn the child. Let a child from a year old be taught to fear the rod and to cry softly; from that age make him do as he is bid, if you whip him ten times running to effect it . . .' This reflects the attitude of his own mother to the Wesley children. The justification for this attitude stemmed from the Biblical proverb: 'He that spareth the rod hateth his son'. Wesley's paraphrase of this is: 'Break his will now, and his soul shall live, and he will probably bless you to all eternity'.

These words now sound remote and alien to our ears. They seem to come from a very distant time, and serve to remind us of the increasing sensitivity which has developed in adult attitudes towards children in the past century. Another voice from the eighteenth century is that of Rousseau: 'let us speak less of the duties of children and more of their rights', but it is salutary to remember that he abandoned all his own children and showed no concern at all over their rearing and education.

Reference has already been made to the Poor Law Relief Act of 1601, in the last years of the reign of Queen Elizabeth I of England. It marked an important stage in the transition from feudal and ecclesiastical organization of society to something more approaching the modern secular state provision. The relief was initially based on local parishes, with the Justice of the Peace as the main administrative figure. The Parishes were empowered to collect rates for the relief of their own helpless, needy and poor, and from this money to provide for hospitals and the relief of those in need.

For the first time legislation defined the liability of parents for children, or of children for parents, depending upon age; it is one of the most important milestones on the path to the recognition of the parents' responsibility for the child. Children were cared for on outdoor relief or in the Work House as this provision developed over the centuries; later special Foundling Hospitals and

Schools were instituted. Before any relief was given the responsibility of parents for young children, or of self-supporting children for ageing or ailing parents had to be investigated, and later this responsibility was extended to grandparents also. The Poor Relief Act was the first formal and national recognition in Western Europe of this kind of responsibility by the state since the days of the Roman Empire, and its importance can never be overstated. Despite modifications it remained intact for well over two centuries, and parts of its provisions were operative into this century in England.

Two factors during the later part of the eighteenth century tended to bring about alteration in the attitude towards children, even though these effects were marginal consequences of the events themselves; the gradual change characterized as the Industrial Revolution in England, and the more abrupt, though less disruptive in terms of ultimate consequences, French Revolution.

The Industrial Revolution changed men's thinking in many ways, especially in respect of time and the resources of nations, just as the French Revolution, more conspicuously, proclaimed new attitudes and proselytized new ideas. The action, reaction and interaction of these two key events in the development of western history brought about many changes in the lives of children during the nineteenth century. The French Revolution thrust the state and national concerns into the forefront of modern thinking, despite its claims on the part of the individual; it was a Revolution of the cities and towns. In the same way the concentration of population in the industrial towns of England brought new attitudes and concerns to the fore.

The mass armies of Napoleon, based on the earlier experiments of Frederick the Great of Brandenburg and Prussia, made the male population an important resource, if only in terms of recruits to the armies in the field. The industrial armies of England were also seen as an important part of the national wealth and resources. The infants who were to grow to take their places in these armies assumed a new and different significance in the eyes of government.

Both Frederick the Great and Napoleon issued edicts against infanticide. Frederick was moved to change the method of execution for infanticides; where they had once been sewn into a sack and drowned they were now to be beheaded. He did not wish anyone to misunderstand his motives in bringing about this change: 'Heaven knows that I do not, for one moment, excuse this horrible act of these Medeas, who, cruel to themselves and the voice of blood, kill the future race'. The classical references and mention of blood and race reverberates backwards and forwards in time disconcertingly.

Kant possibly presents the best evidence of the change that was beginning to take place, although his voice is still that of the Enlightenment which preceded and overlapped both the Industrial and French Revolutions. He confronted the 'child as property of the parents' proposition directly. Parents do not 'have the right to destroy (the child) as if it were their own property, or even to leave it to chance, because they have brought a being into the world, and they have placed that being in a state which they cannot be left to treat with indifference, even according to the natural concept of right. .... From the fact of personality in the children it further follows that they can never be regarded as the property of their parents, but only as belonging to them by way of being in their possession, like other things that are held apart from the possessions of all others and that can be brought back even against the will of the subjects.'

Children looked at as a national resource either from a military or economic point of view, become necessarily the concern of the state, and the state has some part in them. The lives of the children concentrated in English industrial towns and working in factories and mines came under more searching scrutiny. What had happened in the fields and homes for centuries when children were put to work now became more the subject of examination as the children were put to work in the factories and mines.

The factory and mine, as places of employment were removed from the home, and the children were subject to disciplines other than parental. The emergent claims of working men and artisans to decent wages and conditions of work also began to shine a light into the darker areas of children's conditions of employment.

The First Factory Act in England in 1802 was a measure to protect orphans and poor children who had become subject to the Poor Law Acts. It extended minimum protection to a particularly vulnerable class of children, who lacked natural protection through their parents, and was intended to save them from gross exploitation and extreme forms of abuse. It is the first legislation designed specifically to protect a particular group because of age.

Ironically it gave protection to the worst circumstanced children, the orphaned and abandoned, but it did not extend the same protection to children whose parents were still living and exercising control of them. This was because the child was still regarded in law as the possession of the parents and the rights of property prevented the state intervening between the owner and his possession. Thus the 'ordinary' child was left subject to the abuse and long hours of factory work, which the 'workhouse child' was, in theory at least, protected from. Parents continued to place their children in employment at an age and under conditions which many reformers deplored.

The Poor Law Amendment Act of 1834 required that the conditions in the workhouses should be such as to deter anyone applying to come into them. This resulted in conditions of the kind which Dickens had described so graphically. But one consequence of the Act was important for it made discrimination between various types of pauper; able bodied male: able bodied female: children: aged and impotent. These different categories were to be separated for the first time, and the children in the workhouses were to be taught to read and write.

The fate of the children in the workhouses continued to arouse concern, however, and a further amendment in 1848 provided for the removal of the children from the workhouses into Poor Law Schools. This was the first formal acceptance by the national government of a measure of responsibility for the rearing and education of children, for the Poor Law was now subject to overall national control, even if its administration was local. The conditions of work for children were also subject to governmental regulation as a result of successive Factory Acts during the whole of the nineteenth century.

The second half of the century was marked by a whole series of voluntary movements by individuals and societies to try to cope with the problems of pauperism and criminality, which came to be seen increasingly as related. The Society for the Prevention of Pauperism and Crime developed into the Charity Organisation Society for The Relief of Mendacity and Prevention of Crime, whose very title savours of the age and its attitudes. There was also a strong moral element of disapproval in the Victorian attitude; poverty was sin or close akin to sinfulness and all those seeking help from the charity were divided into 'deserving' and 'undeserving' categories.

A degree of discrimination of another kind began to be shown in respect of the child offender, whose identity was recognized by the law. Until 1847 the law made no distinction between child offenders and others. Indeed it took pride in the fact that all were equal before the law even if, in fact, over centuries it had employed other criteria, such as benefit of clergy, to make discrimination. The situation for children was the same as for all other offenders; if they were charged with an indictable offence they had the right to trial by jury at the Assizes of Quarter Sessions. For non-indictable offences (these were usually, but not invariably, less serious) they were tried summarily before a bench of magistrates.

This meant that children were subject to the full range of penalties provided by the law; they could be and were hung for theft, along with others much older than they. In the eighteenth century, a great hanging period, nine out of ten of those hung were under the age of twenty-one. Those who escaped hanging were sent to serve long sentences in prison where conditions were harsh, brutal and corrupting. There was only one escape from the rope, by transportation. This was a device often used by the judiciary to avoid the death sentence for young offenders. It is important to remember, however, that no person could be transported until they were fourteen, which meant that many youngsters spent years in the hulks waiting the proper age to be shipped overseas. What they must have endured in the hulks as the tide of desperate men and women passed through beggars belief and defies the imagination. The fact that such young children endured this torment is substantiated by the Superintendent of the Hulks when he gave evidence to a Select Committee of Parliament, where he said that the youngest of his charges at the time was 'nine years old and deemed incorrigible'.

Other evidence of the treatment of youngsters emerges from the Second Report of the House of Commons Committee on the State of Police in the Metropolis. It reveals that in one year there were 399 convicted felons received in the new prison in Clerkenwell aged from nine to nineteen. These youngsters were flogged on admission and flogged again on discharge, and then 'without a shilling in their pockets, turned loose upon the world more hardened in character than ever'.

No provision for the separation of young offenders was made until 1838, when Parkhurst, which had till that time been a military hospital, was converted for the reception of young offenders up to the age of eighteen. But later commentators indicted Parkhurst for its repressive regime and brutal discipline, characterized by frequent beatings and floggings and the chaining and manacling of the young inmates, who were guarded by warders who carried rifles and whips. The Youthful Offenders Act of 1854 authorized the setting up of Reformatory Schools, which were to be organized by voluntary societies, but subject to inspection by the Home Office and needing a certificate of approval from that body. The young offenders were still required to spend six months of their sentence in an ordinary prison alongside adult offenders before they could be moved on to these special institutions. Parkhurst ceased to be a young offenders' prison in 1864, but is still with us today as a prison for adults.

Meanwhile the Summary Jurisdiction Act of 1847 had allowed young offenders charged with theft to be tried in a Magistrates' Court and not before a higher court; since the powers of the Magistrates' Court were limited, this removed young offenders from the harshest penalties which could be applied to adults. This reform came about because the authorities realized it was almost impossible to obtain a conviction of a young offender before the higher court; juries, knowing full well what the penalties were likely to be, were reluctant to convict youngsters of tender years, and many victims were unwilling to bring to the notice of the police the delinquencies of young offenders.

The Summary Jurisdiction Act of 1879 enlarged the provisions of the Act of 1847, so that offenders under the age of sixteen could be tried summarily for all indictable offences. These measures achieved two things; they reduced the number of juveniles held in prisons, and they simplified the trial process for young offenders. In practice they reduced the penalities that young offenders were subject to, because of the limited powers of the lower courts. But many children still found themselves in prisons and, of course, they still appeared in the lower courts alongside adult offenders.

The next advance in this field did not come until the wave of reforms initiated by the Liberal Governments in the 1900s. A whole range of acts reflected new approaches and thinking. The first was the Probation of Offenders Act of 1907 which allowed an offender to remain in the community under the supervision of an officer of the court in an effort to prove his ability to stay out of trouble. This was of major importance for children and young offenders, but the Children Act, 1908 was primarily directed to their concerns. This Act laid down for the first time the principle that young offenders should be dealt with entirely separately from adults, and to ensure this the Juvenile Courts were established.

Offenders under the age of sixteen had to be tried in a Juvenile Court. This court was a court of summary jurisdiction, and the legislation made it statutory that children should be tried in a separate building where possible and, if this was not possible, on a separate day from adult offenders. This was intended to protect the child from the squalid circumstances of the lower reaches of the courts crowded with drunks, prostitutes and other types of adult offender.

Under the same act imprisonment of children under fourteen was abolished, and those aged between fourteen and sixteen were subject to imprisonment only under exceptional circumstances. The emphasis in the treatment of young offenders move decisively away from punishment towards reformation, and the act allowed a degree of 'welfare' concern in the disposal of youngsters brought before the court. The working of this act and the Probation Act brought a new insight into the problems of children who were also offenders.

During the same period the work of such pioneers as Dr Barnardo had begun to make an impression on the care of children who were orphaned or abandoned, or for whom the family, where it existed, could not provide. A whole group of voluntary organizations provided a wide range of Industrial Training Schools, Orphan Homes, Ragged Schools, Children's Homes and Reformatories for children who were in need through poverty or deprivation or because of delinquent behaviour.

All these institutions were subject to inspection of one kind or another by central government, thus emphasizing the interest that the state has assumed in respect of these children. At the same time the state had intervened decisively in another area. This intervention came about as a consequence of the Infant Life Protection Acts, the first of which was passed in 1872. Prior to this, in 1868, the Boards of Guardians, the bodies now charged with the administration of the Poor Law, had been given powers to prosecute parents who wilfully neglected their children, but this power only applied to children who had already become the concern of the local authority; it was an effort to prevent parents forcing their children into the care of the Boards of Guardians and abusing the Poor Law Provisions.

The 1872 Act was the first direct intervention on the part of the law on behalf of children who were still nominally at least, seen as part of a functioning family unit. This legislation came about because of a wide-spread scandal to do with the burial clubs and insurance practices of the day; many youngsters were insured or entered into burial clubs, and then either allowed to die or done away with; thus the extra mouth was removed and a payment of money was received at the same time.

The first challenge to the absolute legal right of parents over children in the Anglo-Saxon legal tradition came in the United States in New York in 1870. This is a much told story, but the case of Mary Ellen still bears telling to illustrate the condition of the law in respect of children a little more than a century ago. A church missionary was called to visit a dying immigrant woman of German origin in the Hell's Kitchen district of New York. The dying woman asked the missionary to do something about the treatment of a child in a neighbouring family, whom she had heard beaten and abused unmercifully night after night as she lay dying. The missionary tried to intervene, but when she called upon the family she was driven away with threats and abuse.

The missionary made approaches to the police and various welfare authorities, but all to no avail. She was driven by the promise she had made to the dying woman, and would not give up. All the authorities explained to her that no outside body had the right to intervene between a parent and child. Finally she went to Henry Bergh, the founder of the New York Society for the Prevention of Cruelty to Animals; he was moved by the story she told him. He, and various of his friends, studied the statutes for some law which would give them the right to intervene. They discovered there were laws which gave protection to animals but none to give protection to children.

They were dismayed at first, but not without wit and resourcefulness; finally they produced the child in court, wrapped in a horse blanket, and claimed that the child was technically a member of the animal kingdom. They were able to demonstrate to Justice Lawrence the terrible injuries inflicted upon the child, and those present in court were so moved that the motion was allowed and the parents were duly convicted and imprisoned. A society for the protection of children was founded in New York and others were quickly established in other American cities.

As a result of connections between the cities of North America and Liverpool, a similar society was founded in Liverpool in 1883, and in 1891 thirty-one such societies amalgamated in England to form the National Society for the Prevention of Cruelty to Children, with Queen Victoria as Patron. It is an irony that still prevails to this day, however, that the society founded to protect animals is a Royal Society, but the society for the protection of children remains still a national society, despite its first royal patron.

In the year of the amalgamation of the various societies, the National Society won its first most important battle, the passage of a bill through Parliament which has always been described as the Children's Charter. As a result of the Act the law was empowered to intervene effectively on behalf of children to protect them from their own parents. Parents could be imprisoned or fined for cruelty or neglect of their children, and the courts were empowered to remove children in order to safeguard their future from homes where they were at risk. The first secretary of the National Society for the Prevention of Cruelty to Children wrote: 'The Act thus gave power to the Police Courts to act on behalf of injured children as (the Court of) Chancery has long acted on behalf of children with property. This is one of the most drastic changes in the law'.

The other form of intervention of the state between parent and child developed in the field of education. After the first secularization of education in the sixteenth century most provision for education had reverted into the hands of the churches and other denominations. The first active measure taken by the government was in 1833 when grants from central government were made to help various voluntary societies build schools in areas of need, and following on this involvement a system of centralized inspection was inaugurated. Nothing further was done until 1870 when the Elementary Education Act, always associated with the name of Forster, was passed. This, as its name suggests, only made provision for elementary education, and the provision was not free. It was intended to fill gaps in provision left by the voluntary bodies. School boards were appointed who were required to administer the new schools which were financed from public funds.

In response to the sensitivity of the various church organizations a clause was inserted; 'no religious catechism or religious formulary which is distinctive of any particular denomination shall be taught in the school'. Under this act education did not become compulsory, showing also sensitivity to the rights of parents; there was still no emphasis of the right of a child to education.

In 1876 an Elementary Education Act was passed; this placed a duty on the parents to see that children received sufficient education of an elementary kind and, perhaps more significantly, a clause prohibited employers from offering work to children during the hours school was open if the children lived within ten miles of a school. But this still failed to work and in 1880 compulsory education for all children up to the age of ten years was introduced. In 1899 the age limit was raised to twelve and the system became universally free.

The state had thus made a decisive intervention in the relationship between child and parent, but in educational matters this came much later in England than in some continental countries and in the United States. By the end of the century the state had intervened in the field of education, child care and the treatment of delinquency and had created new institutions whose working began to throw up more information and to define new areas of concern and identify specific needs related to children.

Part of this process arose from the study of psychology and theories of perception and learning which focused attention upon the young child and its development to maturity; the work of Freud and others in the field of therapy was also of importance in developing a new view of the condition of childhood. This is part of the development which is not strictly related to the emergence of the child as a legal entity, but its influence during the present century had been of immense significance.

The twentieth century has been marked by a spate of legislation which has gradually prescribed the rights of parents over children; this has been a gradual process, and many of the advances have been spasmodic, in response to specific needs and situations.

The Children and Young Persons Act, 1933 was the great landmark in this area, bringing together concerns from all three fields. For the first time the lower age of criminal responsibility was fixed at eight. The most important statement in the Act was as follows: 'Every court, in dealing with a child or young person who is brought before it, either as an offender or otherwise, shall have regard to the welfare of the child or young person and shall in a proper case take steps for removing him from undesirable surroundings, or for securing that proper provision is made for his education or training'.

Apart from the limited reference made in the Guardianship of Infants Act of 1925, this was the first and most comprehensive statement of the rights of children in English statute.

The first section of the Act was specifically concerned with 'Prevention of cruelty and exposure to moral danger'. This included the following categories: wilful assault, ill-treatment, neglect, abandonment, or any act which is likely to cause unnecessary suffering or injury to health, any injury to any organ of the body or any form of mental derangement'. Neglect was seen as any omission which resulted in the failure to provide adequate food, clothing, medical aid or lodging. It would seem to be completely comprehensive and cover all eventualities.

The 1963 Act of the same title provided for local authorities to undertake preventive work in order to prevent children suffering ill-treatment or neglect, and to avoid deprivation. This would enable local authorities to intervene before the child had made any appearance in court, and was a further prescription of the rights of parents, and an assertion of the rights of children. But this preventive work was not made statutory, and a large number of local authorities made no finances available to carry out any part of such work.

The major change in society's view of the child finds definition in a White Paper, 'Children in Trouble', which was a discussion document preceding the Children and Young Persons Act, 1969.

'A child's behaviour is influenced by genetic, emotional and intellectual factors, his maturity and his family, school, neighbourhood and wider social setting. It is probably a minority of children who grow up in ways which may be contrary to the law. Frequently such behaviour is no more than an incident in the pattern of a child's normal development. But sometimes it is a response to unsatisfactory family or social circumstances, a result of boredom in and out of school, an indication of maladjustment or immaturity, or a symptom of deviant, damaged or abnormal personality. Early recognition and full assessment are particularly important in these more serious cases. Variety and flexibility in the measures that can be taken are equally important, if society is to deal effectively and appropriately with these manifest aspects of delinquency. The measures include supervision and support of the child in the family: the further development of facilities for short-term and long-term care, treatment and control, including some which are highly specialized.'

The Act set out the tests for the taking of what are called 'care proceedings' in the juvenile court. The court must be satisfied:

1. That the child's development is being avoidably prevented or neglected, or his health is being avoidably impaired or neglected, or he is being ill-treated;

or 2. That similar conditions as indicated above have been proved in respect of another child in the same household;

or 3. He is exposed to moral danger;

or 4. He is beyond the control of his parent or guardian;

or 5. He is truanting when of compulsory school age;

or 6. He is guilty of an offence in law, excluding homicide.

As can be seen the law now covers comprehensively most of the conditions likely to bring a child to the attention of the authorities for any reason. It is also interesting that deprivation and delinquency are, by and large, seen as manifestations of a related set of circumstances, and that the law deals with both in the one act. It sees delinquent behaviour in the young as likely to arise from the ill functioning of the family group or the local community, and sees the child against the whole background of these conditions. The welfare concept has incorporated concepts of child protection to the point where the child is not only protected against others, but also against himself.

The juvenile court, in this legislation, had also changed its role and status. It still has the power to punish, but it has extremely powerful rights of intervention in the life of the child and the rights of the parents. It can order supervision of the child in its own home by the local authority under a Supervision Order; it has the right also to extinguish completely the rights of the parents over the child until it is seventeen, by means of a Care Order, where the local authority is given the full rights of parents, and the parents themselves are removed from the processes of care of the child.

The court also has another duty, that of the protection of the rights of the child, in that in effect it has become the licensing authority; the court determines how far and in what way society can intervene in the life of the child. It limits the intervention of the local authority social workers by its orders, and it requires certain conditions to be proved, in a proper legal setting, before it will allow such intervention at all. In this way it is concerned to safeguard the rights of the parents, but also of the child, for any intervention is a diminishment of the freedom of the child. This is a point which is often overlooked, but which is of great importance when we talk about the rights of children.

Nowhere does any statute specifically define in comprehensive fashion what the rights of children are. As a society we have come to accept the right to life itself, to education, to proper medical care, to protection from exploitation, cruelty, ill-treatment and abuse, and we have established minimal conditions for childhood which we feel are acceptable in a civilized society. We have taken powers to intervene both positively and negatively on behalf of the child in a variety of ways where we feel these minimal conditions are not being met. But most of the rights we would now say children enjoy are not defined in any positive fashion; they are defined negatively, by a series of prescriptions of what must not be done to a child and what a child must not be allowed to suffer.

We have recognized the special individuality of the child, and made a careful catalogue of its special needs; we have not faced the more difficult task of a positive definition of what a child is, mainly because we have not given the child full status as an entity in law. Until we address ourselves to this task we will always fail a number of children, and they will suffer neglect, ill-treatment and other forms of damage of many kinds, and some, tragically, will be killed.

Through historical time the face of the child has slowly emerged as a recognizable individual likeness; we have, by prescription, blacked out much of the background in which the outlines of the head were lost. We still have not inserted the features in the outline face, other than the most obvious. The final work will have to be the joint effort of many disciplines. That job remains to be done, to make the child a recognizable entity, especially in the eyes of the law.

Appendix

J. E. OLIVER

INTRODUCTION

This Appendix is a Review of the World Literature on the Extent of Child Abuse, prepared by Dr J. E. Oliver. It was conceived in conjunction with Chapter 5 (Part II). The referencing for this Appendix is detailed at the end of Chapter 5.II. There may be important omissions, particularly in respect of research not published in the English language. Papers have been published on child maltreatment from the Communist and Third Worlds, but few attempt the overall numerical estimates given in studies from the UK, America, Australia and West Germany. This Appendix is mainly concerned with the Western World, because parts of the Western World provide attempts at National Statistics, and individual researchers have prepared some reasonably good local statistics on child victims.

A References	B Age Range	C Types of Abuse	D Death Rate	E Special Features of the Study
British Isles				
British Medical Journal Editorial (1973). Deliberate injury of children[1]	Mostly under 4 years	'Serious Assaults'	Unspecified	Editorial review
British Paediatric Association. Evidence presented to the Select Parliamentary (UK) Committee on Violence in the Family. June (1976)[62]	Unstated — (children under 16, but mostly concerned with pre-school children under 5 years)	A broad range — homicide, serious injuries, minor injuries. Cruelties associated with emotional deprivation and neglect. See col. J for residual defects to the brain and eye	(a) 97 English Authorities recorded 40 fatal cases from 5700, in the last $\frac{3}{4}$ of 1974 (0.7% mortality rate). (b) The BPA reported 869 cases and 60 deaths (6.9% mortality rate)	A broad but disciplined review, with recommendations for changes to be made at National level. (Under-diagnosis is usually attributable to pressure of work in General Practice and in Accident and Emergency Depts., and the reluctance of Doctors to question and pursue the incidents)
Beswick *et al.* (1976). Child abuse and general practice[63]	Under 10 years	(a) Inflicted injuries (b) 'At risk children', assaulted or neglected or in danger from their parents	No deaths recorded	Preventive social medicine by the family doctor and team
Castle, R. L. and Kerr, A. M. (1972). A study of suspected child abuse[3]	Children under 4	Fractures, head injuries, internal injuries, burns and soft tissue damage. There is also consideration of highly suspicious but unconfirmed cases	3 in 292	Emphasis on referral patterns to the NSPCC, with a strong case made for central registries

F Type of Population	G The Abusers	H Ascertainment	I Limitations of Study	J Extent of Child Abuse
UK and USA	No detail. Parents tend to aid and abet each other in attacking their child(ren)	Quotes from papers and reports in UK and USA. 4600 child assault victims per year in UK. 6 children per 1000 live births become battered babies. 10% of all casualties under 2 years, and 25% of all fractures under 2 years, attributable to child abuse		
(a) England (b) UK and Eire	No details	(a) Official sources — Local Authority Social Services Letters. (b) Special BPA survey. Members saw an average of four (serious) cases each per year; *but some dealt with up to 80 per year, but only reported a few of these to the survey*	Undefined cases, or variable definitions. See col. H(b), which suggests that some paediatricians were reporting 'classical' battered babies only, in contrast to others who earmarked a wider range of cruelty cases	(a) 5700 cases in the last $\frac{3}{4}$ of 1974. (b) Four (serious) cases per paediatrician per year (but see cols. H and I). Some paediatricians saw 80 per year. For the '869 cases for whom the outcome was accurately known there were 60 deaths . . . 92 children left with brain damage . . . and 48 with visual defects . . .'
Didcot, Oxfordshire	As above	By the family doctor and others associated with his team (e.g. health visitor)	Many cases (including some severe ones) might not 'surface' into general practice	(a) 12 abuse cases in 4 years from 1841 children under 10 years (b) An additional 30 cases for 1841 children, in March 1976
England and Wales	Not stated	Working referrals from the NSPCC field workers to the research team as the incidents occurred	See col. H. Scant returns with few or no records from certain populous areas. This study must also have missed large numbers not known to the NSPCC field workers	292 in 50 million in one year

A References	B Age Range	C Types of Abuse	D Death Rate	E Special Features of the Study
Chesser, E. (1951). Cruelty to children[4]	(a) Children under 15	(a) Bad neglect, or ill-treatment, or maladjustment associated with parental ill-usage	(a) Unspecified	(a) 'Cold Facts', rather than projections
	(b) Children under 15	(b) As above	(b) Unspecified	(b) 'Cold Facts', rather than projections
	(c) Children under 15	(c) Children suffering (at least one) harmful experience from parent or guardian, which experience has potentially life-long implications	(c) Unspecified	(c) Projections throughout childhood. Comparison of recorded incidents of ill-usage, with overall NSPCC statistics
	(d) Children under 15	(d) As for (a) above, but with repetition(s) of incidents	(d) Unspecified	(d) 'Hard Core' cases
Clegg, A. and Megson, B. (1968). Children in distress[5]	School age approx. 5–15	Broad and all embracing categories considered. Children under severe distress in the home, usually as a result of parental stress, neglect, cruelty, or incompetence. 'Children who are wretchedly unhappy because of the strain put on them at home'	Not considered	A consideration of the extent of distress to children. Direct observations and analysis by educationalists

F Type of Population	G The Abusers	H Ascertainment	I Limitations of Study	J Extent of Child Abuse
(a) England and Wales	(a) Unspecified. Either parent or guardian	(a) NSPCC annual report for 1950 — no reference to other sources		(a) One child in 100 in 1 year (1949) is *known* to be a victim (see cols. C, H and I)
(b) England and Wales	(b) Unspecified	(b) NSPCC annual reports 1945—50. The author believed that most cases of child cruelty were ascertained by the NSPCC, but this seems unlikely nowadays (see text, Chapters 5 and 6)		(b) 100 000 new children per year (from total child population of nearly 11 million) brought to the attention of NSPCC on account of ill-usage
(c) England and Wales	(c) Unspecified	(c) Projections based on NSPCC figures for children abused or neglected *at any time* in their lives up to the age of 15. The significance of the figure given in col. J is uncertain, but under-ascertainment here is less likely than in (b) above. Chesser's observations and deductions imply family clustering of disorders — compare subsections of (Chapter 6, Part I), Oliver[17, 18] and Newcombe[131]		(c) 6 or 7% of all children (see cols. C, H and I). One child in every 16 is brought to the attention of the NSPCC at some time during childhood
(d) England and Wales	(d) Unspecified	(d) Discussion of 'case closures' and repeated episodes of neglect and ill-usage in certain families		(d) 50% of referrals to NSPCC in 1949—50 involved victims who had previously been ill-used within the family setting
United Kingdom, particularly Yorkshire	Biological and substitute parents. Several chapters on different types of rearing failures by families	Via observations from schools on the distress of pupils. Also projections of official statistics. Substantiation of certain of the findings of the Plowden Committee, with quotations from the Plowden Committee, the Newsom Report, and the work of D. H. Stott	Unclear separation of distress caused to children by cruel or selfish parenting, and children suffering from other social or medical handicaps	30 000 out of 300 000 school age children in W. Riding of Yorkshire 'live through extremes of wretchedness', or need 'preventive help'. 15% need special care from their schools at some time in their school life because of the difficulties they face at home'

A References	B Age Range	C Types of Abuse	D Death Rate	E Special Features of the Study
Cooper, C. (1975). 'The doctors dilemma' — a paediatrician's view[6]	Predominantly children of 3 years and under	Battered babies. Surface injuries; fractures; intra-cranial bleedings, etc.	14 deaths in 136 cases (10.3%)	30% of followed-up cases rendered permanently brain damaged
DHSS Publication (1970). *The Battered Baby*[64]	(a) Deaths under 5 years due to homicide and injury purposely inflicted by another person		(a) 71 deaths in 1967 (50 million population)	
	(b) Deaths between 4 weeks and 1 year resulting from *proven wilful violence*		(b) 40 infant deaths per year known* to result from wilful violence (50 million population)	
Fairburn et al. (1975). Child abuse, a scheme of interdisciplinary linkage and coordination[11]	Mostly children under 3 years	Specification involves known inflicted injuries, fractures, bruising and death, but also usage of data from linkage of family information	Unspecified	Multi-agency cooperation in the consideration and surveillance of the local abusing and potentially abusive families
Hall, M. H. (1972). Non-accidental injuries to children[65]	Mostly children under 3 years	Only 'true battered' children considered	Two deaths in 20 children in 1970	The problems of severe child abuse as viewed from the casualty dept., with detailed con-siderations of the patterns of injury

F Type of Population	G The Abusers	H Ascertainment	I Limitations of Study	J Extent of Child Abuse
Newcastle-on-Tyne	Unspecified. Either parent or guardian	Direct firsthand observations by the local paediatricians	Study not designed to look at total numbers in a given population. The authoress recognises under-estimation, particularly in respect of older children	148 episodes of severe injury to 136 children in Newcastle between 1965 and 1971. (From 124 families)
England and Wales	Unspecified. Either parent or guardian	(a) Returns from the Registrar General	(a) Only the most blatantly obvious cases 'surface' in the official numbers	(a) 71 deaths in 1967 (50 million population): but see col. I
England and Wales	Unspecified. Either parent or guardian	(b) Projection from a study of 679 post-natal deaths	(b) Limited spectrum considered (see cols. B and C). Non-recognition of shaking as a cause of death	(b) 40 infant deaths per year known to result from wilful violence; but see col. I, and letter to the *B.M.J.*[112]
City of Bath	Unspecified. Either parent or guardian	The Bath team was an active referral point for all professional people likely to encounter child abuse	This system is influenced by the drive and ability of team members. The data is prepared in a way which makes it hard to compare with other studies	At any one time, 12 battering adults, and 20–30 high risk (battering likely) families in the City of Bath (86 000 population)
Preston and environs. (Also projections applying to Great Britain)	Unspecified	Diagnosis made at first hand in Preston emergency dept.	Ascertainment limited to those cases which present to the doctor in one emergency dept.	45 cases in two years for a population of 300 000. (The department sees 32 000 new patients per year)

A References	B Age Range	C Types of Abuse	D Death Rate	E Special Features of the Study
Hession, M. (1976). Memorandum to the Select Committee on Violence in the family (UK Parliament), presented by the Institute of Child Psychology[66]	Unstated	(a) Child victims of violence in the home seen in connection with the work of the institute (b) As above, but including children *witnessing* inter-parental violence (c) Unacceptable violence in the home (all children)	Unspecified	An attempt to portray rearing failures in London in the 1970s with recommendations to improve the situation of child victims. Sub-normal, mentally ill, physically ill, personality disordered and stressed parents discussed
Holman, R. R. and Kanwar, S. (1975). Early life of the battered child[67]	Children 3 years and under	'Battered babies' fractures, surface and other injuries, but also two cases of severe deprivation	Unspecified	'Social factors' emphasized in a poor area of London
Jackson, G. (1972). Child abuse syndrome: 'The cases we miss'[14]	(a) 100 records of children under 12 scrutinized, but all abused children actually under 2 (b) Unspecified	(a) Fractures, bruising, scalds, lacerations, cerebral haemorrhage, and internal injuries (b) Unspecified child abuse	(a) 2 out of 18 (b) Unspecified	Diagnostic failures discussed, with details given
The Lancet Editorial (1971). Violent parents[68]	Unstated	(a) Assaults (unspecified) (b) Injured or seriously deprived	(a) 10% of the assaulted children die (b) At least 40 babies under 1 year are killed in UK	Quotations and projections based on reports in USA and UK

F Type of Population	G The Abusers	H Ascertainment	I Limitations of Study	J Extent of Child Abuse
London children (compare with Clegg and Megson, on Yorkshire children)	No detail given	(a) and (b) Child psychiatric assessment, diagnostic and treatment services, social service depts and community homes in London boroughs (c) Projected estimates to the London population	The evidence projects data from distressed children being treated, to the London population as a whole. The 1 in 10 figure represents deviation from an undefined norm	(a) At least 20% of the 500—700 children seen per year. (40% of discovered cases of serious injuries come from families with one parent with an IQ lower than 75) (b) 40% of the children seen (c) Physical violence beyond a generally accepted norm occurs in about 10% of families in the general population
London Borough of Lambeth	Unspecified	Official 'Battering' reports from the Lambeth Directorate of Health Observation Handicap Unit. Also a variety of other sources, medical and social	The authors recognize incomplete ascertainment (many cases unrecognized or unreported)	2 Battered babies per 1000 children aged 3 years or under
London children	Unspecified	Study not designed to look at total numbers in a given population (a) 100 random children's case records of physical injury from King's College Hospital examined (b) Known cases of child abuse under treatment by the K.C.H. Paediatric Dept., at time of investigation		(a) 18% of all children under 12 seen with physical injury at K.C.H. were victims of abuse (b) 70 known cases of child abuse under treatment at the time of the survey, at K.C.H.
(a) USA (b) UK	Unspecified	Estimates based on Kempe[34] and Dept. of Health and Social Security[64]	Little recent original work cited. See cols. E and H	(a) Not stated (b) At least 3000 infants and children are injured or seriously deprived in Britain per year

A *References*	B *Age Range*	C *Types of Abuse*	D *Death Rate*	E *Special Features of the Study*
MacKeith, R. (1974). Speculations on non-accidental injury as a cause of chronic brain disorder[69]	See cols. C, E, J. Mostly children under 1 year considered	Attacks on young children leading to brain damage	1.3–13% of the assaulted children die	Skilful projections based on 16 recent papers. Mortality related to morbidity
Okell, C. (1971). Childhood accidents and child abuse[15]	Children under 3	(a) Physical abuse (b) Neglect	Unspecified	Careful scrutiny of the (unselected) families showed unawareness by professional staff of the probability of child abuse
Oliver, J. E. *et al.* (1974). Severely ill-treated young children in north-east Wilts.[18] (See also Chapter 6, Part I especially for additional prospective data)	Children under 5	Detailed stringent criteria (see Text). Emphasis on active physical abuse an essential requirement for inclusion in total numbers. Subsequent data showed high incidence of neglect, etc. in the ascertained group	4 out of 38 killed (1965–1971) Fatality data on the 1972–73 cases given in the text in Chapter 6, Part I	Combined epidemiological and clinical survey. Detailed family and personal histories obtained by searching methods. Severely (but often subtly) pathological family histories thereby revealed. Also detail on types of injury, (including much serious head injury), reinjuries and repetitions. This study is partly retrospective and partly prospective
Ounsted, C. *et al.* (1975). Aspects of bonding failure: the psychopathology and psychotherapeutic treatment of families of battered children[19]	Unspecified, but mostly babies and toddlers	'The battered child syndrome.' More than half the cases seen had been injured on a number of occasions before the diagnosis had been made	Unspecified	A clear and original account of treatment of failures in parent child bonding

F Type of Population	G The Abusers	H Ascertainment	I Limitations of Study	J Extent of Child Abuse
UK, USA, France, Sweden	Unspecified	Mortality figures on child abuse related to likely morbidity. Morbidity figures from brain damage related to child abuse figures. References to studies directly relating child abuse to brain damage		400 new cases in UK per year of chronic brain damage due to child abuse
London children	Unspecified	Children attending two casualty depts with a history of accident	Study not designed to look at total numbers in a given population	(a) 6.7% and (b) 8.9% children attending the two casualty depts
N.E. Wilts, England. Mixed rural and urban, with recent immigrants from London and elsewhere. Also including three large military establishments	Female parent, 82%. Active complicity of female parent, 9%. No involvement of female parent, 9%. Male parent, 40%. Active complicity of male parent, 20%. No involvement of male parent, 40%. In over $\frac{3}{4}$ of families, married (or re-married) natural parent(s) were responsible	Personal ascertainment by members of the team through all agencies and individuals in N.E. Wilts. connected with children. Principles of ascertainment of total numbers (and of linking family and personal data) included prompt recording of verbatim information, comparisons of different records and a sceptical approach to apparently negative information	Small area, small numbers (only 60). The methods of ascertainment tended to select the most deteriorated families. The criteria were too stringent to encompass quite large numbers of cases which would undoubtedly have been included in other surveys but which were not written up in this report (see text)	Rising ascertainment, 1970–73. One new case referred per 1000 children under 4 years old, per year. For England and Wales, this rate would entail referral of over 3000 (very severe abuse) children (aged 0–3) each year. Four children per 1000 live births per annum suffer very severe abuse by closely defined criteria
Oxford and environs	Unspecified	Firsthand diagnoses at a unit which specializes in treating abusive families in which there are bonding failures. (Park Hospital, Oxford)	Study not designed to look at total nos. in a given population. The authors reject the use of statistical data on certain aspects of the problem	110 battered children per 1000 (paediatric) referrals (but see col. H). 19 000 new cases likely per year in England and Wales (Extrapolation from Kempe's 1972 USA data[132])

A References	B Age Range	C Types of Abuse	D Death Rate	E Special Features of the Study
Rose, N. et al. (1975). NSPCC registers of suspected non-accidental injury[70]	Children under 4	Patterns of injury indicating unjustified and excessive parental violence	0.03 per 1000 per year (Manchester) 1 child died out of 35 battered	Large scale use of central registers, with considerations of re-battering and re-injury
Scott, P. D. (1973). Parents who kill their children.[71] (See also 'Fatal battered baby cases'[133])	Children under 16	Children killed by parents	Only dead children considered	Type description and classification of the killing parents. This is to be compared with Scott's subsequent article[133]
Skinner, A. E. and Castle, R. L. NSPCC Publ. (1969). 78 Battered Children. A Retrospective Study[23]	Children under 4	Injuries serious enough to warrant medical intervention	One in 78. (Some more re-battered children died after 1969)	Comprehensive details on the patterns of injury, the victims, the re-injury rate, and the families
Smith, S. M. and Hanson, R. (1974). 134 Battered children: a medical and psychological study[72]	Children under 5	Battered young children. Bruises, burns, scalds, fractures, intra-cranial and intra-ocular damage	21 out of 134 children died	A controlled definitive study with detailed medical and psychological assessments. 20 children had permanent neurological sequelae
Sills, J. A. et al. (1977). Non-accidental injury. A two year study in central Liverpool[73]	All children under 6, more than half under 2 years	Battered babies, with 48% suffering bruising to the face and head; only 14 out of 76 children did not have a record of assaults prior to the main battering. See col. E	No fatalities, but see col. E	Increase in case conferences designed to fore-stall the more severe cases of multiple injury. Multiproblem families with much criminality, psychiatric illness, etc. Sibs often injured previously (two killed by parents)

F Type of Population	G The Abusers	H Ascertainment	I Limitations of Study	J Extent of Child Abuse
Leeds and Manchester Metropolitan Districts	Unspecified; but 30% of the natural fathers were absent	A broad spectrum of agencies supplied data for the Registers (see Ref. [70] for details)	The functioning of the Registers depends on the efficiency, conscientiousness and extra effort by those working in the area	A minimum of 1.2 per 1000 children under 4 are battered, in metropolitan Leeds and Manchester each year. (3500 p.a. projected to England and Wales)
England and Wales	Fewer men murderers kill their *own* child ... than do women (15% men, 69% women)	This study shows the very small numbers ascertained by formal legal methods. 'Every year in England and Wales about 130 murders are known to the Police, and about $\frac{1}{3}$ of these are murders of children under 16 years of age. Over $\frac{3}{4}$ of these child murders are by the parents.'		
England and Wales	42 female, 33 male	Initial information only from questionnaire sent to NSPCC field workers	See col. H. Scant returns, with few or no records from certain populous areas. This, like the 1972 NSPCC study[3] cannot claim to tackle the problem of numbers of abuse cases in a given population	78 in 50 million in one year (July 1967—June 1968) 60% known re-battering rate
Catchment area of Birmingham Children's Hospital	See Ref. [134] Where identified, mothers responsible for at least $\frac{3}{4}$ of the cases	Data direct from Birmingham Children's Hospital and immediate sources	Study not designed to look at total numbers in a given population	134 children (under 5 years) from Birmingham and its environs (approx. 1$\frac{1}{2}$ million) in 2 years
Central Liverpool	Mothers (54%). Fathers or male cohabitees (50%) (22% of males *not* the father of the injured child)	Collated case conferences of the Royal Liverpool Children's Hospital, 1973—4. Rising ascertainment rate	Study not designed to look at total numbers in a given population	76 battered children from 73 families, in 1973 and 1974, from central Liverpool

A References	B Age Range	C Types of Abuse	D Death Rate	E Special Features of the Study
Tunbridge Wells Study Group (1973). Non-accidental injury to children[74]	No clear specification, but mostly children under 4 years considered	No clear specification, but special emphasis given to shaking and brain injury	700 deaths per year for the UK (50 million)	400 children rendered sub-normal from brain damage or battering per year in the UK (estimate)
United States of America				
Adelson, L. (1961). Slaughter of the innocents[75]	Most under 10. All pre-adolescent	Homicides. Infanticide excluded	Only dead children considered	Children easier to kill, their homicides much easier to conceal, than in adult cases. Autopsies on dead children always essential
Akbarnia, B. *et al.* (1974). Mani-festations of the battered child syndrome[76]	More than three-quarters of the children under 3 years	'Battered child syndrome'	Not stated	A descriptive article, mainly from the ortho-paedic standpoint, on the injuries of battered children
Blumberg, M. L. (1974). Psycho-pathology of the abusing parent[77]	Mostly under 3 years	Unspecified. Mainly physical abuse, but some figures include neglect cases	Unstated	Parental characteristics and treatment possibilities discussed. The problem is reaching 'epidemic proportions'
Bryant, H. D. *et al.* (1963). Physical abuse of children. An agency study[78]	Half the children under 7. Three-quarters under 13	Serious physical abuse to the extent that the child needs pro-tection from a source outside the family	3 out of 180 children	Physical abuse of children by their parents is a serious and wide-spread problem in Massachusetts
Ebbin, A. J. *et al.* (1969). Battered child syndrome at the Los Angeles County Gen. Hospital[28]	Children under 16. Most were under 2 years	Fractures, lacera-tions, subdural haematoma, bruises, poison-ing, or burns inflicted by parent, some-times with growth retarda-tion attributable to parental ill-usage	3 out of 106 died	Detailed Medical findings carefully described. Un-stable families with a high rate of parental previous criminal convic-tions, mental ill-ness or alcoholism Previous injuries to index children and sibs

F Type of Population	G The Abusers	H Ascertainment	I Limitations of Study	J Extent of Child Abuse
United Kingdom	Unspecified. Either parent or guardian	Co-ordination of the knowledge of national experts with firsthand clinical, or other direct experience	See cols. B and C. Most figures projected from predominantly medical sources; estimates from clinical practice, rather than planned surveys	4600 cases per year in the UK (50 million). For same population 700 killed, 400 rendered brain damaged per year
Cuyahoga County, USA	18 Fathers 12 Mothers 3 Other relatives	Homicide victims from the Cuyahoga Coroner's office and Dept. of Pathology	The limitations of ascertainment make the group here considered not comparable with the other papers	44 in 17 years in the Cuyahoga jurisdictional area. See col. C
Philadelphia and environs	Incomplete data	Cases and records from St Christopher's Hospital for Children, Philadelphia	Study not designed to look at total nos. in a given population	231 young children in 8 years admitted to St Christopher's Hospital for Children in Philadelphia, with classical battering
USA, especially New York	Mothers responsible in 70% of cases	Figures from official sources discussed along- side personal observations	Study not designed to look at total nos. in a given population. Advice based on indefinite criteria	60 000 cases of child abuse were reported in the USA Press in 1972 (Senator Mondale). 3000 per year reported to the New York central register
Massachusetts	86% of abuse by the parents, fathers and mothers about equally	1. Series of Seminars among welfare committee members. 2. Questionnaire to 18 district offices of Massachusetts SPCC	Unclear specifi- cations. This study obtained data pre- dominantly from non-medical sources	200 children from 134 direct reports, and 180 children from 115 confirmed case reports in one year in the state of Massachusetts
Los Angeles and its environs	Parents or parent surrogates. 30% of the children lived with both parents; 50% with mother only 16% with other relatives, foster parents or un- defined adults; 4% with father only	Cases admitted to the Los Angeles Hospital, and ascertained directly by two of the investigators	Study not designed to look at total nos. in a given population. The authors recognized under- reporting	106 battered children from 1 hospital in Los Angeles in 1 year

A References	B Age Range	C Types of Abuse	D Death Rate	E Special Features of the Study
Elmer, E. (1967). Children in jeopardy[79]	56% of the children were under 10 months. at time of fractures. Eldest child 8	Detailed radio-logical criteria emphasizing broken bones associated with assaults and/or gross neglect	7 out of 50 sub-sequently died	Detailed follow-up of previously battered babies. More than 25% either died or ended in institu-tions. The remainder suffered much dysfunction, including neuro-logical impair-ment and mental handicap
Fontana, V. J. (1971). The maltreated child[29]	Variable and unspecified	(a) Unspecified child abuse	(a) 1 in 4	Review of the situation in the USA
		(b) Unspecified	(b) 1 in 10	(b) 1 in 15 brain damaged
		(c) Unspecified	(c) Unspecified child abuse	
		(d) Physical abuse	(d) Unspecified	
		(e) Unspecified	(e) Unspecified	
		(f) Unspecified child abuse (g) 'Abused, neglected or harmed' (h) Abandonment and neglect	(f) Unspecified (g) Unspecified (h) Unspecified	(f, g, h) Private agencies report much higher than the official sources
		(i) Battered children	(i) 78 in 749 died	(i) 114 in 749 suffered per-manent brain damage
		(j) Unspecified	(j) Unspecified	(j) Very poor reporting by the hospital staff noted
Fontana, V. J. (1971). The diagnosis of the maltreatment syndrome in children[30]	Unspecified	A range of abuses discussed, including assaults, nutritional deprivations, etc.	Unspecified	Discussion of diagnostic con-siderations in ascertaining mal-treated children. Huge rise in ascertainment in New York City between 1966 and 1970

F Type of Population	G The Abusers	H Ascertainment	I Limitations of Study	J Extent of Child Abuse
Pittsburgh	Unspecified. Usually the mother	See col. C. Hospital sources only. Only consideration of X-ray evidence in the initial ascertainment	Study not designed to look at total numbers in a given population	50 admitted to the Pittsburgh Children's Hospital over 13 years. See cols. H and I
(a) USA	(a) Unspecified. (Parent or guardian)	(a) Children's division of the American Humane Society; ascertainment solely from newspaper reports		(a) 662 in 1962 in USA reported in newspapers. Projected true estimate — up to 6000+ per year
(b) USA	(b) Unspecified	(b) Children's bureau — sources unspecified		(b) 447 in 6 months
(c) Chicago and its environs	(c) Unspecified	(c) From County Family Court		(c) 100 cases per month from Chicago Family Court
(d) Chicago and its environs	(d) Unspecified	(d) Cook County Hospital, Chicago		(d) 10 cases per day
(e) New York State	(e) Unspecified	(e) Official reports		(e) 2169 in 1969
(f) New York City	(f) Unspecified	(f) Bureau of Child Welfare		(f) 1674 in 1969
(g) Manhattan, Bronx, Brooklyn	(g) Unspecified	(g) Bronx County Society for the Prevention of Cruelty to Children		(g) 15 772 in 1969
(h) New York City	(h) Unspecified	(h) Official figures, and (h2) Children's Court cases		(h) 2000 awaited placement in 1962. (h2) 5000 dependency and neglect cases in 1962
(i) USA	(i) Unspecified	(i) A nationwide survey of hospitals and law enforcement agencies, but with very incomplete returns		(i) 749 in one year
(j) Massachusetts	(j) Unspecified	(j) Massachusetts Society for the Prevention of Cruelty to Children		(j) 200 cases reported to the Massachusetts SPCC in 1960
New York City	Unspecified, usually the biological parents	New York Central Registry	Study not planned to look at total numbers in a given population, consequently under-estimations	Children attacked by their parents in New York City. 1968—956: 1969—1500: 1970—3000 children neglected by their parents in N.Y.C. 1968/70—35 000

A References	B Age Range	C Types of Abuse	D Death Rate	E Special Features of the Study
Furst, W. D. (1975). The medical profession and child abuse in Texas[80]	Unspecified	Reported and confirmed cases of child abuse	104 children died of abuse in 1974 in Texas	Alerting features, the need for reporting, and treatment of families all emphasized
George, J. E. (1973). Spare the rod: A survey of the battered child syndrome[81]	Variable specifications	Variable specifications. Predominantly-active physical abuse	700 children killed per year in USA (from Kempe[35])	A lengthy review of the literature on child abuse (mainly USA)
Gil, D. G. (1970). Violence against children. Physical child abuse in the United States[82]	'Children under 18'	Prior specifications encompass physical assaults with 'Intent of perpetrator', but also include acts of omission such as 'Intentional with-holding of food', etc.	Approx. 3.4% of recorded cases were fatal. The author recognizes under-representation of fatalities, especially in certain states	Massive survey providing a broad analysis on which a typology of child abuse and conceptual framework are based. *REPORTED RATES FOR EACH STATE IN USA GIVEN*
Gil, D. G. (1968). Incidence of child abuse and demographic characteristics of persons involved[83]	(a) Unspecified (b) Under 18 (c) Unspecified	(a) Unspecified (b) Complex definition; mainly deliberate physical injury, but also 'Deliberate omission, such as "starvation", etc' (c) Unspecified	(a) Unspecified (b) 1.4% of abuse incidents led to death (c) 164 out of 504 were fatalities	(a) Questionnaire population of eliciting know-abuse incidents (b) Detailed pilot ornia described in book. This can with the report-other states and parts of the USA the same book (c) Press clipping results with prev-American Hum-

F Type of Population	G The Abusers	H Ascertainment	I Limitations of Study	J Extent of Child Abuse
Texas, USA	Unspecified	Official reporting, including the Texas State telephone reporting system to the Dept. of Public Welfare	No amplification of the State figures. Un-critical accept-ance of unproven family 'treatment programmes'	In Texas in 1973, 4000 cases of child abuse were reported and 2500 confirmed, out of 4 million children. See also col. D
USA	Unspecified	Comparisons of C. H. Kempe's and D. G. Gil's figures. 5 cases of battering admitted to Colorado General Hospital per week; 15% of children under 5 who come into the emergency room fall into the battered category (Kempe). In USA 2.53–4.07 million suspected child abuse incidents per year (from replies to questionnaire sent to small sample; projected estimate relating to 190 million adults); however only 6000 confirmed cases per year for 200 million people in USA (D. G. Gil[125]).		
Nationwide survey of USA	47.6% mother or mother substitute. 39.2% father or father substitute. 12.1% other relative	Data from Central State registries. Parallel data from sample cohorts the screening of press reports, the Bureau of Vital Statistics and other agencies	Marked inter-state variation indicates variable quality of basic data. Over-whelming (but inevitable) reliance on data from 'Official Sources' when these were known to be adequate	5993 children for 1967. 6617 children for 1968 from all USA Central registries (population of 200 million)
sent to a sample adults in USA, ledge of child	(a) Parents or caretakers details not specified	(a) Between 2.53 and 4.07 million adults (out of 110 million adults) in USA know of families involved in incidents in which children were deliberately physically injured or killed by their parents or other persons caring for them		
study from Calif-Appendix A of be compared ing rate for 13 4 cities in other in Chapter 2 of	(b) As above	(b) 1174 reported incidents of physical child abuse during first year of legal reporting in California (Partial extra-polation). Less than one-third this number fulfilled Gil's criteria		
survey, comparing ious survey by the ane Association[126]		(c) 412 incidents of child abuse, involving 504 children, were reported in the press throughout USA in 6 months		

A References	B Age Range	C Types of Abuse	D Death Rate	E Special Features of the Study
Green, F. C. (1975). Child abuse and neglect[84]	Discussed in text. Generally children under 18	'Physical and mental injury, sexual abuse, negligent treatment or mal-treatment which indicate that the child's health and welfare is harmed or threatened . . .' (Green also discussed other expanded concepts)	1. See col. E 2. 200–400 deaths attributable to child abuse occur per year in USA 3. One child per week is killed by a parent (or care-taker) in New York City	'An abused child returned to his home without proper thera-peutic precautions being taken "runs a 50% chance of repeated abuse and a 10% chance of death" '. Green opposes the 'Cultural tolerance' of cruel rearing practices
Hall, D. A. (1974). Protecting the abused child in Maine[85]	Children under 16	(a) Unspecified child abuse (b) Complaints of neglect and abuse requiring child protective services. (c) Confirmed physical abuse	Unstated	A brief paper emphasizing the physicians' duties, and widespread under-reporting by doctors
Helfer, R. E. and Pollock, C. B. (1968). The battered child syndrome[86]	Half the children under 3. One quarter under 1 year	'Severe injury'	5% of the assaulted children killed	General article, with both first-hand data, and data from other sources
Hudson, P. et al. (1975). (Special article from New Jersey, USA). The Health professions and child abuse and neglect[87]	Unspecified	Children suffering any type of abuse or neglect	220 children died from abuse or neglect in New Jersey alone in 1973–74	The need to report cases is emphasized and detailed criteria are given in the article. In 1973–74 only $\frac{1}{5}$th of the total cases were reported

F Type of Population	G The Abusers	H Ascertainment	I Limitations of Study	J Extent of Child Abuse
Children in the USA, but some figures derive from Washington DC (part of col. J)	Mothers and female caretakers abuse most frequently but fathers and male caretakers cause most serious injuries	The estimates are largely based on other studies, in the light of Green's own experience. Some figures are deduced by the comparison of reports from public agencies with other sources	See col. H. There is a mixture of original data, data from other sources, and deductions, with varied criteria	(See also cols. D and E) 250 000–400 000 cases of child neglect and abuse in USA per year. 10% of Emergency Room Trauma in children under 3 is non-accidental. 30% of fractures in children under 2 are non-accidental. 50% of established abuse cases have suffered previously
(a) USA (b) & (c) State of Maine	No detail given	Maine Dept. of Health and Welfare. Less than 10% of total cases were referred by doctors or hospitals in Maine (b) and (c)	This article is more concerned with alerting, than with epidemiological detail	(a) 250–300 reports per million per annum (USA) (b) 1700 per annum (Maine) (c) 170 per annum (Maine)
USA	Unspecified	Sources of estimates not clearly given — partly based on surveys and projections by D. G. Gil	See col. H	In 1900 at least 10 000–15 000 children in USA were severely injured by abuse. Of these, 5% were killed and 25 to 30% permanently injured
New Jersey	No details specified	Data prepared by the New Jersey Division of Youth and Family Services in conjunction with Medical Sources	Few details are given on the bald statements from which the information in cols. D and J is derived	25 000 children in New Jersey alone suffered abuse and neglect in 1973–74. See also col. D

A References	B Age Range	C Types of Abuse	D Death Rate	E Special Features of the Study
Jaffe, A. C. et al. (1975). Sexual abuse of children[88]	Variable. Sexually abused children aged 2–15, mean age 10.7 years	(a) Sexual Abuse (b) Physical Neglect (c) Physical Abuse (d) Battered Child (e) Infanticide	(a) 2 from 2400 (b) 5 from 5000 (c) 10 from 600 (d) 7 from 60 (e) 5 All over a 10 year period	Sexual abuse compared with other forms of child abuse. Details and discussions on types of child molestation
Kempe, C. H. et al. (1962). The battered child[34]	No prior definition. Mostly children under 3 years	A spectrum of abuse is considered ranging from a single episode, to severely and repeatedly battered babies	Cases reported by hospitals 33 out of 302 children died. District Attorneys reported that 45 out of 447 children died	Highlighting, diagnosis and differential diagnosis of battered children. 114 children suffered permanent brain damage. This study was the landmark in generating awareness
Kempe, C. H. (1969). The battered child and the hospital[35]	Variable; mostly children under 5	Variable specifications. Active attack(s) specified and 'failure to thrive' discussed	700 children killed each year in USA by parents or parent surrogates	Treatment of battered parent strongly emphasized. About 3 out of 10 'failure to thrive' babies are in this state simply as a result of not being properly fed or not being emotionally cared for
Kempe, C. H. (1971). Paediatric implications of the battered baby syndrome[36]	No prior definition. Mostly children under 3 years	A spectrum of abuse is considered ranging from 'Mild bruising' to 'repeated serious injuries'. See col. I	Not stated	Highlighting of the identification of child abuse in families, not appearing to be socially 'Bad', and in parents not clearly 'mentally ill'

F Type of Population	G The Abusers	H Ascertainment	I Limitations of Study	J Extent of Child Abuse
Minneapolis, USA	(a) All male mostly unrelated to child (b)–(e) no details specified, but references given	Minneapolis, Police Dept. (plus Hospital) records (incest cases recorded by local hospital and welfare dept, where Police had problems in proceedings)	Inadequate information given on relation-ships between victim and offender. Unlike the other papers in this table this seems *not* to be mainly concerned with parents or caretakers	(a) 2400 (291 in 1970) (b) 5000 (c) 600 (d) 60 (e) 5. (a) Derives from Minneapolis Police records only, but (b)–(e) from Hennepin County Medical Centre. All 1964–1973 incls
Denver, USA. Also data obtained from other hospitals and District Attorneys in USA	No details on identification of actual abuser but usually parent or close relative	This paper deals with direct original observa-tions, and with data from legally reported cases and diagnostic returns from several hospitals in USA	Study not designed to look at total numbers in a given population over a given period of time	302 cases from 71 hospitals. 447 cases from 77 District Attorneys
Colorado and Rochester NY in USA	Unspecified. Parent or guardian	Direct clinical observations are combined with data from other (hospital) sources	Data on families is not clearly 'married up' with statements on prognosis	15% of all children under 5 seen in the emergency room have been battered. See also col. E for 'failure to thrive' cases, and col. D for deaths in USA
Denver, USA. Also data from New York and Pittsburgh quoted	No details on identification of actual abuser	This paper deals with direct original observa-tions, and with data from legally reported cases and diagnostic returns from several hospitals in USA	Early descrip-tions of the 'battered baby syndrome' are not clearly 'married up' with the total numbers projected by Kempe, nor with the prognostica-tions on treatment	6 in 1000 live births (projected estimate). 175–225 reports per million population per year (Denver and New York). 10–15% of all trauma to chil-dren under 3 due to abuse. 25% of all fractures to children under 2 due to abuse. Denver has 40 new abuse cases per year seen by Kempe's team

A References	B Age Range	C Types of Abuse	D Death Rate	E Special Features of the Study
Kempe, C. H. (1974). Duty to report child abuse[37]	Unspecified	'Significant physical abuse' (see col. D)	'The initial mortality is 5%; permanent brain damage due to subdural haematoma occurs in another 5%'	Strong medical, moral, and legal (in USA) reasons for doctors to report and act on cases of child abuse
Lauer, B. et al. (1974). Battered child syndrome. Review of 130 patients with controls[89]	Children under 10. 63% were under 2 years old	Children hospitalized because of physical injuries inflicted by parent, caretaker, etc. (many also neglected and previously abused)	6 out of 135 children died	During last 3 years of study, 3% of total admissions to wards were abuse cases. Rising rate of child battering. 53% of sibs maltreated
Light, R. J. (1973). Abused and neglected children in America. A study of alternative policies[38]	'Children under 18'	(a) 'Physical abuse' (b) 'Severe neglect or sexual abuse'	(a) Not stated	Several sources of data are used to estimate the incidence of child abuse. Three potential social policies are analysed in detail. Family size data suggest that widespread family planning education might help prevent child maltreatment
Merrill, E. J. (1962). Physical abuse of children. An agency study[90]	Half the children under 7 years, three-quarters under 13	Severe physical assaults, illustrated by selected case descriptions	3 in 200	A broad but clear early study with case descriptions, dealing with data on 115 families with 180 children. A classification of abusive parents is described

F Type of Population	G The Abusers	H Ascertainment	I Limitations of Study	J Extent of Child Abuse
USA	No detail	Official reportings? No detail	This report gives figures on incidence, etc. but no detail on ascertainment	'The current number of children reported for significant physical abuse in the United States is 380 per million population per year (70 000 children annually)'
San Francisco and environs	Unspecified	San Francisco General Hospital medical records, including the hospital social service records	Predominantly medical sources. Study not designed to look at total numbers in a given population	135 children, in 6 years, admitted to San Francisco General Hospital. 3% of all admissions (1969–71) to paediatric ward were for abuse
USA 67 million children considered	Biological parents are more likely to abuse than step-parents, adoptive parents or foster parents	(a) and (b) Projected estimates, based on official state data and published studies	The statistical projections are complex. There are so many stages of argument that conclusions could well be vulnerable to criticism at several points	(a) Estimated yearly number of cases: 200 000. Upper bound 500 000. (b) Estimated yearly number of cases: 465 000. Upper bound 1 175 000. (a) and (b) 1 in 100 (at least) children in USA are physically abused, sexually molested or severely neglected. 4–10 per 1000 families with children under 18 have physically abused at least one of their children
Massachusetts	Abuse committed by mothers and fathers (mostly young). 86% of abusers the biological parent	Referrals to the Massachusetts Society for the Prevention of Cruelty to Children	Study not designed to look at total numbers in a given population over a given period of time	In 1960 'well over 100 cases' investigated by the Massachusetts SPCC 'involving 200 children'

A References	B Age Range	C Types of Abuse	D Death Rate	E Special Features of the Study
Mindlin, R. L. (1974). Child abuse and neglect: the role of the paediatrician and the academy[91]	(a) Unspecified	(a) Unspecified physical abuse — neglect excluded	(a) Unspecified	(a) Figures from D. G. Gil in 1967
	(b) Unspecified	(b) Unspecified physical abuse — neglect excluded	(b) Unspecified	(b) More recent figures from nationally reported cases
	(c) Unspecified	(c) Unspecified	(c) Unspecified	(c) Estimates from C. H. Kempe
	(d) Unspecified	(d) Unspecified abuse and neglect	(d) Unspecified	(d) Estimates from D. G. Gil[82] and R. J. Light[38]
Morse, C. M. et al. (1970). A 3 year follow-up study of abused and neglected children[92]	Children under 6	Broad criteria. One or more episodes of active abuse and illnesses due to neglect	? Excluded in the design of the study	Detailed follow-up of a sample of 25 children, from 23 families including re-injuries, sequelae etc. 70% of the ill-used children judged to be 'outside the normal range' of intellectual and other CNS/ social function
Nazzaro, J. (1974). Child abuse and neglect[93]	Unspecified	Unspecified abuse and neglect	Unstated	A broad report on current trends in 1974
Schloesser, P. T. (1964). The abused child[94]	Children under 14, but 70% under 3 in the main survey, and 32% under 6 months	Fractures, surface injuries, strangulation, starvation, and severe neglect	14 out of 85	An epidemiological survey, with clear methodology and apt comments. Many children died or suffered permanent CNS trauma. Child abuse worsening in Kansas

F Type of Population	G The Abusers	H Ascertainment	I Limitations of Study	J Extent of Child Abuse
(a) USA	(a) Unspecified	(a) Compilation of reports from state central registries, by Gil in 1967	(a) Not new data	(a) 5993 cases in USA in 1967
(b) USA	(b) Unspecified	(b) Official returns from USA registries in 1972	(b) Unclear statement on the new data, see col. J	(b) The above figures 'more than double' by 1972
(c) USA	(c) Unspecified	(c) Kempe 1972[127]	(c) No details given	(c) 60 000 children severely abused in USA in 1972
(d) USA	(d) Unspecified	(d) Estimates by D. G. Gil in 1970 and R. J. Light in 1973	(d) No details given	(d) 0.5 to 2.5 million children abused and/or neglected in USA in 1972
Rochester, NY	Unspecified; either parent or guardian, but the follow-up children often had a variety of care after initial abusive episodes	Cases presenting and diagnosed at a general hospital emergency department	See col. C. A very varied group of families, and seemingly a rather attenuated sample from the earlier study[33]	20% of children seen for injuries in the hospital emergency department had suffered these as a result of abuse or neglect by parents
Figures quoted for Florida	Unspecified	'Hot line' telephone calls from private individuals and public agencies	Not an 'in depth' study. A journalistic-cum-technical presentation of assorted data	30 000 cases of abuse and neglect in Florida in $1\frac{1}{2}$ years reported via the 'Hot line'. 40—50% confirmed
Kansas	From 85 cases, the adults responsible were: 31 Unstated or undetermined. 30 Mothers 11 Fathers 5 Stepfathers 4 Other relatives 4 Unrelated	Questionnaire survey of physicians in co-operation with child welfare committee of the Kansas Medical Society	Incomplete ascertainment, from predominantly medical sources. The authoress discusses under-reporting	85 cases in the state of Kansas, USA, in 1962 and 1963. It was also noted that 15% of 310 dependency and neglect cases *in one Kansas Juvenile Court* involved beaten 5—10 year olds

A *References*	B *Age Range*	C *Types of Abuse*	D *Death Rate*	E *Special Features of the Study*
Silver, L. (1968). Child abuse syndrome: A review[95]	Variable specifications	Several specifications given. Battered babies. Child neglect. General ill-usage	33 out of 302 battered babies died. 85 received permanent injury. (From C. H. Kempe, 1962[34])	Review of known studies, mostly from USA
Simons, B. *et al.* (1966). Epidemiological study of medically reported cases[44]	Children under 16. More than two-thirds were under 5	No prior specification 'Cases involving medical care or corroboration'. Beatings, 'battered child syndrome', burns, dehydration, malnutrition, sexual molestations, etc.	16 out of 313 died, mostly children under 2	Most abused children from multi-problem families with multi-agency involvement. Broad spectrum of abuse/neglect patterns
Solomon, T. (1971). History and demography of child abuse[96]	At age 4. Most under 2 years	Limited specifications in relation to the nos. given. Average time of exposure to battering 1–3 years	5–25%	Discussion of the problems of standardizing the statistics in USA
Weston, J. T. (1969). Pathology of child abuses. The battered child[97]	(a) All under 13 months (b) All but 2 under 4 years	(a) Death by neglect. (b1) Death by single episode of trauma. (b2) Death by multiple episodes of trauma	Only dead children considered. (a) 13 deaths (b1) 13 deaths (b2) 23 deaths See col. J	Detailed analysis of deaths by neglect, by single episode of trauma, and by repetitive multiple traumatic episodes
Zalba, S. R. (1966). The abused child: a survey of the problem[98]	Variable specifications	Severe physical injuries such as to endanger the child's life or health	12 children died out of 56 cases followed up	Review article giving a broad scan of existing literature (1966)

F Type of Population	G The Abusers	H Ascertainment	I Limitations of Study	J Extent of Child Abuse
New York City. California. Colorado. Denver	Mostly child's own parents. Fathers and mothers more or less equally responsible in the references cited	All quotes from other writers, who in turn were themselves sometimes citing others. 200 000–250 000 cases of child abuse in USA each year. 302 battered children in 71 hospitals in 1962[34]. Improved recognition raised the recorded number in one hospital from 0 in one year to 50 the following year! 4000 cases of child neglect came to the attention of the courts in New York City in 1962[128]. A minimum of 20 000 children per year need protective services in California[129]. 100 cases of child abuse referred monthly for protection, to the Denver Public Welfare Department[130]		
Inhabitants of New York City	33% Unidentified 29% Mothers 19% Fathers 14% Sibs, Cohabitees or Babysitters	Child Abuse Registry. A legal requirement for medicals to report, since July 1964. Supplementary data from Welfare Department	Incomplete medical reporting. No standard data from protective agencies, school, police, neighbours, etc. *Low professional awareness in the first year* of the registry	313 children from 293 families in one year, in a city of 7 840 000. See col. I
(a) USA (b) New York City (c) USA	Unspecified	(a) & (b) American Humane Society. Only 11 cases reported by medical and dental practitioners. Introduction of central register in New York increased reportings by 549%. (c) Extrapolated data from California and Colorado		(a) 10 000 cases reported in 1969 (USA) (b) 2600 cases reported in 1969 (New York) (c) 200 000–250 000 children in USA per year need protective services; 30 000–37 000 badly injured
Philadelphia	Details of ascertainment by forensic pathologist and medico-legal sources. Assailants in group (b) as follows — mothers 12, fathers 10, step-parents and cohabitees 3, sibs 5, foster parents and babysitters 3, unknown 3		Only dead children considered. Many of the suspicious deaths may have evaded autopsy	In 5 years, for 212 394 births there were 60 children shown to be killed by abuse and neglect. (But see col. I)
Mainly USA, but interesting comments on an early (1952) UK book by Chesser[4]	Unspecified. Either parent or guardian	Consideration of a variety of papers and books, mostly from USA. Extrapolated from California, Colorado and England	No original data. Projected estimates from a variety of studies	Nearly $\frac{1}{4}$ million children per year in USA (population 200 million) require protection. Approx. 35 000 suffer serious physical abuse (see col. H)

A References	B Age Range	C Types of Abuse	D Death Rate	E Special Features of the Study
Australia				
Birrell, R. G. and Birrell, J. H. W. (1968). The maltreatment syndrome in children: a hospital survey[58]	9 and under. Mostly under 4 years	25 — physical violence only. 10 — physical violence and neglect. 7 — gross neglect only	Unstated	$\frac{1}{4}$ of the children were rendered mentally retarded. More than $\frac{1}{4}$ of the children had congenital defects. High rate of parental mental disorder and chaotic social environments
Colclough, I. R. (1972). Victorian governments' report on child abuse. A reinvestigation[59]	Variable specifications. Children mostly under 2 (at time of early assaults)	No prior specifications, but case histories given. Some cases of gross neglect included	6 died out of 26 cases	An individual finds many cases that a Government Committee failed to ascertain
Dawe, K. E. (1973). Mal-treated children at home and overseas[99]	Mostly under 3	Variable specifications, from bruises and other surface injuries, to the classical battered baby	A minimum of 16 died out of 261 cases	A broad examination of maltreated children and their families
Canada				
Dawe, K. E. (1973). Child abuse in Nova Scotia[100]	Unclear prior specification. Mostly under 5 years	'Battered' and 'Maternally deprived' children, officially or otherwise reported	Not specified	A combined attack on the problem in Nova Scotia by medical, legal and social workers
Fried, C. T. (1973). Child abuse is a family social disease[101]	Unspecified. Mostly babies and young children	Active abuse, and defects in mothering lead-ing to neglect and malnutrition	Unspecified	Diagnosis and medical aspects considered in relation to social principles

F Type of Population	G The Abusers	H Ascertainment	I Limitations of Study	J Extent of Child Abuse
31 from Melbourne. 11 from country areas around Melbourne	Incomplete data	From one hospital only. Medical records, Medical Social Work Dept., ward sister, and personal involvement by the investigators	Data predominantly from hospital sources only. Study not designed to look at total numbers in a given population	42 children in 31 months from the Royal Children's Hospital, Melbourne
State of Victoria	Unspecified. Either parent or guardian	See col. E. An elective survey conducted through the case records, and interviews, at 16 hospitals	Inadequate specifications of population. Data only obtained from certain hospitals	50 or more cases between 1960 and 1967, from 16 hospitals in the Australian state of Victoria. 26 cases surveyed in detail
Melbourne area	No detail given	Cases known to the hospital medical social workers (20% of all 'failure-to-thrive' cases result solely from 'deficiency of mothering')	Study not designed to look at total numbers in a given population. Variable criteria. Much derived from sources in the USA	A minimum of 261 children in 6 years at the Royal Children's Hospital, Melbourne. (See also col. H)
Nova Scotia	Incomplete data	Official reports, but most data came from hospital records. A retrospective study	'Vital information was not being obtained by physicians or social workers . . .'	A minimum of 59 in 5 years in Nova Scotia (See col. I)
Alberta	Unspecified, usually parent	See col. I. All numbers quoted derive from sources in the USA	A general, broad article which does not give details of sources	25% of all trauma in children admitted to the hospital emergency room was non-accidental. 15% of all fractures in children are non-accidental

A References	B Age Range	C Types of Abuse	D Death Rate	E Special Features of the Study
McRae, K. N. et al. (1973). The battered child syndrome[102]	No prior definition. 78% of the children under 3 years	Battered young children, bruising, fractures, intracranial damage, but also children presenting initially as 'Medical' problems	8 died out of first 88 children. High rate of 'Infant crib deaths' amongst sibs	Detailed descriptive medical study. 'Failure-to-thrive' was the presenting feature in 8 battered babies out of 132. *12 children of 34 followed up were mentally retarded*
Rodenberg, M. (1971). Child murder by depressed parents[103]	Children under 16 (mostly 1–5 years)	Children killed by parents	Only dead children considered	Comparisons of murders of children by parents, and by others

International Publication (from Switzerland)

Underhill, E. (1974). The strange silence of teachers, doctors and social workers in the face of cruelty to children[53]	Variable.	Predominantly battering and active cruelty	Britain: 700 young children killed by parents each year. Canada: 100 children killed each year from ill-treatment	An international 4600 young of 60 000 van Stolk Secretary of murder, between

South Africa

Irwin, C. (1974). Specialists on child battering[55]	Unspecified. Babies mainly considered	'Baby battering', and shaking of babies	Unstated	A strong emphasis on the need for better family planning. Rising ascertainment levels

West Germany

Trube-Becker, E. (1971). Autopsy of children who have died suddenly[104]	Children under 6	Deaths caused by homicide, neglect, and (sustained) maltreatment	Only dead children are considered	Autopsies essential for all children who die suddenly, to ascertain neglect or abuse as a cause of death
Trube-Becker, E. (1973). Child abuse and its consequences[52]	Mostly under 3 years	Battered babies. A variety of severe traumata, often with severe neglect accompanying	100 young children per year die of maltreatment in West Germany	Post-mortem examination essential after the death of any small child. Most subdural haematomas of uncertain origin in children are due to repeated ill-treatment

F Type of Population	G The Abusers	H Ascertainment	I Limitations of Study	J Extent of Child Abuse
Catchment area of Winnipeg Children's Hospital, Canada	Mother figure 31.8% Father figure 27.2% Either parent 10.6% Unknown 22%	Data direct from Winnipeg Children's Hospital and immediate sources	Study not designed to look at total numbers in given population	88 children (1967–1969, plus first half of 1970). 44 in second half of 1970 and 1971, from Winnipeg and its environs. See col. E
Canada	8:7 ratio. Mothers to Fathers responsible for the killings	Small numbers ascertained by formal legal methods. In Canada from 1964–68 there were 141 incidents of child murder. 74 (54%) of these were caused by the parents. Many killing parents committed, or attempted suicide		

review highlighting complacency about cruelty to young children. A. White Franklin (Britain) reports that children are battered in Britain per year (Population 50 m.). *Newsweek* reported a minimum figure children wilfully beaten, burned, smothered or starved per year in USA (Population 200 m.). Mary estimates 4810 incidents of child abuse per year in Canada (Population 21 m). Dr Bayerl, State, reports that well over 3000 people were convicted of cruel ill-treatment of children, including 1969 and 1971 in West Germany (Population 62 m.).

F Type of Population	G The Abusers	H Ascertainment	I Limitations of Study	J Extent of Child Abuse
Johannesburg	Unspecified	Cases presenting at Johannesburg Children's Hospital. Hospital ascertainment only	Only limited details given, particularly in relation to epidemiological data. Under-ascertainment	6 cases in 1972. 20 cases in 1973. 30 cases in the first 10 months of 1974. These figures represent 'Only the tip of an iceberg'
Dusseldorf	Not stated	By autopsy. In West Germany the magistrate may order a post-mortem if the death certificate has the statement 'unexplained cause of death'	Only dead children considered, and many of the suspicious deaths may have evaded autopsy (see col. H.)	From 1385 autopsies, 78 (5.6%) were due to homicide; 54 (3.9%) were caused by neglect; 35 (2.5%) were the result of (sustained) maltreatment, in children under 6 years
West Germany	Unspecified. Usually the mother	Predominantly from autopsies, or from legal and medical records	Incomplete ascertainment, (see col. H)	4500 people sentenced in 1 year in West Germany (population 62 million) for endangering the physical and mental well-being of 6500 children

Index

abandonment   123, 141, 194
abortion   5, 6
abuse
  adaptation to   102, 154, 155
  aetiology   75
  age of child   129, 130, 140, 154, 159, 171
  biological aspects   178–180
  Canadian studies   245–315
    House of Commons recommendations
    267–269
  child's viewpoint   1–8
  clinical features   16–39, 130–133
  definition   205, 222, 223, 252–255, 317,
    327, 332, 342
  diagnosis   12–14, 54, 58–61, 65–67, 122,
    277–280
  detection   15
  emotional   48, 169, 258, 274, 275 see
    also psychological abuse
  epidemiology   95–119, 121–153, 144–
    148, 158, 205, 206, 273
  frequency of injuries   18, 171
  historical aspects   4, 95–99
  in care   40, 41
  management   83–94, 194–196, 238–240,
    309, 310
  medical aspects   9–68
  prevention   10–15, 83, 90, 91, 93, 94,
    102, 301, 306
  psychological   60, 205–219, 221–223,
    258
  radiological and pathological aspects
    69–81
  sexual   see sexual abuse
  sex incidence   17, 129, 130, 189, 207
  Wiltshire study   121–174

adoption   298 see also fostering
autopsy   77–81
baby farming   353
battered child syndrome   78, 175, 190, 194
  definition   176, 177, 205, 222, 223
    252–255
  see also   abuse and neglect
battered wives   176, 193, 194, 235
behaviour   abnormalities   in   battered
  children   38, 231
bites   23, 76, 78
  saliva test   23
bonding   233, 361
  failure   101, 149, 155, 225, 286
  father and baby   14
  mother and baby   33
    development of   13, 14
bone injuries   26–28, 122, 175
  differential diagnosis   60, 61, 65–67
  joint swelling   28
  long bone fracture   27, 71
  radiological features   27, 69–74
  rib fractures   27, 63, 80
  skull fracture   28, 72, 78, 122
  spiral fracture   27, 71
Bowlby's theory   2
  overview and criticisms of   353–364
brain damage
  clinical features   28, 168
  incidence   107, 122, 133, 257
breast-feeding   15, 187, 303
bruising
  black eye   22, 23, 30
  cheek   22, 23
  ear   22
  fingertip   20, 21, 77, 78

frequency 20
differential diagnosis 60, 76
mouth 22
petechial 21, 22, 24
subcutaneous 21
see also haematoma *and* skin injuries
burns *see* skin injuries
case conferences 87, 88
case histories 160–167, 295–298, 383–385
case history method 206
sexual abuse 329–345
child labour 96, 97, 405, 406
Church, attitude to children 396–399
cot death 33, 34
courts *see* law
death
autopsy after 77–81
case history 281, 282
cot death 33, 34
incidence 18, 75, 109, 111, 122, 130, 133, 146, 147, 206, 221
relation to age 17
relation to sex 17
deprivation, maternal *see* Bowlby's theory
doctor
medical–legal difficulties 293–295
role in child welfare 15, 61, 62, 85, 265, 266
under-reporting by 262
drowning 33
drug abuse, relation to child abuse 101, 317–350
dwarfism
deprivation 36–39, 47, 48, 54–56, 109, 168, 223, 232, 253
differential diagnosis 60, 76
education
historical development 402, 403, 410
parentcraft 10–12, 240, 241, 250, 251, 266, 273, 299, 379, 380
sexual 7, 8, 379
environment 182, 183
epidemiology 95–119, 121–153, 144–148, 158, 205, 206, 273
Africa 105
Asia 105
Australia 105
Canada 245–315
England 108, 112, 113
Holland 107, 111, 112, 114
North-East Wiltshire 121–174
UK 105, 106, 107, 109, 111, 112, 113, 114
USA 105, 106, 111, 112, 114
West Germany 106, 109
examination, physical 49–52, 77–79, 180–182
eye damage *see* vision

failure to thrive *see* dwarfism
family characteristics in child abuse cases 134–138, 147, 148, 288–290
see also parents
fostering 55, 56, 89, 200, 201, 291, 298, 300, 388
fractures *see* bone injuries
'funny turns' 34, 49
haematoma, subdural 17, 28, 29, 65, 78, 122
see also bruising
health visitor, role in child welfare 84, 301, 307
historical aspects of child abuse 4, 95–99
history-taking 41–49, 127, 282, 283
hospitalization 51, 52, 86, 90, 280
role of paediatric unit 52–56
incest *see* sexual abuse
illegitimacy, relation to child abuse 130, 188, 207, 224, 341, 353
infanticide 98, 122, 190, 191, 247, 394, 395, 399, 404
information
collection 156–158
interviews 209–211
questionnaires and tests 210, 211, 213, 214, 218, 302
record-keeping 374, 375
typology 214, 215
see also history-taking
injury
assay of 77–79, 180, 182
see also poisoning, skin, bone, brain, vision, internal, psychological intelligence
child's 212
see also mental handicap
parents', relation to child abuse 102, 106, 114, 211, 212, 216
internal injury 30
language, importance of 229, 236
law
medical–legal difficulties 293–295
role in child abuse cases 15, 61, 62, 85, 291–293, 325–327, 334, 335, 336, 339, 346–348, 374, 412, 413
the child as a legal entity 393–413
literature on child abuse 105–119, 415–446
maladjustment 231
management of abuse 83–94, 194–196, 238–240, 309, 310
Medea complex 183, 188, 198
mental handicap following brain damage 122, 168–173, 212, 223
Alaskan study 170
see also brain damage
mercy killing 188

midwife, role in child welfare 84
Mongolian blue spot 24, 61
native Canadians, child abuse in 304, 305
needs of children 221–243
  psychological 227–230
neglect 141, 156, 169
  definition 123, 252–255, 317, 327, 332, 342
  medical aspects 61–68
  types of 172
  see also abuse
neuroticism, parental 210, 211, 217
  see also parents
notification of abuse 125, 262–267
  failure 345
  under-reporting 147, 262–264
NSPCC see voluntary organizations
nurse, district, role in child welfare 3
paediatrics see doctor
paedophilia 320
parentcraft see education
parents
  age 182, 216
  attitude to abnormal children 198
  see also mercy killing
  background 48, 101, 102, 134, 179, 182, 279
  collaboration between 184, 185
  characteristics 140–144, 193, 194, 195, 199, 215, 279, 283, 290, 291
  expectations 100, 212, 226
  inadequate 225
  IQ see intelligence
  personality disorders 102, 208–211
  see also psychopaths and neuroticism
  problems 34, 35, 182, 183
  see also stress
  provocation see provocation
  social class 146, 216
  violence, patterns of 223–227
  see also family
pathology of abuse 74–77
poisoning 32, 33, 223
police, role in child abuse cases 57, 58, 85, 87, 88, 364–367
  see also law
pornography, child 7, 321–345
postnatal depression 179
prediction of child abuse 301
  prediction scales 215–217
prevention of abuse 10–15, 83, 90, 91, 93, 94, 102
  see also education
prostitution, child 318–321
provocation 283
  from baby 187, 191–193, 234
  from husband 183, 184
  from wife 184

psychiatrist
  role in child abuse 4, 6, 33, 57, 88, 200, 286–288
  viewpoint of 175–203
psychological abuse 205–219, 221–223, 258
  differential diagnosis 60
psychopaths 194, 226
psychosis, parental 210
psychotherapy 19, 357
punishment 192, 247, 248, 266
radiology see bone injuries
registers of abused children 90, 263, 264, 265, 269, 375
rehabilitation, family 84
rejection, maternal 36–39
  effects of 233, 234, 304
reporting of abuse see notification
rights of children 260, 261, 275–277
  see also needs and law
role reversal 193, 208, 216
Samaritans see voluntary organizations
separation, postnatal, effect of 179, 187, 303, 355–360
  see also Bowlby's theory
sexual abuse 7, 39, 40, 48, 49, 79, 189, 317–350
  incest 155, 305, 323, 325–327, 338, 343
  physical injury in 320, 324
  see also prostitution and pornography
shaking 29, 168, 223
siblings
  abuse in 136, 138, 139
  emotional stress in 222
skin injuries
  cigarette burns 26
  differential diagnosis 61
  grasp marks 23
  lacerations 25
  ligature marks 24
  scalds 25
  weals 24
social agencies
social class, relation to child abuse 146, 216
  future problems of 376–388
  historical development of 351–353
social worker
  influence of Bowlby's theory on 361–364
  problems 381–383
  relationship with police, teachers and voluntary bodies 364–369
  role of 283–286, 307, 351–391
  society's expectations of 370, 371
  training of 371–376
societal care 249, 250
stress, parental 12, 208, 283

suffocation   123, 223
  see also cot death
teachers, role in child abuse cases   367, 368
television violence, effect on children   251, 252, 266
typology   214, 215, 217
vision damage in child abuse   30, 31, 79, 80, 122, 168

voluntary organizations
  Canadian   269–274, 308
  role in child abuse   92, 368, 369, 377
  Odyssey   327
wives
  battered   176, 193, 194, 235
  working   246
  see also parents
young offenders treatment of   406–408